U0294016

疑难皮肤病彩色图谱

Color Atlas of Difficult Skin Disorders

第 3 版

主　编　朱文元　倪容之

河南科学技术出版社

·郑州·

内容提要

本书在第 2 版的基础上修订而成，共收集疑难和少见皮肤病 475 种，图片 1383 张，按其主要病因分类编排。每种病除有典型的临床表现外，还配有相关的组织病理、免疫组化和真菌培养等实验室检查照片。内容新颖，资料珍贵，图片清晰，同时有图片的中英文说明，第 3 版对部分图片英文说明做了修正。便于读者查阅国外文献和国际交流。国内尚无类似专著。提供图片的第一作者共 283 人，因此本图谱是集体智慧的结晶，具有较强的原创性、理论性和实用性，是国内外皮肤科和相关科室临床医师必备的重要参考书，亦可作为医学图书馆珍贵的典藏书。

图书在版编目（CIP）数据

疑难皮肤病彩色图谱/朱文元，倪容之主编. －3 版. －郑州：河南科学技术出版社，2018.1

ISBN 978-7-5349-9056-4

Ⅰ.①疑… Ⅱ.①朱… ②倪… Ⅲ.①皮肤病－疑难病－图谱 Ⅳ.①R751-64

中国版本图书馆 CIP 数据核字（2017）第 309107 号

出版发行：河南科学技术出版社
北京名医世纪文化传媒有限公司
地址：北京市丰台区丰台北路 18 号院 3 号楼 511 室　　邮编：100073
电话：010-53556511　010-53556508

策划编辑：杨磊石
文字编辑：黄栩兵
责任审读：邓　为
责任校对：龚利霞
封面设计：吴朝洪
版式设计：王新红
责任印制：陈震财
印　　刷：三河市春园印刷有限公司
经　　销：全国新华书店、医学书店、网店
幅面尺寸：185 mm×260 mm　　印张：27　　字数：597 千字
版　　次：2018 年 1 月第 3 版　　2018 年 1 月第 1 次印刷
定　　价：248.00 元

如发现印、装质量问题，影响阅读，请与出版社联系并调换

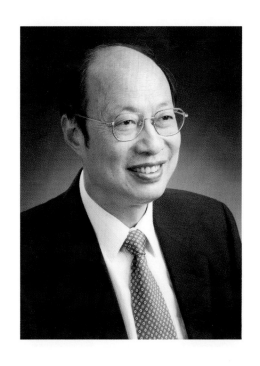

朱文元　　1960 年上海第一医学院医学系毕业,同年至北京协和医院皮肤科工作。1966 年起在南京医科大学第一附属医院皮肤科工作。现任皮肤科主任医师、教授、博士生导师,《临床皮肤科杂志》主编,美国皮肤病杂志 *Archives of Dermatology* 国际编委。国内 5 种专业期刊编委,亚洲色素细胞研究会理事。1989～1991 年在美国迈阿密大学医学院作高级访问学者。发表论文近 300 篇,英文论文 49 篇。主编《荨麻疹》、《白癜风与黄褐斑》、《痤疮》、《毛发疾病》等专著 7 部,参编《Cosmetic Formulation of Skin Care Products》等书 8 部,主审《现代皮肤性病学进展》等专著 3 部。承担国家、部和省级科研课题 16 项,黑素细胞研究 3 次获国家自然科学基金资助。获省、厅科技进步奖 7 项。"外阴部脂溢性角化病含人乳头瘤病毒"获美国皮肤科学会金质奖。指导博士研究生 15 名。1992 年享受国务院特殊津贴,荣获江苏省有特殊贡献专家和高校先进工作者称号。1998 年被评为全国优秀教师,2000 年被评为江苏省优秀研究生导师。2004 年《临床皮肤科杂志》荣获江苏省期刊一等奖,全国二等奖。

Zhu Wenyuan, MD.

Chief Physician, Professor, and supervisor of PhD candidates. Dermatology Department of the First Affiliated Hospital of Nanjing Medical University. Dr. Zhu is the editor-in-chief of Clinical Journal of Dermatology and a member of 6 editorial boards including the Archives of Dermatology and has authored a total of 300 publications including 49 English papers and 7 books. Dr. Zhu was the visiting scholar of Medical College of Miami university in 1989 to 1991.

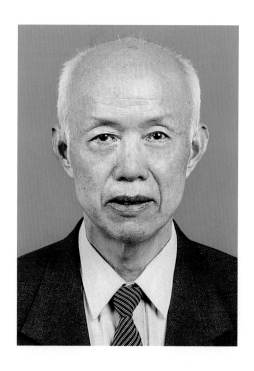

倪容之　　历任南京军区南京总医院皮肤科主任、主任医师、教授。南京大学医学院临床学院教授,上海第二军医大学兼职教授。中华医学会江苏省皮肤科分会副主任委员、中西医结合学会江苏省皮肤科分会副主任委员、江苏省制冷学会常务理事、解放军医学科学委员会皮肤科学会常委。南京军区医学科学委员会委员兼皮肤科专业组组长。《临床皮肤科杂志》副主编、《中华皮肤科杂志》常务编委、《中国皮肤性病学杂志》编委、《美中皮肤科杂志》编委、《人民军医》杂志特约编委。主编的专著有《现代皮肤病治疗学》、《药疹》,参加编写著作 8 本。曾获国家卫生部三等奖、江苏省科技成果三等奖、南京军区科技成果三等和四等奖。荣立三等功 1 次,曾被授予"军中名老医学专家"称号。

Ni Rong-zhi　MD.

Dep. Dermatology. Nanjing General Hospital of Nanjing Military Command.

School of Medicine，Nanjing University

Medical College，Second Military Medical University.

Associate Chief Editor of Journal of Clinical Dermatology.

Editor of Chinese Journal of Dermatology.

Editor of the Chinese Journal of Dermatovenereology.

编(译)者名单

主　编　朱文元　倪容之

副主编　侯麦花　谭　城　张汝芝

英文翻译　侯麦花　朱文元

英文审核　Theodora M. Mauro，Kevin Zhu

秘　书　马立文

编　者　(以第一作者论文数或姓氏笔画为序)

朱文元	谭　城	马东来	张汝芝	侯麦花	常建民	肖　尹	鲁　严	李　丽	
李　雪	王大光	王宏伟	王　雷	闫　洁	陈思远	陈仁贵	陆　原	翟志芳	
孙建方	马慧军	王　刚	关　杨	刘玉峰	刘跃华	朱学骏	李春阳	李顺凡	
李　颂	杜　娟	狄　梅	吴　艳	宋志强	张　卉	杨　敏	杨　岚	杨希川	
陈柳青	姜　薇	胡　瑾	赵　娟	赵　广	徐　斌	夏明玉	郭生红	晋红中	
彭少文	蔡　林	廖文俊	鞠　强	Rigopoulos D		马立文	万　川	万东芳	
于娜沙	尹志强	方木平	方　晶	孔庆云	尤海燕	韦应波	王文岭	王迎林	
王爱琴	王铃艳	王惠琳	王　涛	王　磊	王　娣	王家璧	王鹰鹰	甘　戈	
甘吉洪	舟玉平	石仁琳	左亚刚	皮肖冰	田中华	龙福泉	闫　言	朱小红	
朱国兴	朱铁山	朱家洪	朱晓浚	刘广仁	刘　方	刘升云	刘　安	刚　怡	
刘建军	刘　玮	刘金耀	刘春平	刘　栋	孙志平	孙国钧	孙秀坤	孙　嬛	
孙　青	孙　莹	邢有兰	邢传平	乔树芳	吕淑琴	庄殿英	任　英	邢　颖	
毕新岭	陈连军	陈　坚	陈　征	陈小娥	陈　龙	陈晓红	陈　敬	陈　晨	
陈珺怡	吴　迪	吴绍熙	吴建华	吴　梅	吴　凤	吴信峰	吴黎明	汪　晨	
张　红	张建中	张　贤	张　武	张金松	张勇枚	张春香	张春敏	张桂秀	
张峻岭	张　浩	张　倩	张晓梅	张淑环	张理涛	张继玲	张超英	李文海	
李　卉	李　军	李会申	李　利	李　波	李　明	李　莉	李恒进	李晓杰	
李诚让	李　敏	李　峰	李葆春	李　萍	李　澄	宋志新	宋佩华	苏向阳	
苏金发	苏忠兰	肖家诚	沈征宇	沈剑鸣	何　弘	汪　盛	严淑贤	邱丙森	
林自华	林　彤	林　挺	林建华	金慧玲	武小红	杨光河	杨　励	杨　玲	
杨玉花	杨雪源	杨　健	杨恩品	杨淑欣	杨慧兰	周春丽	周存才	周冼苁	
周建华	周辉谱	郑艳红	郑云燕	郑　敏	郑优优	宫立民	金　江	罗迪青	
庞晓文	范光明	岳学状	苗　青	赵小东	赵　亮	赵淑肖	姜一化	姜红浩	
姜祎群	姚志远	项力俭	钟桂书	相广才	祝永航	郝　进	贾雪松	高　洁	

高　亮	高瑛瑛	顾有守	徐益明	徐春兴	徐美萍	徐　磊	徐素芹	袁华刚
袁小英	袁肖海	袁　姗	唐　珊	唐　莉	郭小艳	陶晓苹	郭志飞	钱坚革
敖俊红	梁建平	宿　斌	曹发龙	曹元华	曹　蕾	曹鸿玮	曹　扬	曹碧兰
崔炳南	黄　敏	黄淑琼	渠　涛	康定华	戚丽华	普雄明	谢　忠	谢作刚
谢　慧	谢　勇	傅志宜	阎　衡	彭　军	曾建英	童燕芳	景红梅	葛　峥
蒋　献	韩春雷	虞瑞尧	赖声正	雷山川	谭升顺	谭　琦	谭立恒	蔡　林
蔡　梅	廖万清	熊　霞	潘健楷	潘　敏	潘德海	樊翌明	樊平中	黎兆军
翟立新	霍亚兰	戴迅毅	薛筑云					

Tong、LIN Ting、LIN Jian-hua、JIN Hui-ling、WU Xiao-hong、YANG Guang-he、YANG Li、YANG Ling、YANG Yu-hua、YANG Xue-yuan、YANG Jian、YANG En-pin、YANG Shu-xin、YANG Hui-lan、ZHOU Chun-li、ZHOU Cun-cai、ZHOU Sheng-yi、ZHOU Jian-hua、ZHOU Hui-pu、ZHENG Yan-hong、ZHENG Yun-yan、ZHENG Min、ZHENG You-you、Gong Li-min、JIN Jiang、LUO Di-qing、PANG Xiao-wen、FAN Guang-ming、YUE Xue-zhuang、MIAO Qing、ZHAO Xiao-dong、ZHAO Liang、ZHAO Shu-xiao、JIANG Yi-hua、JIANG Hong-hao、JIANG Yi-quan、YAO Zhi-yuan、XIANG Li-jian、ZHONG Gui-shu、XIANG Guang-cai、ZHU Yong-hang、HAO Jin、JIA Xue-song、GAO Jie、GAO Liang、GAO Ying-ying、GU You-shou、XU Yi-ming、XU Chun-xing、XU Mei-ping、XU Lei、XU Su-qin、YUAN Hua-gang、YUAN Xiao-ying、YUAN Xiao-hai、YUAN Shan、TANG Shan、TANG Li、GUO Xiao-yan、TAO Xiao-ping、GUO Zhi-fei、QIAN Jian-ge、AO Jun-hong、LIANG Jian-ping、SU Bin、CAO Fa-long、CAO Yuan-hua、CAO Lei、CAO Hong-wei、CAO Yang、CAO Bi-lan、CUI Bing-nan、HUANG Min、HUANG Shu-qiong、QU Tao、KANG Ding-hua、QI Li-hua、PU Xiong-ming、XIE Zhong、XIE Zuo-gang、XIE Hui、XIE Yong、FU Zhi-yi、YAN Heng、PENG Jun、CENG Jian-ying、CHENG Li-xue、TONG Yan-fang、JING Hong-mei、GENG Zheng、JIANG Xian、HAN Chun-lei、YU Rui-yao、LAI Sheng-zheng、LEI Shan-chuan、TAN Sheng-shun、TAN Qi、TAN Li-heng、CAI Lin、CAI Mei、LIAO Wan-qing、XIONG Xia、PAN Jian-kai、PAN Min、PAN De-hai、FAN Yi-meng、FAN Ping-shen、LI Zhao-jun、ZHAI Li-xin、HUO Ya-lan、DAI Xun-yi、XUE Zhu-yun

"三个一百"原创出版工程

证　书

中华人民共和国新闻出版总署

"三个一百"原创出版工程

证　　书

人民军医 出版社：

　　你社出版的《　　　　疑难皮肤病彩色图谱　　　　》一书
入选新闻出版总署第二届"三个一百"原创图书出版工程。

　　特颁此证。

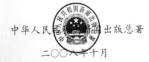

中华人民共和国新闻出版总署

二〇〇八年十月

第 3 版前言

《疑难皮肤病彩色图谱》出版后深受广大医师好评,2008 年获中国新闻出版总署"三个一百"原创图书出版工程奖。在第 2 版中,我们删除了部分重复和一般的皮肤病。新增加疑难皮肤病 125 种,图片 317 张。第 3 版图谱共有疑难皮肤病 475 种,图片 1383 幅,并对部分图片英文说明作了修正。希望《疑难皮肤病彩色图谱》第 2 版能成为皮肤科医师的良师益友。光阴荏苒,皮肤病的新病种和新表现将会不断出现。我们将继续收集、整理,并把它们汇编成图谱,为皮肤病的教学任务,尽一份微薄之力。

南京医科大学第一附属医院皮肤科教授

朱文元

2017 年 10 月

Foreword to the third edition

After publication of *the Color Atlas of Difficult Skin Disorders* has been praised by the majority of the physicians, which wan outstanding book award of the China General Administration of Press and Publication in 2008. In the second edition of the atlas we deleted some duplication and general dermatological disease (60 and pictures 195), and added 125 additional skin disease and 317 images. The third edition atlas includes 475 total skin disease and 1383 pictures. Some of the pictures in English description have been corrected I hope that atlas' first episode of the third edition to be a dermatologist mentor. Time unknowing passing, new diseases and new manifestation of the skin disorders will appear constantly. We will continue to collect and put them on color atlas .In order to the teaching task of dermatology, we will try our best to the meager strength.

Zhu Wen-yuan M.D.

Professor of Dermatology, The First affiliated Hospital, Nanjing Medical University
October, 2017

第 1 版序一

皮肤病的诊断与其他学科一样,都是要根据病史、体检、各种实验室检查及影像学检查等而确定。但是皮肤病的形态学在皮肤病诊断中仍然占有十分重要的地位,因此皮肤病图谱对皮肤科医师有很大的帮助,特别是一些疑难少见的皮肤病,它可起到"看图识病"的效果。

有鉴于此,朱文元教授在担任《临床皮肤科杂志》主编后,注意收集疑难与少见的皮肤病病例,并且添加了朱教授多年来积累的疑难病例,将之汇编成册,予以出版。这本书共收集疑难病例 414 例,图片 1264 帧,不仅有临床照片,同时还有组织病理、免疫组化,以及一些必要的检查,为确诊提供了依据。这些图片图像清晰,色彩逼真,印刷质量高,不失为一本高质量的图谱。它为广大皮肤科临床医师提供了一本有价值的参考书与教材。

本书的另一特点是图解说明采用中英文两种文字,并且同时向国外发行。这在国内出版的图书中还是首次。它可使国外的皮肤科医师对我国的皮肤病有所了解,从而扩大了国际间的学术交流,也增进了与国外皮肤科医师间的相互了解,有利于我国皮肤科事业的进步与发展。

我对朱文元教授和倪容之教授主编的这部图谱的出版表示祝贺。

中国医学科学院皮肤病研究所教授　徐文严

Foreword to the First edition

Professor Zhu Wenyuan is the editor-in-chief of Journal of Clinical Dermatology, he is rich in clinical exprience. After collecting the pictures of difficult, complicated and unusual cases published on the Journal and from his clinical practice, he compiled and edited the atlas.

The atlas consists of 414 cases and 1264 pictures including clinical, histopathological and other labolatory findings. The pictures are clear, true to life, and sufficiently big. It is really a color atlas of high quality, and provides a valuable reference and textbook for the dermatologists.

Another feature of the atlas is that the explanations of the atlas are bilingual, both in Chinese and English, besides the atlas will be distributed to other countries, this is the first time for dermatologic books. It enables the dermatologists of other countries easy to read, and understand the dermatology in China, what are the difficult and complicated skin diseases, how are they manifested etc. The result will broaden the international academic exchanges, enhance mutual understanding between the Chinese dermatologists and their foreign counterparts, and promote the development of dermatology of China.

I warmly congratulate the publication of the atlas edited by Professor Zhu Wen-yuan and Professor Ni Rong-zhi.

Xu wenyan, MD
Professor of Dermatology
Institute of Dermatology
Chinese Academy of Medical Sciences

第 1 版序二

　　我一直热切盼望着这本关于中国皮肤疾病的重要图书的出版。对西方皮肤病医生而言，中国人群的皮肤结构和皮肤疾病在很大程度上仍是个未知数。我们相信所有的常见病都会出现在这个人口众多和多样化的民族中，此外必定还有许多常见病的少见变异型以及罕有病种的存在，而在中国以外的地方少见或不为所知。这本图谱将告诉我们期待已久的中国人群的皮肤结构和皮肤疾病。近年来贸易合作的加强，旅游业的普及以及定居各地中国人群亲属间的探访活动，造成亚裔人群在美国人口比例升高，因此这本著作意义尤显重大。在与亚裔人群越来越多的接触中，西方皮肤病医生能拥有这本图册在手作为参考很有用。不仅能提高诊断能力，还能对以往不能处理的常见或少见病的病人提供新的治疗选择。因此，再次祝贺本书的出版。

Peter M. Elias，M.D.

美国加利福尼亚大学医学院旧金山分校皮肤科

Foreward to the First edition

　　I am eagerly awaiting and anticipating the publication of this most important volume on skin diseases in the Chinese population. For Western dermatologists, the world of chinese skin and skin diseases is still largely a mystery. We know that all of the common diseases must occur in this huge and diverse population, but there must be many unusual variations on the common, as well as many unusual and rare disease entities that are still uncommon or unknown outside of China. Therefore, the images in the atlas will tell the longawaited story of Chinese skin and skin disease to the outside world. The importance of this work is further underscored by the considerable intermingling of our populations that has occurred in recent years due to intense commercial interactions, ever-more common tourism, visitations among relatives of Chinese in all part of the world. It will be important for the Western dermatologist, therefore, to have this volume close at hand as a reference work during his/her increasingly frequent interactions with these groups of patients. Finally, increased awareness will not only improve diagnostic capabilities, but also open up new treatment options for formerly-isolated patients with both common and rare skin diseases. Therefore, I must once again congratulate you on this important effort.

Peter M. Elias, M. D.

Professor of Dermatology

University of California San Francisco

&. Dermatology Service and Research Unit (190)

Department of Veterans' Affairs Medical Center

4150 Clement Street

San Francisco, CA 94121-1545

第 1 版前言

中国有 13 亿人口、56 个民族和 960 万平方公里土地，她是有五千年历史的文明古国。根据报道中国人和外国人皮肤病的患病率基本相等。因此可以推算中国的皮肤病患者绝对人数应是世界第一，一定有很多少见病、疑难病。中国地理环境和气候差异很大，因此同一种病可能有各色各样的临床表现和曲折多变的转归。我深信绝大多数国外新发现的皮肤病都会在中国出现；我也深信中国人患的皮肤病中有尚未被认识的新病种。

据 1995 年中华医学会皮肤科学会公布的资料，全国共有 11 144 名皮肤科医师，其中主任医师 446 人，副主任医师 1105 人，主治医师 4069 人，住院医师 5524 人。他们分布在全国 28 个省、自治区各级医院内。随着人民生活水平的不断提高，患者保健和求医意识的增强，许多少见和疑难皮肤病不断被报告。《临床皮肤科杂志》创刊于 1980 年，办刊宗旨是面向临床，主要刊登病例报告、临床研究和治疗的文章。初为季刊，后改为双月刊。2002 年改为月刊，采用全彩版印刷，图片更清晰。发表了很多高水平的少见和疑难皮肤病，对广大年轻皮肤科医师受益匪浅。应国内外读者的要求，我们将近 6 年来在本刊上发表的疑难皮肤病图片汇集成册，其中还添加我 46 年临床实践中所积累的照片和十余年来指导博士研究生报告的疑难病例。共计有 414 个疑难皮肤病例，1264 张照片编成图谱。本图谱有下列特点：①均为少见和疑难皮肤病；②除临床照片外还同时有组织病理、免疫组化和相关检查，能提供确实的诊断依据；③为增强和扩大学术交流，图解说明采用中英文两种文字；④图片清晰，色彩逼真，图片较大，真实反映了皮肤病的原貌，便于读者学习；⑤本图谱是集体智慧的结晶，编写人员即提供图片的第一作者共计 278 人，他们为图谱提供了很多精美图片。本图谱能顺利出版，我衷心感谢"临床皮肤科杂志"全体编辑和人民军医出版社杨磊石主编的支持。感谢徐文严教授为本书作序。特别感谢美国加利福尼亚大学医学院旧金山分校皮肤科 Theodora M. Mauro 教授在百忙中为图片英文说明审校。该科国际知名教授 Peter M. Elias 为图谱作序。他们的帮助和支持使图谱更加精彩。图片中英文说明由我和副主编侯麦花博士编写。由于时间仓促，疏漏谬误之处，恳请海内外读者不吝赐教，以备再版时修正，渐臻完善。

《临床皮肤科杂志》主编

南京医科大学第一附属医院皮肤科教授

朱文元

2007 年 10 月

Foreword to the First edition

China has a population of 1. 3 billion, 56 nationalities and 9. 6 million square kilometers of land, and represents an ancient nation with a 5000 year history. According to reports, the morbidity of skin disease is basically equal between Chinese and foreigners. Therefore, the absolute population of Chinese patients with skin diseases is the highest in the world, and certainly China has many rare and difficult skin diseases. The geographical environment of China and the climate differences are very unique. Therefore, identical diseases may have assorted clinical manifestations and outcomes. I strongly believe that the overwhelming majority of skin diseases recently discovered overseas should soon appear in China; I also deeply believe that the Chinese have the new skin diseases which are not yet known or well described.

The China Academic Association of Dermatology announced data regarding dermatology in China in 1995. The nation altogether has 11,144 dermatologists,446 physicians-in-charge (i. e. Professors), 1105 assistant director doctors (i. e. Associate Professors), and 4069 doctors-in-charge (i. e. Assistant Professors), 5524 residents. These various individuals are distributed in different hospital levels all over China. As the living standard, patient healthcare, as well as, seeking medical help consciousness is improving, many rare and difficult skin diseases will be consistently reported. The "Clinical Journal of Dermatology" began publication in 1980; the Journal objective is to publish mainly case-reports, clinical research and articles about patient treatment. Initially, it was a quarterly publication, but later changed to a bimonthly publication. In 2002, the Journal changed to a monthly publication with the entire Journal published in color, with enhanced quality. The Journal published many articles about rare and difficult skin diseases. At the request of many domestic and foreign readers, the pictures of difficult skin diseases that were published in the last six years of the Journal and included clinical pictures from my 46 years of clinical practice published in a single monograph. This totaled some 414 difficult skins cases and 1,264 pictures to create an atlas of Dermatology. This atlas has the following characteristics:①It includes rare and difficult skin diseases;②In addition to the clinical pictures, histopathology has been organized along with immunopathology and related examinations to help provide a more accurate diagnosis;③In order to strengthen and expand the academic exchange, Figure legends are provided in both Chinese and English languages;④The photoimages are clear, color, life-like and large sized to help reflect the original skin disease condition, which is advantageous for the readers to study and review;⑤This atlas is the culmination of collective wisdom in dermatology, combing clinical images previously published by many individual dermatologists, 278 of which were the first author. Each of them provided many fine images for the atlas, making this publication readily possible. My heartfelt thanks to all Editors of the "Clinical Journal of Dermatology" and to the Chief Editor Yang Leishi of the People's Military Medical Publishing House for supporting this work. and to the professor XU Wenyan for writing the foreword of the atlas. Specially, the authors thank Professor of Dermatology, Theodora M. Mauro, School of Medicine, University of California in San Francisco for editing English text that accompanies the images. In addition, the authors thank internationally-renown Professor, Peter M. Elias who wrote the foreword for the atlas. Their help and support allowed the atlas to be more splendid. Due to the time constraints, the explanations for the pictures in both Chinese and English were compiled by vice-Chief Editor, Dr. Hou Maihua, and myself. We would appreciate if readers would notify us of any oversights and/or mistakes, such that a revised edition can be greatly improved.

ZHU Wenyuan M. D.

Editor-in-Chief of Clinical Journal of Dermatology

Professor of Dermatology, The First Affiliated Hospital, Nanjing Medical University

In October, 2007

目录 CONTENTS

1

第6章　寄生虫、昆虫及动物性皮肤病
Parasitic Infestations, Stings, and Bites

第 7 章　性传播性疾病 Sexually Transmitted Diseases

第 8 章　物理性疾病 Dermatoses Resulting from Physical Factors

第 9 章　变态反应性皮肤病 Hypersensitivity Diseases

第 10 章　职业性皮肤病 Occupational Disease

第 11 章　结缔组织病 Connective Tissue Diseases

第 12 章　与皮肤有关的免疫缺陷病
Skin Related Immunodeficiency Disorder

第 13 章　角化性皮肤病 Keratoderma

第 14 章　红斑性皮肤病 Erythematous Disease

第 15 章　丘疹鳞屑性皮病 Papule and Scale Diseases

第 16 章 大疱和无菌性脓疱性皮病 Chronic Blistering Dermatoses

第 17 章　真皮弹性纤维疾病 Dermal Elastic Tissue Diseases

第 18 章　萎缩性皮肤病 Atrophy Diseases

第 19 章　皮肤血管炎 Cutaneous Vasculitis

第 20 章　皮肤脉管性疾病 Cutaneous Vascular Diseases

第 21 章　皮下脂肪组织疾病 Subcutaneous Adipose Tissue Diseases

第 22 章　非感染性肉芽肿 Noinfectious Granuloma

第 23 章　皮肤附属器疾病 Diseases of the Skin Appendages

第 24 章　内分泌障碍性皮肤病 Endocrine Skin Diseases

第 25 章 代谢、营养障碍性皮肤病
Metabolic and Nutritional Skin Diseases

第 26 章 色素障碍性皮肤病 Disturbances of Pigmentation

第 27 章　先天性、遗传性皮病 Genodermatoses

第 28 章　黏膜及黏膜皮肤交界处疾病
Disorders of the Mucous Membranes

第 29 章　皮肤肿瘤 Tumors of the Skin

第 30 章　与皮肤病有关的综合征
Cutaneous Syndromes in Dermatology

第1章
病毒感染性皮肤病 Viral Diseases

1. 新生儿单纯疱疹病毒感染
Neonatal herpes simplex virus infection

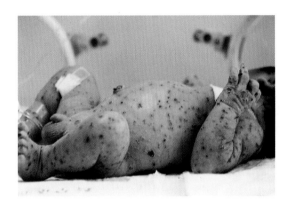

图 1-1-1　全身散在红斑、丘疹、水疱、血疱和结痂

Figure 1-1-1　Generalized lesions all over the body including erythema, petechiae, umbilicated vesicles, and hemorrhagic bullae on the base of erythema

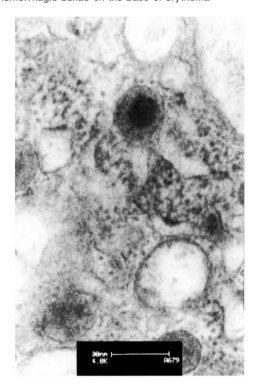

2. 双侧带状疱疹
Bilateral herpes zoster

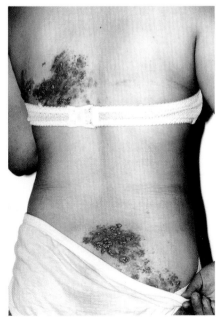

图 1-1-2　透射电镜下单纯疱疹病毒颗粒外观（×20 000）

Figure 1-1-2　Detectable particles of HSV in the biopsied lesion under electron microscope

图 1-2-1　左侧胸背部和右臀部在红斑的基础上有簇集的水疱

Figure 1-2-1　Groups of vesicles are situated on an erythema base on the left chest back and right buttoch

1

3. 巨大寻常疣伴皮角
Giant verruca vulgaris associated with cutaneous horns

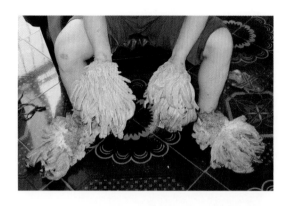 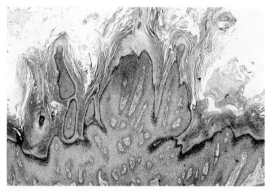

图 1-3-1　双手足数百个密集融合、巨大的坚硬皮角，皮角直径 0.5～5cm,长 0.5～21cm,皮角呈棕黄色

Figure 1-3-1　Hundreds of giant confluent yellowish brown, hard cutaneous horns on both hands and feet. The horn size ranged from 0.5 to 5cm in diameter and from 0.5 to 21cm in length

图 1-3-2　角化过度,棘层肥厚和乳头瘤样增生,表皮嵴延长,两侧向内卷曲(HE 染色,×100)

Figure 1-3-2　Hyperkeratosis, acanthosis and papillomatosis rete ridges elongate and curve inwards at both margins (HE stain, ×100)

4. 外耳道乳头状瘤病
Papillomatosis of external auditory canal

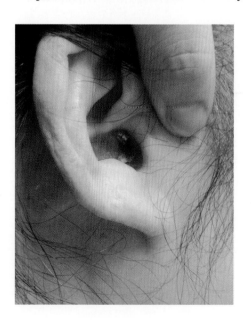

图 1-4-1　二个褐黑疣状丘疹在右外耳道

Figure 1-4-1　Two dark brown verrucous papules in the right external auditory canal

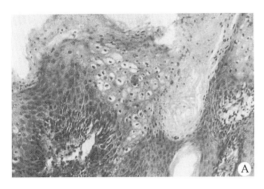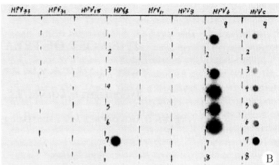

图 1-4-2 A. 病理表现为棘层肥厚和乳头瘤样增生,棘层上部有凹空细胞(HE 染色,×100); B. 聚合酶链检测发现为人乳头瘤病毒 DNA 6 型

Figure 1-4-2 A. Acanthosis and papillomatosis with a few vacuolated cells in the upper stratum Malpighi(HE stain,×100); B. HPV DNA type 6 was detected using polymerase chain reaction

5. 鲍恩样丘疹病
Bowenoid papulosis

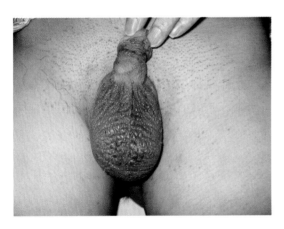

图 1-5-1 阴囊和阴茎有群集扁平,光滑紫红色丘疹

Figure 1-5-1 Grouped flat, smooth, violet red papules on the scrotum and penis

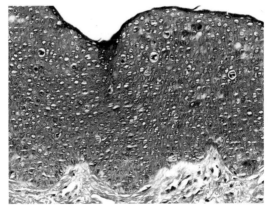

图 1-5-2 部分表皮细胞大,核深染,异形,有不典型核分裂(HE 染色,×100)

Figure 1-5-2 Some of epidermal cells are large, hyperchromatic and pleomorphic and atypical mitoses (HE stain,×100)

6. 非对称性近屈曲部疹

Asymmetric periflexural exanthema

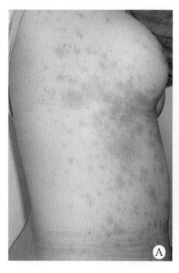
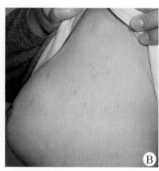

图 1-6-1 A. 右侧胁、胸腹部密集分布红斑、丘疹,部分融合成片;B. 左侧躯干仅少量分布红斑、丘疹

Figure 1-6-1 A. Erythemas and papules were densely distributed on the right thorax and abdomen, some of which tended to becoalesced; B. Similar lesions were sparsely distributed on the left trunk

第 2 章
球菌感染性皮肤病 Bacterial Infections

1. 富尼埃坏疽(暴发性生殖器坏疽)
Fournier gangrene(Severe Fournier gangrene)

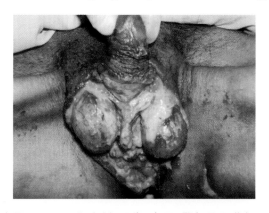

图 2-1-1　肛门左侧、阴囊、会阴、臀部及阴茎根部可见大片溃疡,深达筋膜,双侧睾丸裸露,溃疡潜行,溃疡基底不平,散布黄豆大红色肉芽组织

Figure 2-1-1　Large ulceration on the external genitalia,which involved perianal,and scrotal regions

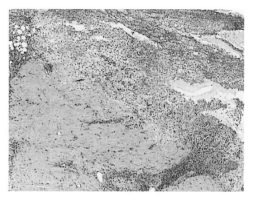

图 2-1-2　真皮浅层血管扩张、水肿,散在或小片状淋巴细胞、组织细胞及浆细胞浸润,真皮下部及皮下组织血管增生扩张,有淋巴细胞、组织细胞及中性粒细胞浸润,可见片状组织坏死(HE 染色,×20)

Figure 2-1-2　Dilated vessels and edema in the superficial dermis and scatter lymphocytes, histocytes and neutrophils infiltrate, with focal necrosis in the dermis (HE stain, ×20)

2. 浅表肉芽肿性脓皮病
Superficial granulomatous pyoderma

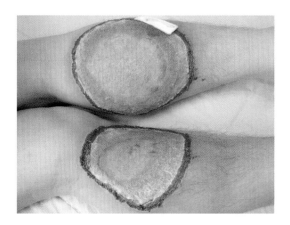

图 2-2-1　双侧小腿伸侧各有红褐色圆形斑块,边缘隆起,中间呈特征性结痂

Figure 2-2-1　Red-brown annular papules and plaques with elevated borders and central scars on the extensors of both calves

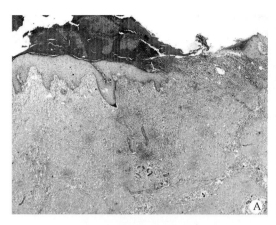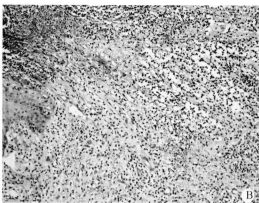

图 2-2-2　部分表皮坏死缺失,真皮浅层部分血管壁纤维素样变性,血管周围淋巴细胞、组织细胞、嗜中性粒细胞及嗜酸性粒细胞浸润(HE 染色,A×40,B×200)

Figure 2-2-2　Partial epidermal necrosis and defect;some fibrinoid degeneration of vessel walls in the upper dermis;Perivascular lymphocyte,histiocyte,neutrophil and eosinophil infiltration (HE stain,A×40,B×200)

第3章
杆菌感染性皮肤病
Mycobacterial Diseases

1. 界线类偏结核样型麻风
Tuberculoid borderline leprosy

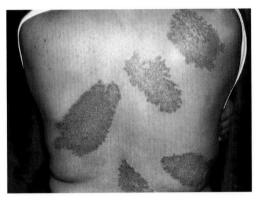

图 3-1-1　背部淡褐色斑块,边界清楚,中央稍萎缩,表面少许鳞屑

Figure 3-1-1　Well-circumscribed, scaly, slight brown plaques with central atrophy on the back

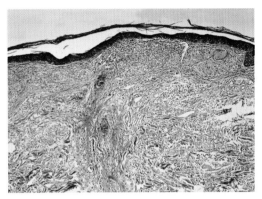

图 3-1-2　表皮萎缩,表皮突变平,真皮浅、中层可见结核样肉芽肿(HE 染色,×100)

Figure 3-1-2　Atrophy epidermis, flat rete ridges, tuberculoid granuloma in the upper and middle dermis (HE stain, ×100)

2. 增殖性寻常狼疮
Proliferative lupus vulgaris

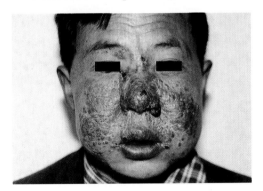

图 3-2-1　鼻、面部暗红色浸润性斑块及结节

Figure 3-2-1　Brown reddish plaques and nodules on the face and nose

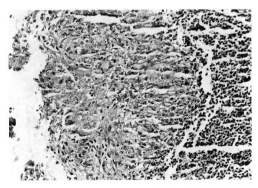

图 3-2-2　真皮网状层可见上皮样细胞团块,周围有淋巴细胞及多核巨细胞浸润(HE 染色,×200)

Figure 3-2-2　Tuberculoid structures consisted of epithelioid cells, giant cells and lymphocytes in the reticular dermis (HE stain, ×200)

3. 疣状皮肤结核
Tuberculosis verrucosa cutis

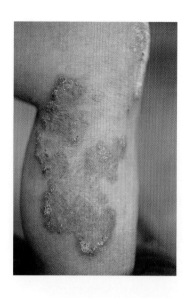

图 3-3-1   左小腿有一大的疣状角化斑块,中心萎缩,周围有炎症红斑

Figure 3-3-1   A large verrucous plaque with an inflammatory border and an atrophy at center on the left leg

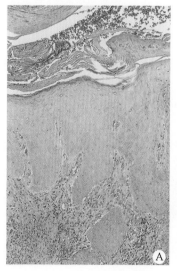
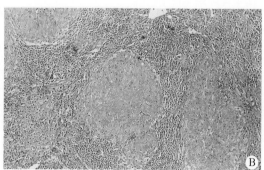

图 3-3-2   A. 真皮内有结核样结节(HE 染色,×40);B. 角化过度和棘层肥厚,真皮浅层有结核样结节(HE 染色,×100)

Figure 3-3-2   A. Tuberculoid granulomas in the dermis(HE stain,×40);B. Hyperkeratosis and acathosis associated with tuberculoid granuloma beneath the epidermis(HE stain,× 100)

4. 游泳池肉芽肿
Swimming pool granuloma

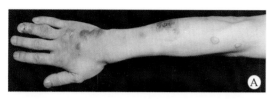 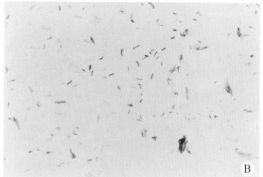

图 3-4-1　A. 右手环指甲周暗红色斑块,同侧手背、手腕、前臂及上臂成串排列的黄豆至蚕豆大小暗红色结节,共 15 个皮损;B. 组织培养分离出海分枝杆菌(Z-N 染色,×1000)

Figure 3-4-1　A. The size of soybean and horsebean dusky red plaques and nodules on the right ring fingers, back of the hands, wrist, forearm and the upper arm, in linear arrangement; B. Identification of Mycobacterium marinum in tissue culture (Ziehl-Neelsen stain, × 1000)

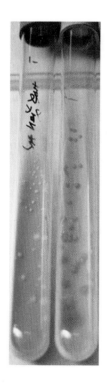

图 3-4-2　海分枝杆菌菌落经自然光照射后产生黄色色素,左侧为照光前,右侧为照光后

Figure 3-4-2　Mycobacterium marinum colony produces yellow color under sunlight, before sunlight(left), after sunlight (right)

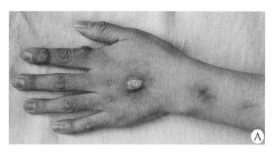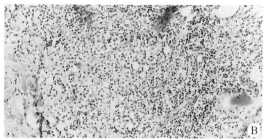

图 3-4-3　A. 左手示指、手背 3 个暗红色结节,腕关节伸侧 2 个暗红色浸润性斑块;B. 真皮大片组织细胞和淋巴细胞浸润,偶见嗜酸性粒细胞,呈感染性肉芽肿改变(HE 染色,×200)

Figure 3-4-3　A. Three reddish nodules on the forefinger and back of the hands, two reddish infiltrative plaques on the back of wrist; B. Multiple histocytes and lymphocytes infiltrate in the dermis with sporadic eosinophil and granuloma formation (HE stain,×200)

5. 皮肤炭疽病
Cutaneous anthrax

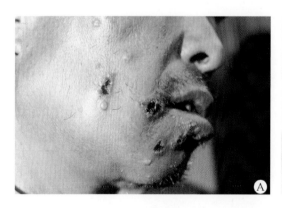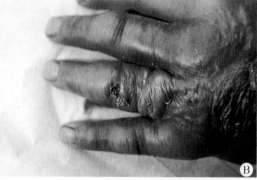

图 3-5-1　A. 右颊部有 4 个被黑色痂的溃疡,周围有水疱和脓疱;B. 左手背有明显弥漫性水肿紫红色斑,中心有溃疡

Figure 3-5-1　A. Four ulcers covered with dark crasts surrounded by vesicles and pustules on the right cheek; B. Intense diffuse swelling and violet red patches undergoing central ulcer on the dorsum of left hand

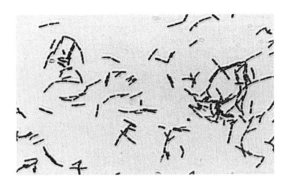

图 3-5-2　炭疽杆菌为革兰染色阳性粗大杆菌（革兰染色，×400）

Figure 3-5-2　Bacillus anthracis are large rod-shaped, gram-positive organism（Gram stain，×400）

6. 窝状角质松解症
Pitted keratolysis

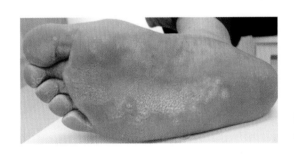

图 3-6-1　跖部有 1～4mm 直径圆形凹坑

Figure 3-6-1　Many discrete round pits in the size of 1 to 4 mm in diameter were on the plantar region

第 4 章
衣原体及立克次体感染性皮肤病
Chlamydiae Diseases

1. Reiter 综合征
Reiter's syndrome

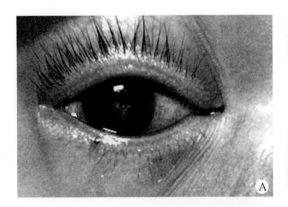
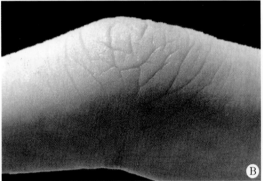
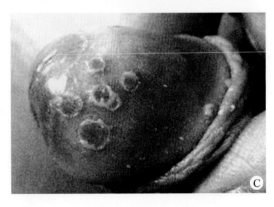

图 4-1-1　A. 右眼结膜充血；B. 右手中指关节肿胀；C. 尿道口红肿，周围可见环状浅表性溃疡
Figure 4-1-1　A. The right conjunctivitis; B. The right middle finger joint swelling; C. Annular superficial ulcers around redness and swelling urethra

第5章
真菌感染性皮肤病 Diseases Resulting from Fungi and Yeasts

1. 成人不典型黄癣
Adult atypical favus

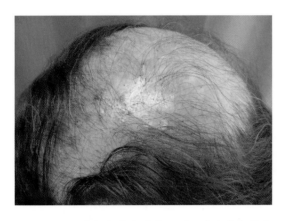

图 5-1-1 55 岁妇女头生秃疮 50 年,头皮有大片光滑薄纸样萎缩斑片,上有鳞屑

Figure 5-1-1 A 55-year woman suffered from baldness for fifty years. A large glossy, thin and paper-white atrophic patch with scales on the scalp

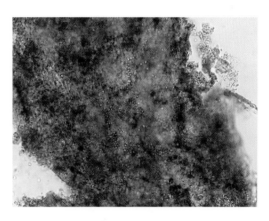

图 5-1-2 光镜下多数发内型孢子

Figure 5-1-2 Numerous microspores of endothrix were found by microscope

2. 猪小孢子菌引起的脓癣
Kerion caused by Microsporum nanum

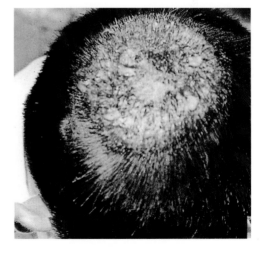

图 5-2-1 头顶有一块溢脓的炎性斑块

Figure 5-2-1 There is an inflammatory plaque exuding pus on the vertex

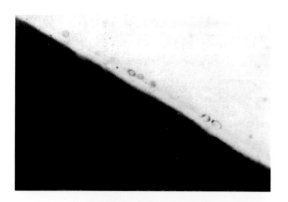

图 5-2-2　病变表面有椭圆形孢子,表面有稀疏突起(×840)

Figure 5-2-2　Ovoid spores with sparse small projections on the shaft of infected hair(×840)

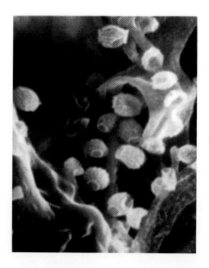

图 5-2-3　扫描电镜下毛干上有许多卵圆形或梨形大分生孢子,表面有稀疏小短突起和颈圈

Figure 5-2-3　Neumerous ovid or pear-shaped macroconidia with spare small projections and collarettes on the shaft by SEM

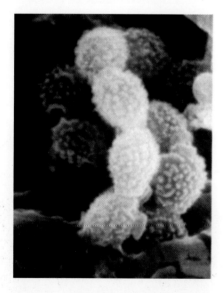

图 5-2-4　扫描电镜下见培养基中的大分生孢子表面稀疏短突和颈圈

Figure 5-2-4　Macroconidia with sparse small projections and collar in culture by SEM

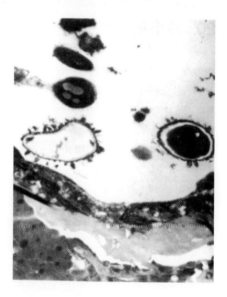

图 5-2-5　透射电镜下见病变表面有大分生孢子,表面有电子致密的绒毛样突起(×8 000)

Figure 5-2-5　Macroconidia has villus-like projections with electrondense areas on the surface of infected hair by TEM(×8 000)

3. 红色毛癣菌致股癣合并龟头癣
Tinea cruris and tinea of glans penis caused by Trichophyton rubrum

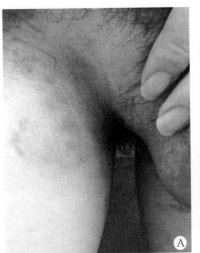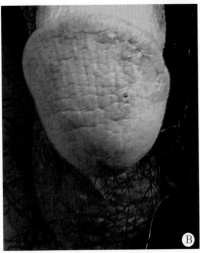

图 5-3-1 股内侧皮肤(A)及龟头(B)处见境界清楚的红斑伴少许鳞屑,边缘微隆起

Figure 5-3-1 Scaly erythemas with clear and raised margins of bilateral groin and the glans of the penis

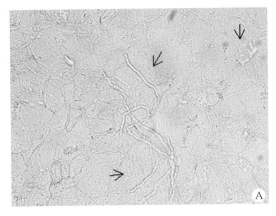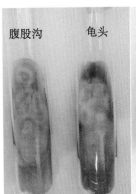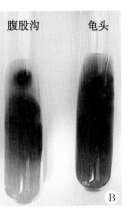

图 5-3-2 A. 真菌镜检见分枝菌丝(×40);B. 沙堡培养基 25℃ 培养 7 天,培养基从白色(左)变成深红色(右)

Figure 5-3-2 A. Branchingmycelium was found by microscope examination (×40);B. The colony was incubated on Sabouraud dextrose agar at 25℃ for 7 days. The color of the medium became port wine color (right) from white (left)

15

4. 红色毛癣菌肉芽肿
Trichophyton rubrum granuloma

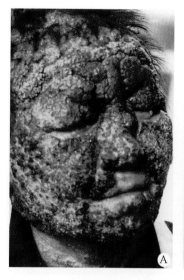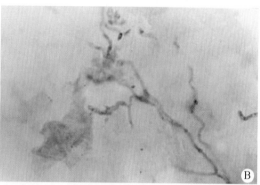

图 5-4-1　A. 头面许多暗红色浸润斑块结痂伴面部疣状结节；B. 镜检查见真菌菌丝

Figure 5-4-1　A. Numerous dark red infiltrate plaques and verrucous nodules associated with crusts on the face and scalp；B. Slide showing mycelium

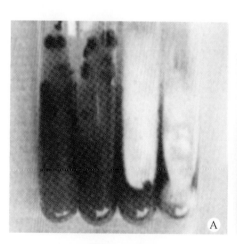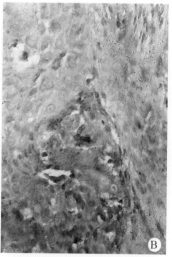

图 5-4-2　A. 培养为红色毛癣菌生长；B. 角化过度，棘层肥厚，真皮内可见中性粒细胞、嗜酸性粒细胞、淋巴细胞、浆细胞、上皮样细胞等非特异性炎症浸润，并见多核巨细胞，见真菌孢子和菌丝（PAS 染色）

Figure 5-4-2　A. Cultures of Trichophyton rubrum；B. Hyperkeratosis and acanthosis, neutrophils, eosinophils, lymphocytes, plasm cell and epithelioid cells infiltrate in the dermis with multinucleated giant cells, fungal spores and hyphae (PAS stain)

5. 皮肤播散性红色毛癣菌病

Diffused dermatophytosis resulting from trichophyton rubrum

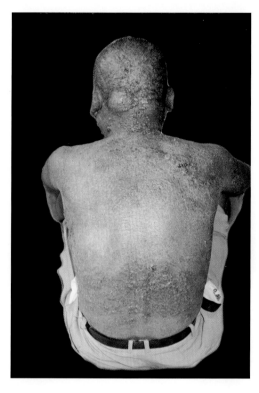

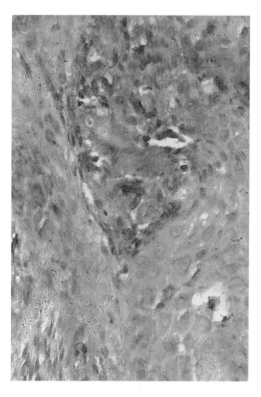

图 5-5-1 毛发稀疏及片状脱发区,头部有明显浸润的暗红斑;枕部两鸡蛋大小的斑块,躯干及肢端有大小不一的斑块及灰色、红色及暗褐色的斑片

Figure 5-5-1 Sparse hair, patchy hair-loss areas, dark erythemas with obvious infiltration appeared on the head; two egg-sized masses presented on the occipital area. Various-sized plaques and gray, red, or dark black patches distributed on the trunk and extremities

图 5-5-2 组织中有孢子及菌丝(PAS 染色,×200)

Figure 5-5-2 The pathological changes of the lesion showed: fungal spores and hyphae in the tissue (PAS stain, ×200)

6. 掌黑癣

Tinea manuum nigra

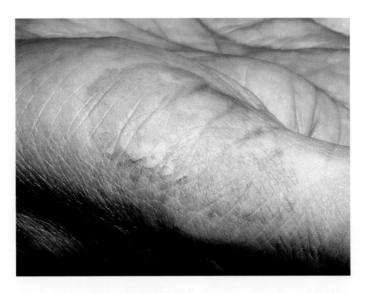

图 5-6-1 右手掌有一个大浅黑色斑

Figure 5-6-1 A big light dark macule on the right palm

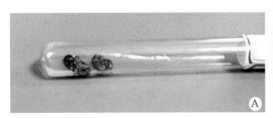
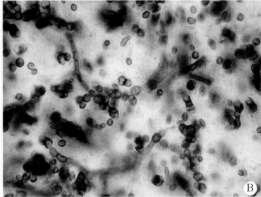

图 5-6-2 A. 培养为黑色酵母样菌落；B. 镜下可见棕色分隔菌丝，大量厚壁孢子(棉蓝染色，×40)

Figure 5-6-2 A. A black yeast-like colony on the medium; B. Brown septate hyphae and lots of chlamydospores under the microscope (cotton blue stain, ×40)

7. 花斑癣
Tinea versicolor

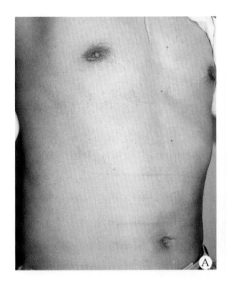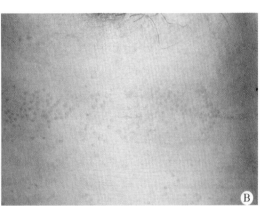

图 5-7-1　右胸部见密集性粟米大小红褐色斑丘疹。皮损沿数个 Blaschko 线群集成 S 形（Blaschko 线 lb 型）

Figure 5-7-1　On the right chest, there were numerous follicular brownish-red maculopapules, giving several S-shaped band-like appearances（type 1b Blaschko's lines）

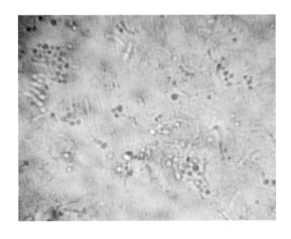

图 5-7-2　显微镜下可见大量短杆状的菌丝和少量聚集的圆形孢子，似意大利面条及肉丸样

Figure 5-7-2　Direct mycological examination showed slender septate hyphae and spores with spaghetti and meatball-like appearance（×40）

8. 皮肤念珠菌性肉芽肿合并念珠菌性颈淋巴结炎
Skin candidal granuloma complicated by candidal cervical lymphadenitis

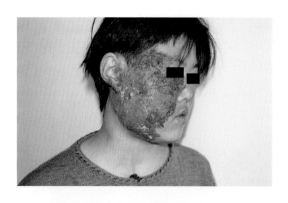

图 5-8-1　右侧面部边缘整齐、棕红色疣赘,结痂性肉芽肿

Figure 5-8-1　Brownish red neoplasm and granuloma on the face

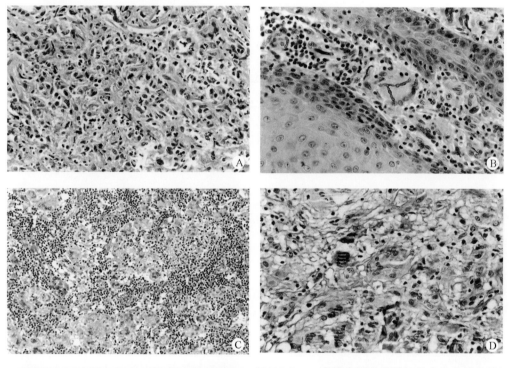

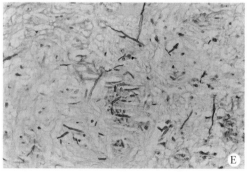

图 5-8-2　A. 黏膜表面肉芽肿组织中见多量菌丝(HE 染色,×200);B. 真皮内见大量炎性细胞浸润,肉芽肿形成,巨细胞内外见大量菌丝(HE 染色,×400);C、D. 淋巴结组织内见大量念珠菌引起的肉芽肿(HE 染色,×100、×400);E. 细胞内外见大量念珠菌菌丝,部分菌丝有分枝(PAS 染色,×100)

Figure 5-8-2　A. Numerous mycelial filament in the granuloma tissue(HE stain,×200); B. Numerous inflammatory infiltrate and granuloma in the dermis,numerous mycelial filament in and outer of giant cells(HE stain,×400);C,D. Numerous candidal granuloma in lymph node (HE stain, C×100, D×400); E.Numerous mycelial filament in and outer of cells(PAS stain,×100)

9. 慢性皮肤黏膜念珠菌病
Chronic mucocutaneous candidiasis

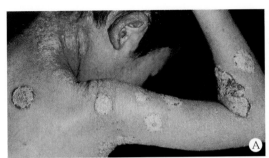
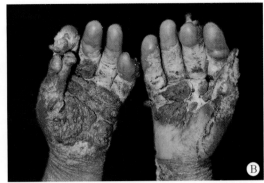
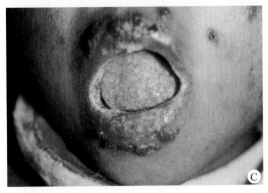

图 5-9-1　A. 右上肢有许多暗红色和褐色斑,表面有结痂和鳞屑;B. 双手掌疣状赘生物;C. 舌和唇有不易脱落的白色假膜

Figure 5-9-1　A. Many duck red and brown patches covered with crusts and scales on the right arm; B. Both metacarprophalangeal verrucous vegetation; C.Moniliasis of the tongue and lips

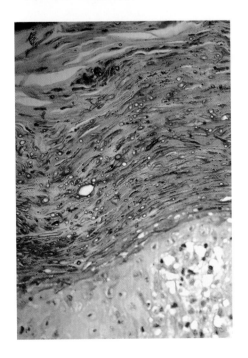

图 5-9-2　表皮角质层内有大量菌丝和孢子(PAS 染色,×400)

Figure 5-9-2　A large of hyphae and spors in keratotic layer of epidermis(PAS stain,×400)

10. 原发性皮肤隐球菌病
Primary cutaneous cryptoccosis

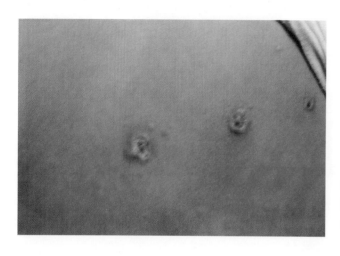

图 5-10-1　背部有 3 个中心呈脐凹状隆起的丘疹和结节

Figure 5-10-1　Three elevated papules and nodules with umbilicated centers on the back

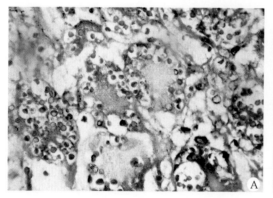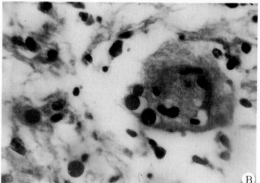

图 5-10-2　A. 真皮多核巨细胞内外有大量真菌孢子(PAS 染色,×400);B. 3 个典型的孢子在真皮中一个多核巨细胞内(PAS 染色,×1500)

Figure 5-10-2　A. A large mass of spores is located in or outer giant cells in the dermis(PAS stain,×400); B. Three typical spores are present in a giant cell in the dermis(PAS stain,×1500)

11. 皮肤隐球菌病
Cutaneous cryptococcosis

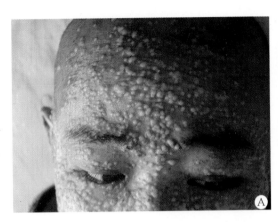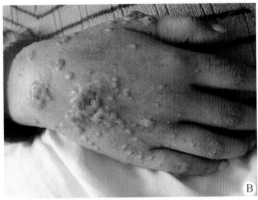

图 5-11-1 面部(A)及手背(B)密集乳白色米粒至黄豆大丘疹或蚕豆大斑块

Figure 5-11-1 Multiple molluscum contagiosum-like skin lesions on the face（A）and forearm（B）

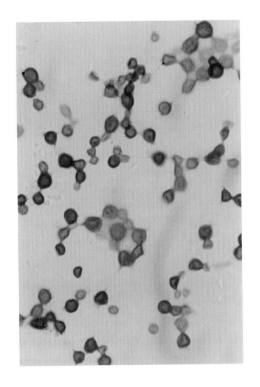

图 5-11-2 真皮空隙内有大量紫红色圆形孢子（PAS
染色，×1000）

Figure 5-11-2 A large of violet red spores in dermis
（PAS stain，×1000）

12. 传染性软疣样皮损表现的播散性隐球菌病
Disseminated cryptococcosis resembling molluscum contagiosum

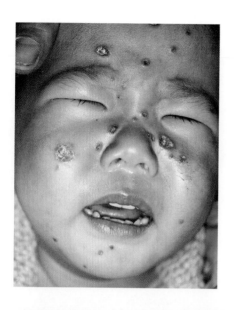

图 5-12-1　面部原发传染性软疣样丘疹,部分继发坏死、溃疡、结痂

Figure 5-12-1　The papules resembling molluscum contagiosum on the face, some of them having necrosis, ulcers and crust

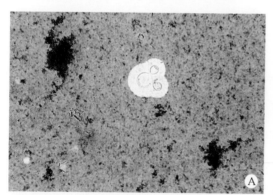

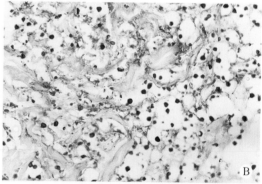

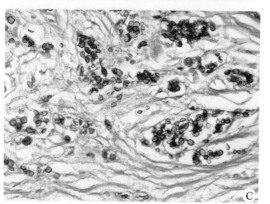

图 5-12-2　A. 脑脊液直接涂片镜检,显示具有荚膜的孢子,部分出芽(印度墨水染色,×40);B. 传染性软疣样丘疹组织病理检查,显示真皮内众多一致性较小圆形嗜伊红孢子,部分孢子出芽(PAS 染色,×40);C. 皮损组织病理显示:经阿新蓝 PAS 复染后,异染孢子呈红色,周围荚膜呈蓝色(阿新蓝-PAS 染色,×40)

Figure 5-12-2　A. Smears from CSF fluid showed the spore surrounded by a capsule, some of them budding (Indian ink stain, ×40); B. Numerous small round eosinophilic spores in the dermis, some of them budding (PAS stain, ×40); C. The alcian blue stain and the PAS reaction combined, the red spores surrounding blue capsule (Alcian blue-PAS stain, ×40)

13. 表现为皮肤溃疡和骨髓炎的播散性隐球菌病
Disseminated cryptococcosis with multiple cutaneous lesions and osteomyelitis

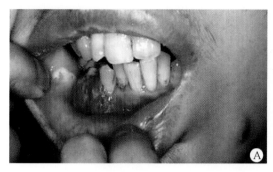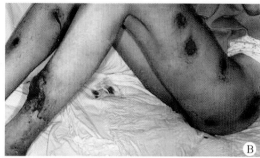

图 5-13-1　A. 下齿龈的右侧一 1.5 cm×2.0cm 的结节,上有溃疡;B. 肢端的结节及溃疡溢脓

Figure 5-13-1　A. A nodule with ulcer sized 1.5 cm×2.0 cm on the right lower gum; B. Nodules and ulcers with discharge on the extremities

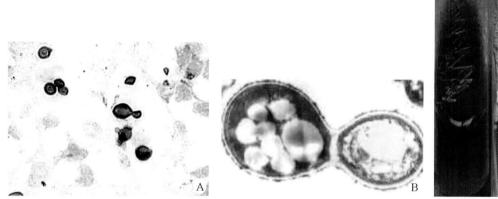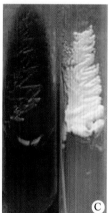

图 5-13-2　A. 组织镜检发现许多菌丝(Gomori 银染色,×1000);B. 透射电镜发现圆形和卵圆形孢子(×12 000);C. 在含 20%尿素的沙堡培养基上 25℃培养 5 天,培养基从白色变为深红色(左侧),而对照组无改变(右侧)

Figure 5-13-2　A. Microscopic examination of the tissue showed numerous budding yeast cells (stained with Gomori's methenamine silver, ×1000); B. Transmission electron microscopy showed the section of spores was round or oval with buds (×12 000); C. The colony was incubated on Sabouraud dextrose agar containing 20% urea of at 25℃ for 5 days. The color of the medium became port wine color from white (left side), while the color of the control did not change (right side)

14. 多发结节表现的孢子丝菌病
Sporotrichosis manifesting in the form of polynodulus

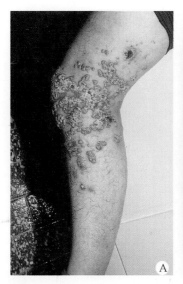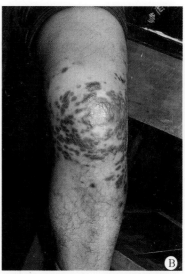

图 5-14-1　A. 膝部多数结节、斑块；B. 治疗 3 周后皮疹基本平坦，部分
瘢痕增生

Figure 5-14-1　A. Multiple nodules and plaques on the knees；B. Lesions flat with scars after treatment for three weeks

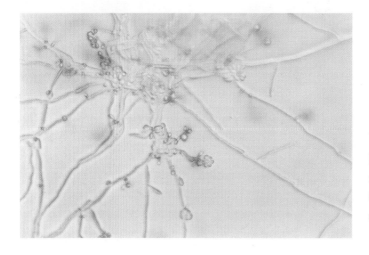

图 5-14-2　培养菌落高倍镜下见直角
分枝梨形孢子(×40)

Figure 5-14-2　Branching pyriform spores in culture(×40)

15. 淋巴管型着色芽生菌病
Chromoblastomycosis with lymphatic spread

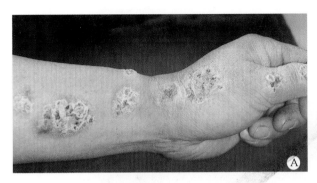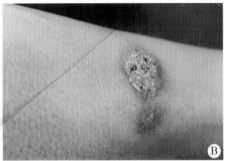

图 5-15-1　A. 皮损自左拇指起结节,呈条状排列伴溃疡结痂;B. 暗红色斑块,上覆黄白色厚痂和散在黑点

Figure 5-15-1　A. The nodules distributed in lines with ulcer and crust from left thumb; B. Wine-coloured plaques covered with yellow-white thickened crust and numerous black speckle

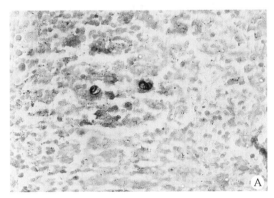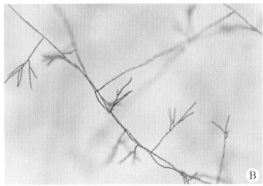

图 5-15-2　A. 组织中见棕色厚壁孢子有隔(PAS 染色,×400);B. 菌落小培养见枝孢型(PDA,×200)

Figure 5-15-2　A. Dark-brown thick-walled oval spores with crosswalls in tissue (PAS stain, ×400); B. Phialophora verrucosa in culture(PDA stain,×200)

16. 蛙粪霉病
Basidiobolomycosis

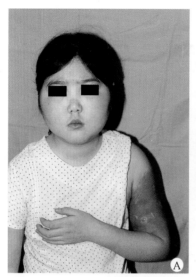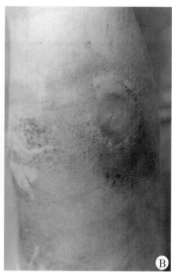

图 5-16-1　左上臂棕色斑块

Figure 5-16-1　The brown mass on the left upper arm

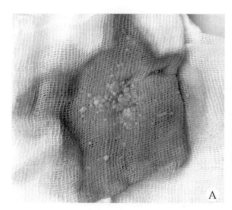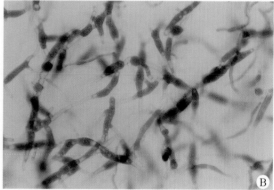

图 5-16-2　A. 柔软的鲜红斑中心破溃,破溃处淡黄色颗粒及脓液溢出; B. 蛙粪霉病的真菌培养,伊曲康唑治疗之前,有隔膜的菌丝生长良好,部分形成孢子(×11 000)

Figure 5-16-2　The flushing erythemas which were softened and broken in the center, the yellowish granules and pus discharged from broken places; B. The observation of fungous culture, before treatment of itraconazole, septate hyphae grew well, some of which expanded to form sporangia(× 100);
(×11 000)

17. 手部放线菌病
Hand actinomycosis

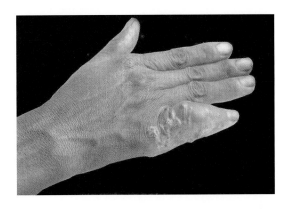

图 5-17-1 小指肿胀表面有多个小脓肿
Figure 5-17-1 Several abscesses in skin of the swelling finger

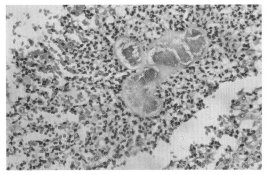

图 5-17-2 小脓肿内见放线菌丛(HE 染色,×100)
Figure 5-17-2 Actinomyces in small abscesses (HE stain,×100)

18. 中型原藻病
Zopfii Protothecosis

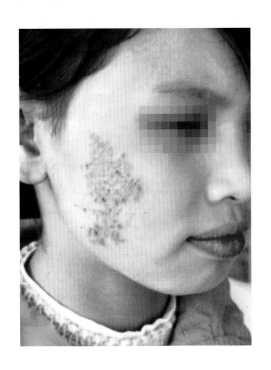

图 5-18-1 左侧面部大片红斑,丘疹,上覆细小鳞屑
Figure 5-18-1 The erythemas,papules and scales are occurred on her right face

29

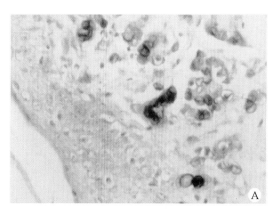
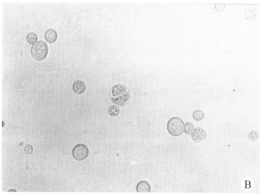

图 5-18-2　A. 真皮浅层,血管和附属器周围少量单一核细胞浸润(PAS 染色,×100);B. 涂片可见散在圆形或椭圆形厚壁孢子,直径 10～18 μm,内含多个直径 3～8 μm 的内孢子(×400)

Figure 5-18-2　A. A few of monocytes infiltrate around the blood vessels and epidermal appendages in the upper dermis(PAS stain,×100);B. A great quanity chlamydospores(diamer 10-18 μm,some diameter 3-8 μm entosporum inside) were discoved in microscope(×400)

19. 奴卡菌性足菌肿
Mycetoma caused bynocardia brasiliensis

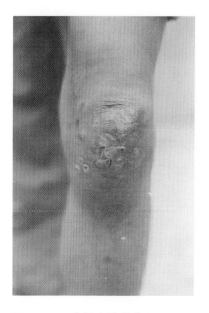

图 5-19-1　膝部皮肤结节和细小窦道,膝上方见一手术切口

Figure 5-19-1　Nodules and small sinus on the knee,a surgical cut on the upside of knee

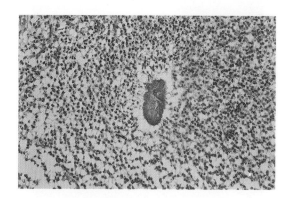

图 5-19-2　大量肉芽性炎症浸润,可见硫黄颗粒(HE 染色,×200)

Figure 5-19-2　Numerous granulomas and inflammatory cells associated with some sulfurate granulas (HE stain,×200)

20. 多变根毛霉引起原发皮肤毛霉病
Primary cutaneousmycormycosis caused by Rhizomucor variabilis

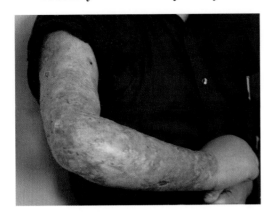

图 5-20-1 右上肢皮肤弥漫性肿胀、斑块、溃疡和结痂

Figure 5-20-1 Diffused swelling, suppurating plaques, ulcer and crust on the right arm

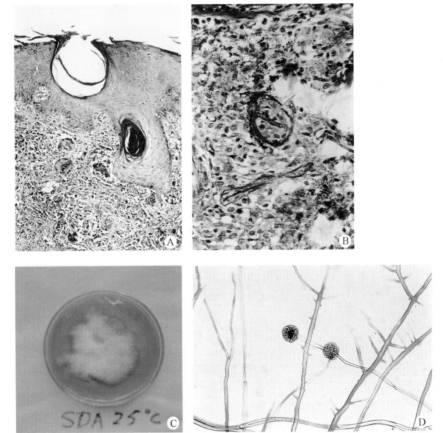

图 5-20-2 A. 真皮内有多数炎性细胞和多核巨细胞浸润(HE染色,×250); B. 血管内和周围有阳性粗长的菌丝(PAS染色,×500); C、D. 多变根毛霉菌菌落形态和大分生孢子

Figure 5-20-2 A. Many inflammatory cells and multinucleated glant cells in the dermis(HE stain,×250); B. A long and wide mycelia(↑),within and around the vessel(PAS stain,×500); C,D. Rhizomucor rariabilis colong and macrospore on the medium

21. 皮肤链格孢霉病
Cutaneous alternariosis

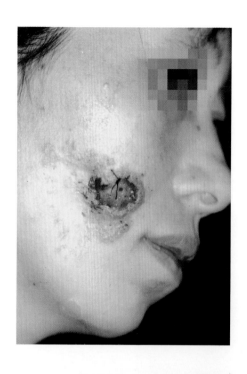

图 5-21-1　右颊部溃疡，边缘呈堤状隆起

Figure 5-21-1　Infiltrative plaques on the right cheek and ulceration in the center

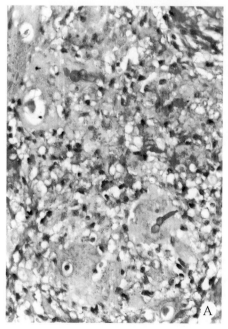

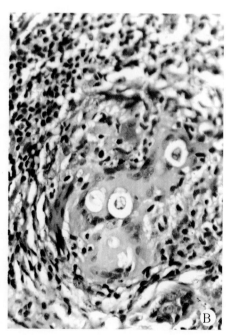

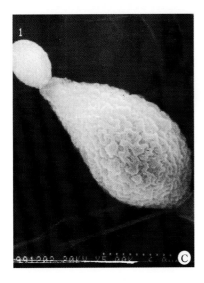
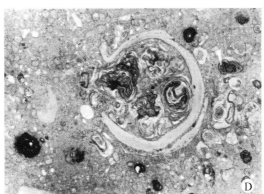

图 5-21-2　A. 巨细胞内大圆形孢子和菌丝(PAS 染色,×400);B. 真皮上部局限性结核样肉芽肿,巨细胞内棕色孢子和空泡样结构(HE 染色,×400);C 链格孢扫描电镜下形态,新生分生孢子(×5000);D. 链格孢透射电镜下形态,巨细胞内较大圆形孢子(×5000)

Figure 5-21-2　A. staining revealed irregular septate hyphae and large round spores inthe giant cells(PAS stain,×400);B. Tuberculoid granulomas with numerous giant cells at the margins of ulceration. Vacuole-like structures and brown septate hyphae and brown spores in the giant cells (HE stain,×400);C. Septate hyphae spores by scanning electron microscopy (×5000);D. Large round spores in the giant cells under transmission electron microscopy (×5000)

22. 镰刀菌皮肤肉芽肿
Skin Fusarium sp. granuloma

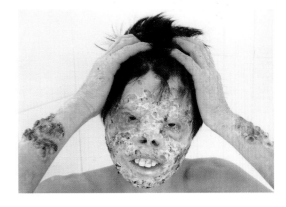

图 5-22-1　面部弥漫浸润性红斑,边缘较清楚,表面有溃烂、结痂、脱屑,双眼睑、鼻翼、耳郭部皮肤溃烂、缺失,睑裂闭合不全,眉毛脱失

Figure 5-22-1　A diffuse infiltrated plaque with ulcers,crusts andscals was on the face. Both eyelid, wing of nose and auricle were destroyed or lost without eyebrow

33

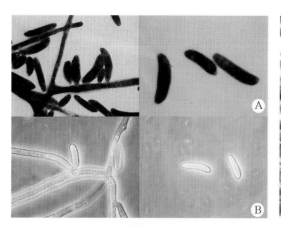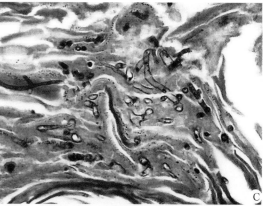

图 5-22-2　A、B. 菌丝分隔、分枝、透明、较粗，小分生孢子呈卵形、椭圆形、肾形，大分生孢子呈镰刀形（A.革兰染色，×5680）；C. 表皮角质层内见真菌菌丝，有分隔（HE 染色，×400）

Figure 5-22-2　A,B. The septate transparent hyphae with branching,oval microspres and sickle like macrospores were present (A.Gram stain,×5680);C. The septate hyphae was present in the horny layer (HE stain,×400)

23. 腋毛菌病
Trichomycosis axillaris

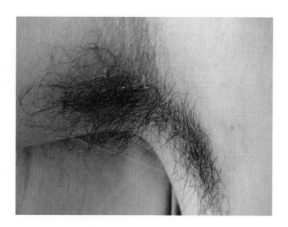

图 5-23-1　受累的腋毛被许多大小不等、形状不规则的结节和细管包绕

Figure 5-23-1　The affected axillary's hair is surrounded by many nodular or tubular concretions in various size and irregular shape

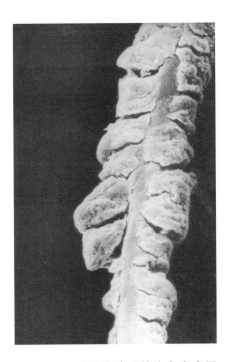

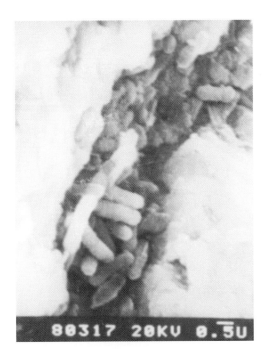

图 5-23-2　受累的腋毛被许多大小不
等、形状不规则的结节和细管包绕
Figure 5-23-2　The affected axillary's
hair is surrounded by many nodular or tubular concretions in various size and irregular shape

图 5-23-3　在凝块表面或凹陷内有粗短的微小
棒状杆菌
Figure 5-23-3　On the surface of the concretions
in their pits there is lots of Coynebacterium Tenuis

第6章
寄生虫、昆虫及动物性皮肤病
Parasitic Infestations, Stings, and Bites

1. 皮肤利什曼病
Leishmaniasis cutis

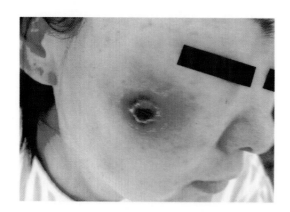

图 6-1-1 左面颊见一个 5 分硬币大溃疡,表面结痂,边缘稍隆起,周边皮肤呈红褐色

Figure 6-1-1 A round ulcer with crust around rufous skin on the left cheek

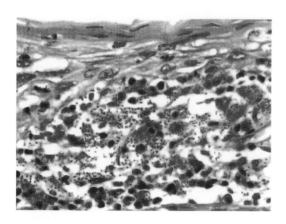

图 6-1-2 真皮乳头层细胞内、外见颗粒状物质(HE 染色,×400)

Figure 6-1-2 Granule-like bodies in the dermis papillaries (HE stain, ×400)

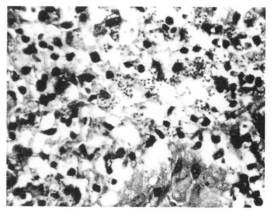

图 6-1-3 利什曼小体内可见到一个较大的紫红色或红色圆形营养核和一个较小的副核(Giemsa 染色,×400)

Figure 6-1-3 A red round nucleus and a smaller rod-like paranucleus in the parasites (Giemsa stain, ×400)

2. 皮肤并殖吸虫病
Skin distoma paragonimiasis

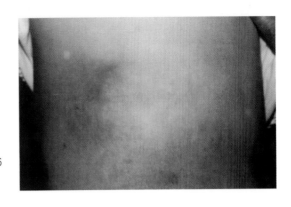

图 6-2-1 腹部有一个 3 cm×6 cm 皮下肿块

Figure 6-2-1 A subcutaneous mass in size of 3 cm×6 cm in diameter on the abdomen

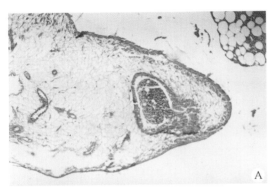 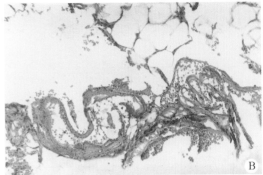

图 6-2-2 在皮下组织有并殖吸虫的肠管部分(A)(HE 染色,×12.5×16)和尾部(B)(HE 染色,×12.5×16)

Figure 6-2-2 Digestine tuke(A) and tail(B) of distoma in subcutis(HE stain,×12.5×16)

3. 匐行疹
Creeping eruption

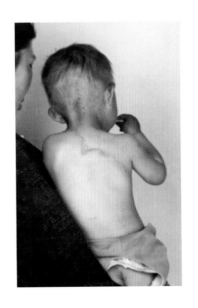

图 6-3-1 枕部、颈部及背部弯曲线状连续性皮疹

Figure 6-3-1 Curve lesions on the occiput,neck and back

4. 皮肤、脑猪囊虫病

Cutis and brain cysticercosis

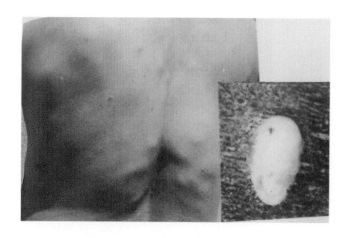

图 6-4-1　背部多个皮下结节

Figure 6-4-1　Numorous subcutaneous nodules on the back

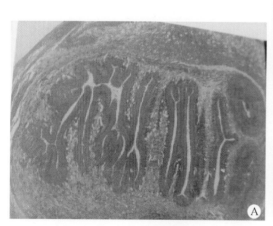

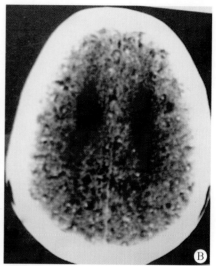

图 6-4-2　A. 皮下有一囊壁,中有圆形吸盘及猪囊尾虫幼的剖面(HE 染色,×40);B. 脑 CT 脑实质中小结节状高密度影,侧脑室体扩大

Figure 6-4-2　A. A parasite in the cystic wall under the subcutaneous(HE stain,×40);B. Computed tomography of the brain showed an enhancing lesion in the cerebral,lateral ventricle of cerebrum dilated

5. 牛皮蝇幼虫所致皮肤蝇蛆病
Cutaneous Myiasis caused by larvae of Hypoderma bovis

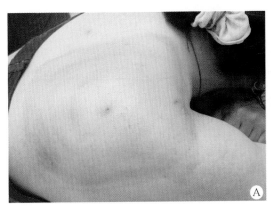
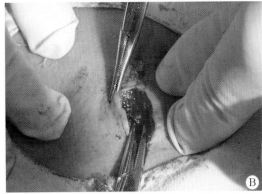

图 6-5-1　A. 肩背部可见三处疖样损害和色素沉着,其中最后发作处皮损且未挤出虫体;B. 活检术中,可见一已与周围组织机化的虫体(下方血管钳所夹、顶端有一黑点)

Figure 6-5-1　A. Three furuncle-like lesions and pigmentation on the shoulder and back(Site C is the most recent lesion with no larva);B. A larva surrounded by tissue (held by vessel forceps with black spot on the top could be seen

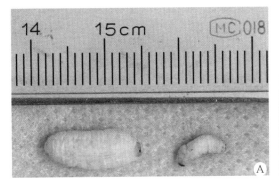
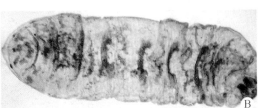

图 6-5-2　A. 虫乳白色,前尖后钝圆柱形,体大者长约 12mm,宽约 5mm;体小者长约 7mm,宽约 2mm;B. 三龄幼虫镜下照片:虫体圆柱形、分节,左为头节,右为腹节(×10)

Figure 6-5-2　A. A cylindrical and milky body with pointed front-end and blunt back-end. The sizes of larvae range from 12mm×5mm to 7mm×2mm;B. Third instar larvae under microscope:The segmented cylindrical body (the left side is scolex and the right side is abdomen) (×10)

6. 眼睑虱病
Phthiriasis palpebrarum

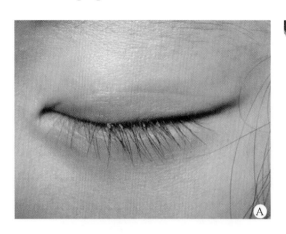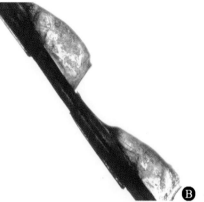

图 6-6-1　A. 左上眼睑睫毛根部可见活动的虫体及密集重叠的灰白色"痂皮"，外观似睑缘炎的鳞屑；B. 头发上的虫卵（×50）

Figure 6-6-1　A. Alive pubic lice and gray white scabs at the roots of the eyelash on the left upper eyelid, mimicking the appearance of the scales in blepharitis; B. The egg is attached to the side of the hair（×50）

7. 蜱叮咬
Tick bite

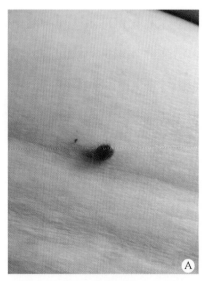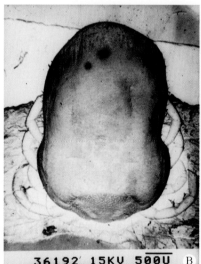

图 6-7-1　A. 腹部有一个蜱叮咬；B. 扫描电镜下有 4 对分节腿，背盾板上有许多刻点

Figure 6-7-1　A. An attached tick occurred on the abdomen; B. The attached ticks had four pairs of segmented legs and a scatum with many punctions was observed by SME

8. 结痂性疥疮（挪威疥）
Norwegian scabies

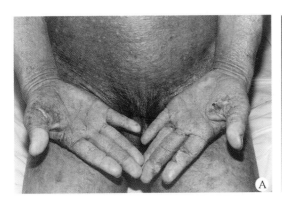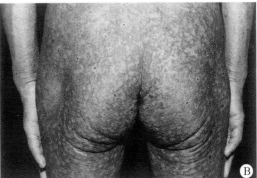

图 6-8-1　A、B. 躯干、四肢散在大量暗红色丘疹、丘疱疹和脓疱，双手掌可见厚积的角化鳞屑斑

Figure 6-8-1　Numerous wine papules, papulevesicles and pustules on the trunk and four limbs, diffuse generalized hyperkeratotic and scale lesions of both palms

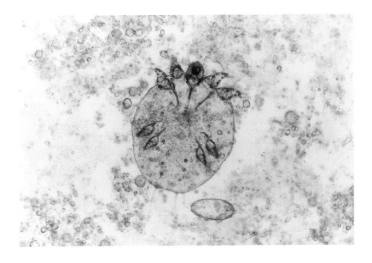

图 6-8-2　手掌鳞屑镜检见大量疥螨和虫卵

Figure 6-8-2　Large numbers of Sarcoptes scabiei mites in the skin scrapings examined by microscope

9. 婴儿蒲螨皮炎
Infant pyemotes dermatitis

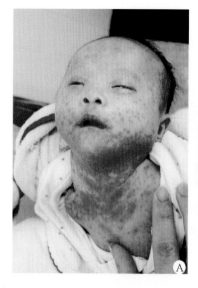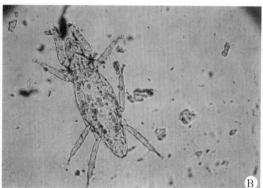

图 6-9-1　A. 头、颈、胸部密集针尖至粟粒大丘疹、丘疱疹；B. 虫体纺锤形，有 4 对足，背面前端有勺状感器 1 对(直接镜检×100)

Figure 6-9-1　A. Dense, pinpoint to millet sized papules or papulovesicle on the head, neck and chest; B. Spindly worm with eight feet, and two scoop receptivity organ on the front of back(×100)

10. 水母皮炎
Jellyfish dermatitis

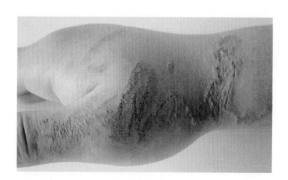

图 6-10-1　手背及上肢鞭打样红斑、水疱

Figure 6-10-1　Erythema and vesicles could be seen on the dorsa of hand and upper limb

第7章
性传播性疾病
Sexually Transmitted Diseases

1. 多发性硬下疳
Multiple chancre

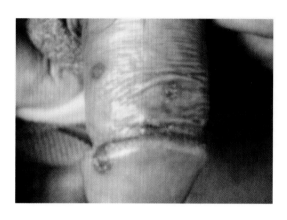

图 7-1-1　阴茎、冠状沟和龟头上有圆形溃疡，边界清，基底清洁，少量渗液，部分表面少量鳞屑

Figure 7-1-1　Well-circumscribed round ulcers with a few extravasate and scaling on the penis and glans

2. 环形疹、扁平湿疣共存的二期梅毒
Secondary syphilis presented with annular syphilid and condyloma latum

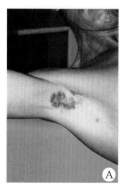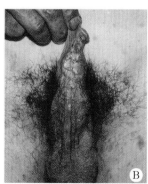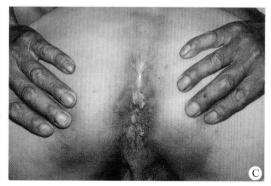

图 7-2-1　A. 双侧腋窝中央环形或半环形丘疹，肉红色，类似"环形肉芽肿"；B. 阴茎干、阴囊环形丘疹，铜红色，表面白色黏性鳞屑，类似"环形肉芽肿"；C. 肛周扁平湿疣

Figure 7-2-1　A. Annular and half-annular wine-colored papules in the both axillae, like granuloma annulare; B. Annular erythematopapulous on the penis and scrotum, with white adhesive scale on the surface, like granuloma annulare; C. Condyloma latum on the perianal

3. 结节性二期梅毒疹
Secondary syphilis with nodular lesion

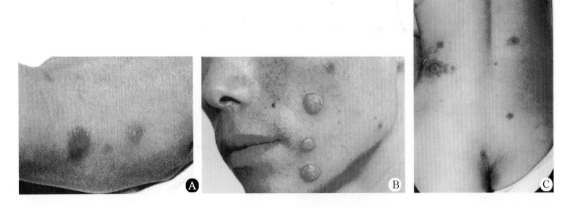

图 7-3-1　A. 腕伸侧直径 0.8～1.5cm 红色结节；B. 面部散在大小不等的暗红色结节和斑块；C. 躯干散在浸润性红斑、丘疹和结节

Figure 7-3-1　A. A Red nodules 0.8-1.5cm in diameter on wrist；B. Erythematous nodules and plaques discrete over the face；C. Infiltrative erythematous, papules and plaques discrete over the trunk

4. 环状红斑样二期梅毒疹
Annular erythema secondary syphilis

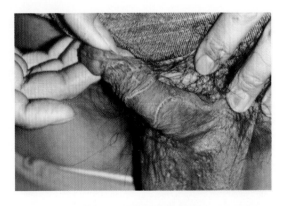

图 7-4-1　阴茎有多个圆形、半圆形及不规则形环状红斑，边缘呈堤状隆起，上覆少许鳞屑

Figure 7-4-1　Multiple round, semicircular and irregular annular erythema with few squamae on the penis

5. 梅毒性脱发
Syphilitic alopecia

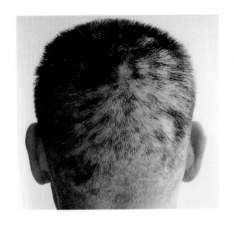

图 7-5-1 头枕部、颞部弥漫性小片状脱发区,毛发参差不齐,外观似虫蚀状,基底可见淡红色斑

Figure 7-5-1 Worm-biting like or diffused small patches, with hyperemia and redness surrounding the follicular orifice in the lesions

6. 扁平型生殖器疣
Flat condyloma

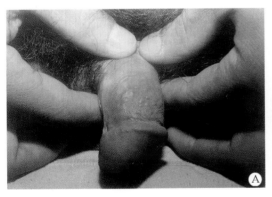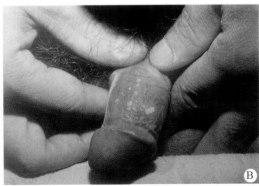

图 7-6-1 A. 包皮内侧健皮色扁平丘疹;B. 经涂 5% 醋酸疣体变白

Figure 7-6-1 A. Flesh-color flat maculopapules on the inferior of his prepuce; B. Positive aceto-white staining

第8章
物理性疾病
Dermatoses Resulting from Physical Factors

1. 火激红斑
Erythema abigne

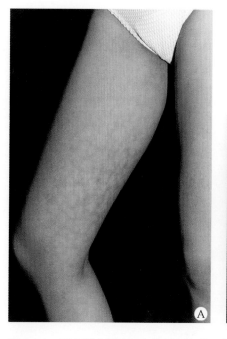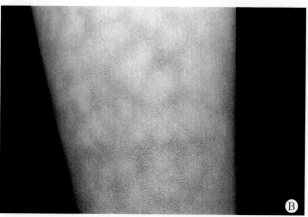

图 8-1-1　两大腿内侧暗红色和深褐色的网状色素斑,界限不清,未见毛细血管扩张、皮肤萎缩和角质增生

Figure 8-1-1　Reticular erythema with pigmentation on the inner of both thigh without definite borderline

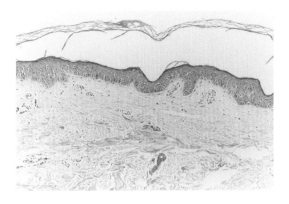

图 8-1-2 表皮角化过度,棘层萎缩变薄,基底层色素增加。真皮乳头毛细血管扩张充血,其周围有少量慢性炎症细胞浸润(HE 染色,×40)

Figure 8-1-2 Hyperkeratosis and epidermis flattened, hyperpigmentation in the basal cells, telangiectasis in papillary dermis,and surrounding inflammatory cells infiltrated(HE stain,×40)

2. 光化性扁平苔藓
Actinic lichen planus

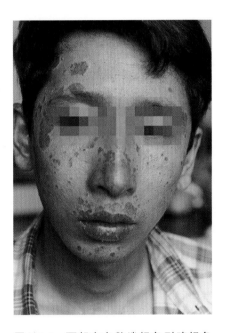

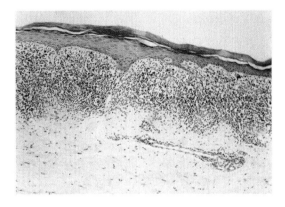

图 8-2-1 面部有多数淡褐色到暗褐色斑,部分边缘隆起

Figure 8-2-1 Numerous light and dark brown patches slightly raised at the edge on the face

图 8-2-2 轻度角化过度和颗粒层增厚,基底细胞液化变性伴带状炎性细胞浸润(HE 染色,×40)

Figure 8-2-2 It shows light hyperkeratosis and increase in thickness of the stratum granulosm. There are destruction of the basal layer and bandlike infiltrate(HE stain,×40)

47

3. 植物光皮炎
Phytophotodermatitis

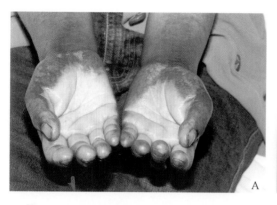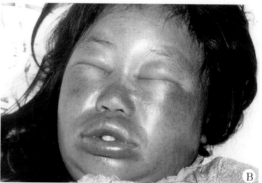

图 8-3-1　双手(A)和面部(B)显著的非凹陷性水肿性紫红色瘀斑,表面紧张发亮,双眼睑肿胀,睁眼受限,口唇外翻,张口困难

Figure 8-3-1　Marked swell, well-circumscribed violaceous petechiae with tensity(A) and shine(B), swollen eyelid opening restricted, and eversion of the lips opening mouth difficult

4. 植物光皮炎伴手指坏疽
Phytophotodermatitis with digital gangrene

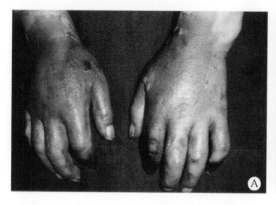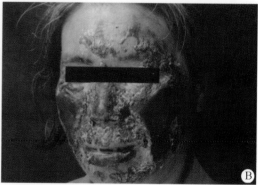

图 8-4-1　患者吃野菜(苣荬菜和蒲公英)后强光下暴晒 2 小时:A. 双手背暗褐色斑,呈非凹陷性肿胀,手指坏疽;B. 双颊、鼻周、口周大片暗褐色痂

Figure 8-4-1　The patient had some edible wild herbs before two hours of sun exposure: A. Dark brown ecchymosis and non-edematous swelling on both dorsal hands, gangrene on the fingers; B. A large dark brown patch with crusts on the face

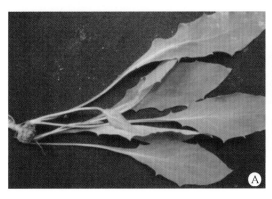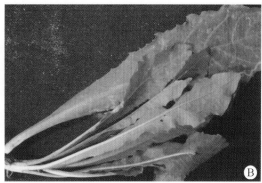

图 8-4-2　苣荬菜(A)和蒲公英(B)

Figure 8-4-2　Souchus bracgcotus dc(A) and Taraxacum Lugubre Hand-Mazz(B)

5. 野胡萝卜煎剂引起的植物日光性皮炎
Phytophotodermatitis due to wild carrot decoction

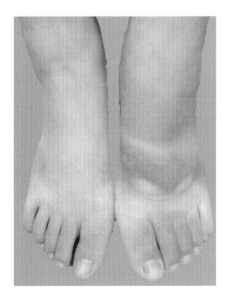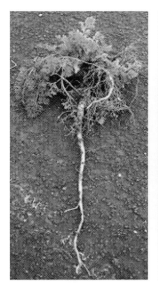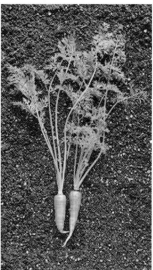

图 8-5-1　左足背和左踝外侧深褐色斑，边界清楚,右足皮肤正常

Figure 8-5-1　Well-demarcated dark brown patches on the dorsum of left foot and anterior aspect of left ankle. The skin of her right foot remained normal

图 8-5-2　野胡萝卜(A)和普通胡萝卜(B)

Figure 8-5-2　An image comparing the wild carrot (A)and ordinary carrot(B)

6. 中药煎剂引起的植物日光性皮炎
Phytophotodermatitis due to Chinese herbal medicine decoction

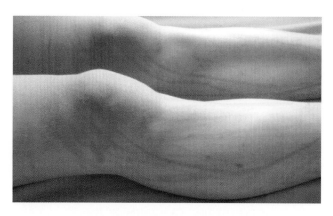

图 8-6-1　股前和小腿伸侧边界清楚的色素沉着线

Figure 8-6-1　Sharply demarcated hyperpigmented lines and curves on the extensor aspects of thighs and legs

7. 胶样粟丘疹
Colloid milium

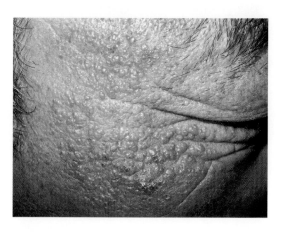

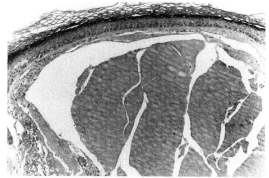

图 8-7-1　右眼外侧散在或融合的粟粒大、半透明淡黄色丘疹

Figure 8-7-1　Translucent, slightly yellow papules on the outer of right eye

图 8-7-2　真皮乳头内可见嗜酸性团块状均质的胶样物质沉积,周围有裂隙(HE 染色,×100)

Figure 8-7-2　Homogenous, fissured masses deposited in the dermal papillaries(HE stain, ×100)

8. 人工皮炎
Factitious dermatitis（Dermatitis artefacta）

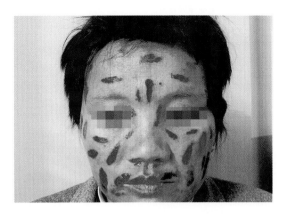

图 8-8-1　面部散在多处楔形条索状红斑，表皮剥蚀，部分覆血痂或渗液，形态规则

Figure 8-8-1　Multiple stripe，regular erythema with epidermis peeling，and partly covered with blood crasts or extravasate

第 9 章
变态反应性皮肤病
Hypersensitivity Diseases

1. 形态罕见的刺激性接触性皮炎
Irritant contact dermatitis with rare type of skin lesion

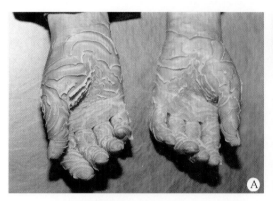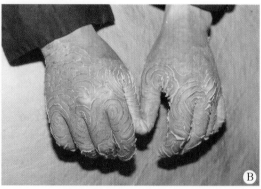

图 9-1-1　A. 掌面腕部至指尖可见多片白色鳞屑环绕手掌，中心类似螺纹状，层次清楚；B. 手背部皮疹
Figure 9-1-1　A. Multiple white scales circling the palms from the wrist to fingertip, arranging whorl in the central clearly；B. Lesions on the back of hand

2. 芒果皮炎
Mango dermatitis

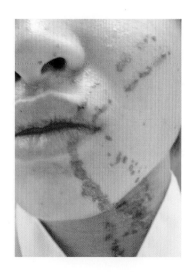

图 9-2-1　左侧面颊及颈部线状红斑、水疱，多数水疱破溃后形成糜烂面及结痂（患者系接触芒果树枝枝叶）
Figure 9-2-1　Erythemas and vesicules arranged in lines on the left face；Formation of erosion and crusts resulting from the breaches of vesicules

3. 水芹菜引起的接触性皮炎
Contact dermatitis caused by bengal waterdropwort herb

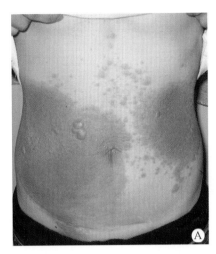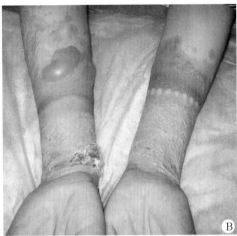

图 9-3-1　A. 下腹境界清楚的水肿性红斑,表面有散在壁薄水疱; B. 双前臂可见境界清楚的水肿性红斑,有大小不一的壁薄水疱,部分溃烂结痂

Figure 9-3-1　A. Well-circumscribed edematous erythema with a few thin-walled vesicles on the lower belly; B. Primary irritant dermatitis: well-circumscribed edematous erythema with a number of thin-walled vesicles,ulcers and crusts on the forearms

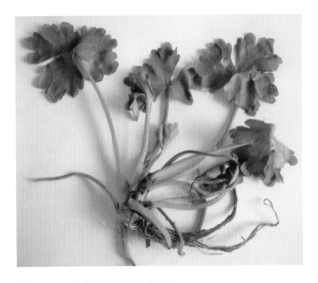

图 9-3-2　水芹菜(俗称鸭脚板)

Figure 9-3-2　Bengal waterdropwort herb

4. Blaschko 皮炎
Blaschko dermatitis

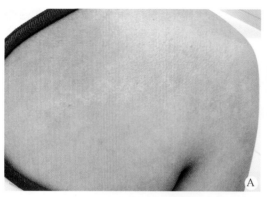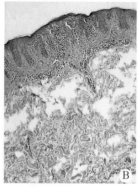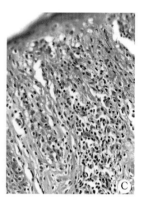

图 9-4-1　A. 肩胛部见带状色素减退斑,表面有红色丘疹、鳞屑; B. 表皮内局灶性角化过度及角化不全、明显海绵水肿,真皮浅层、中层血管周围淋巴细胞浸润(HE 染色,×100);C. 表皮细胞内水肿及海绵水肿,淋巴细胞移入表皮,其下表、真皮交界处可见少量淋巴细胞浸润(HE 染色,×100)

Figure 9-4-1　A. The scapular region presenting with band-like hypopigmented macules with superimposed inflammatory papules and scales; B. Focal hyperkeratosis, dyskeratosis and spongiosis. Lymphocytic infiltration can be found in the superficial dermis(HE stain, ×100). C. Intracellular edema and spongiosis were notable pathological findings, with lymphocytes infiltrated at the junctions between the dermis and epidermis(HE stain, ×100)

5. 创伤后湿疹
Post-traumatic eczema

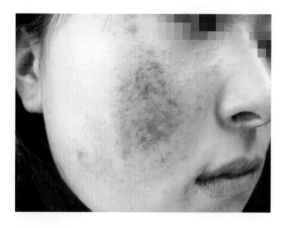

图 9-5-1　放射性核素敷贴 13 年后在右侧面颊原血管瘤处出现红斑、丘疹及轻度渗出,未累及正常皮肤

Figure 9-5-1　Thirteen years after radionuclides application,eczematoid changes with erythema,papules and mild oozing presented on the previous sites of hemangioma on her right cheek,without involvement of the normal skin

6. 晕皮炎

Halo dermatitis

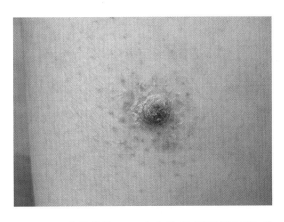

图 9-6-1 左胫前约 8mm 大小丘疹，周围见红斑、丘疹、鳞屑等湿疹样改变

Figure 9-6-1 A 8mm-sized papule presents on the left pretibial skin，with neighboring eczematoid changes as erythema，papules and scales

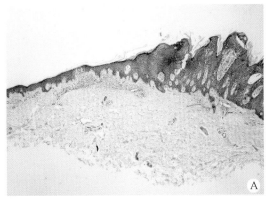 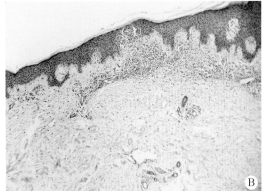

图 9-6-2 A. 角化过度、棘层肥厚及乳头瘤样增生，病变下端界限分明，其中可见角栓。真皮浅层淋巴细胞浸润明显(HE 染色，×40)；B. 脂溢性角化周围病理改变见表皮内局灶性角化不全、海绵形成，其下真皮浅层淋巴细胞沿血管浸润明显(HE 染色，×100)

Figure 9-6-2 A. Hyperkeratosis, acanthosis, keratotic plug and a flat bottom are present. Infiltrating lymphocytes can be seen in the superficial dermis (HE stain，×40)；B. Pathological changes of the skin neighboring seborrheic keratosis show focal parakeratosis, spongiosis and lymphocytes infiltration around vessels in the dermis (HE stain，×100)

7. 记忆性荨麻疹
Recall urticaria

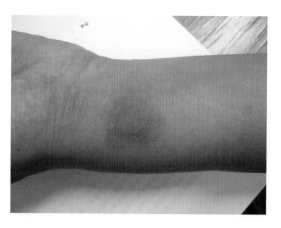

图 9-7-1　左腕关节处可见一圆形风团,局部无色素沉着

Figure 9-7-1　A solitary oval wheal is noted on the right wrist. Localized hyperpigmentation was not obvious

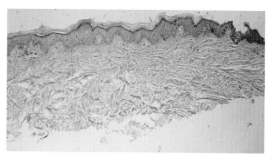

图 9-7-2　表皮大致正常,真皮浅层水肿,毛细血管扩张,周围见少量淋巴细胞浸润(HE 染色,×100)

Figure 9-7-2　Histology of the lesions revealed interstitial dermal edema,dilated venules and a paucity of lymphocytes infiltration(HE stain,×100)

8. 大疱性荨麻疹
Bullous urticaria

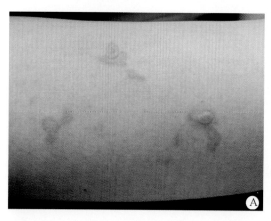

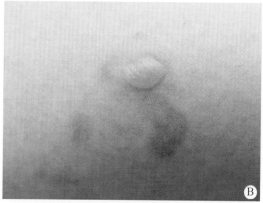

图 9-8-1　A. 右大腿内侧有数个风团,其上有透明水疱;B. 风团上有疱壁紧张的大疱

Figure 9-8-1　A. A few large wheals covered with a transparent bullae occured on the inside of right thigh; B. Large tense bullae arising on wheals

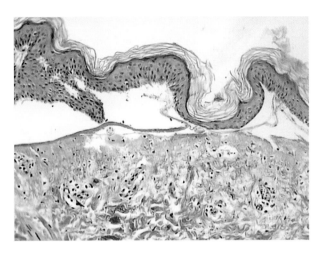

图 9-8-2　表皮下大疱,真皮乳头水肿(HE 染色,×200)

Figure 9-8-2　A subepidermal bulla and papillary dermal e-dema(HE stain,×200)

9. 妊娠瘙痒性荨麻疹性丘疹斑块

Pruritic urticarial papules and plaques of pregnancy

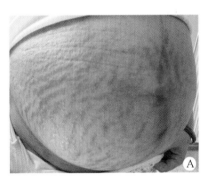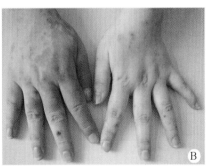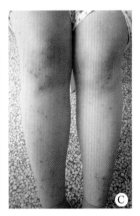

图 9-9-1　A. 腹部妊娠纹处荨麻疹样丘疹和斑块;B、C. 手背、下肢红斑和丘疱疹

Figure 9-9-1　A. Urticarial papules and plaques on the striae distensae of abdomen;B、C. Erythema papulovesicles on the dorsal hands and the lower limbs

10. 泛发性固定性药疹
Extensive fixed drug eruption

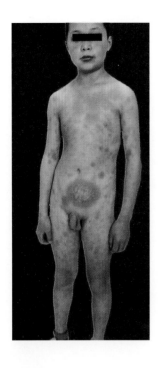

图 9-10-1　颜面、颈部、胸部、腹部、四肢可见散在或密集分布的红斑

Figure 9-10-1　Scattered or grouped erythema on the face, neck, chest, abdomen and lower and upper extremity

11. 环形固定性药疹
Annular fixed drug eruption

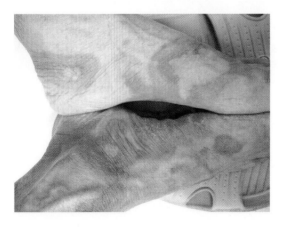

图 9-11-1　数个红色或紫红色环形斑分布在双足背。其中夹杂较小的靶形皮损

Figure 9-11-1　Several well circumscribed annular erythematous and violaceous patches over the dorsal aspects of both feet. In addition, a few smaller targetoid lesions were admixed

12. 掌跖部无色素沉着型固定性药疹
Nonpigmenting fixed drug eruptions affecting the palms and soles

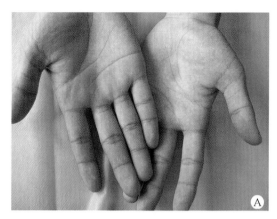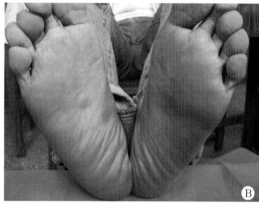

图 9-12-1　掌(A)跖(B)部位对称分布的直径 1～ 3cm 的圆形或卵圆形鲜红斑,边界清楚,中心无水疱及毛细血管扩张

Figure 9-12-1　The round to oval, well-circumscribed bright-red macules symmetrically distributed on the palms(A) and soles(B). The diameter ranged from 1 to 3cm. there is no central blister or telangiectasis

13. 氨苯砜综合征
Dapsone hypersensitivity syndrome

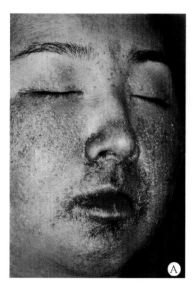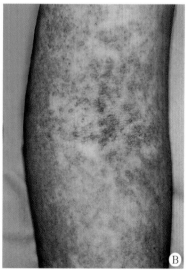

图 9-13-1　A. 面部高度浮肿,有红斑及紫红色的丘疹；B. 前臂红斑及紫红色丘疹

Figure 9-13-1　A. Highly edematous, with erythematous and purple papules on the face；B. Erythematous and purple papules on the arm

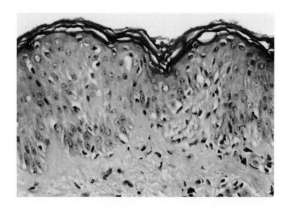

图 9-13-2　轻度角化过度及基底细胞液化变性（HE 染色，×200）

Figure 9-13-2　Mild hyperkeratosis and liquefaction of the basal cell layer (HE stain, ×200)

第 10 章
职业性皮肤病 Occupational Disease

1. 职业性疣赘
Occupational neoplasm

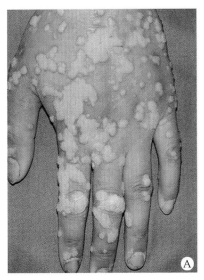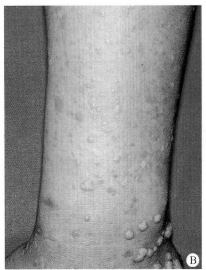

图 10-1-1　A. 手背寻常疣样皮损；B. 前臂寻常疣样及扁平疣样皮损

Figure 10-1-1　A. Verruca vulgaris-like lesions on the dorsal of both hands；
B. Verruca vulgaris and verruca planae-like lesions on the forearm

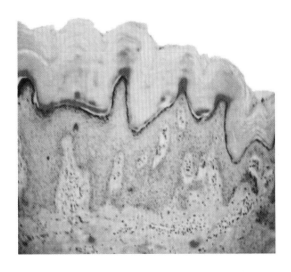

图 10-1-2　角化过度，棘层肥厚，乳头瘤样增生（HE
染色，×40）

Figure 10-1-2　Hyperkeratosis, acanthosis and papillomatous hyperplasia（HE stain, ×40）

第 11 章
结缔组织病 Connective Tissue Diseases

1. 环状红斑型亚急性皮肤型红斑狼疮
Annular erythematous type subacute cutaneous lupus erythematosus

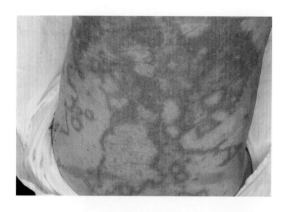

图 11-1-1　背部见不规则环状红斑,多数已融合成多环状,红斑宽约 0.3 cm,边缘略隆起,覆细薄鳞屑

Figure 11-1-1　Annular and polycyclic erythema with thin scale and elevated edge on the back

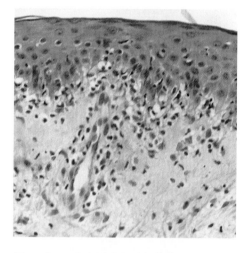

图 11-1-2　表皮突变平,基底细胞灶性液化变性,真皮浅层血管周围有淋巴细胞、嗜酸粒细胞浸润(HE 染色,×400)

Figure 11-1-2　The epidermis is atrophic and liquefaction degeneration of the basal cells, the lymphocytic and eosinophilic perivascular infiltrations in the upper dermis(HE stain,×400)

2. 大疱性系统性红斑狼疮
Bullous systemic lupus erythematosus

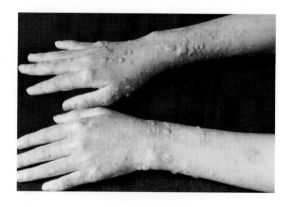

图 11-2-1　双前臂、手背散在多数水疱

Figure 11-2-1　Numerous blisters on the forearms and dorsal of both hands

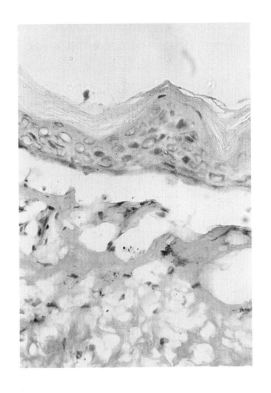

图 11-2-2 表皮下水疱,基底细胞液化变性(HE 染色,×400)

Figure 11-2-2 A subepidermal bulla, liquefaction degeneration of basal cells(HE stain,×400)

3. 肿胀性红斑狼疮

Lupus erythematosus tumidus

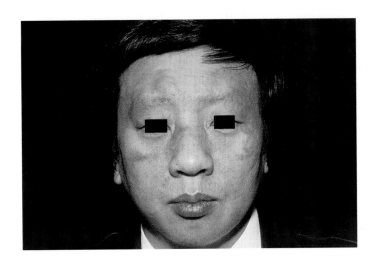

图 11-3-1 前额、双上眼睑、颧部、鼻部散在水肿性红斑

Figure 11-3-1 Edematous erythema on the face

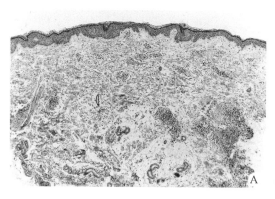
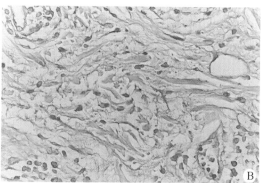

图 11-3-2　A. 真皮浅、深层和附属器周围有中等量淋巴细胞、组织细胞浸润(HE 染色,×40); B. 胶原纤维束间黏蛋白沉积(阿新蓝染色,×400)

Figure 11-3-2　A. Lymphohistiocytic infiltration in the superficial and deep perivasculatures and around appendages of the skin (HE stain×40); B. Alcian blue stain showed abundant mucin deposition in collagen bundles of dermis (Alcian blue stain,×400)

4. 新生儿红斑狼疮
Neonatal lupus erythematosus

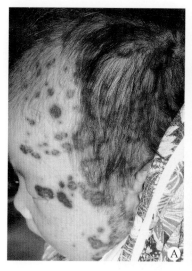
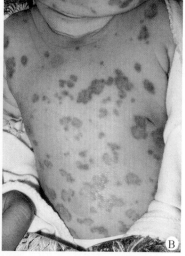

图 11-4-1　A. 头面部紫红色环状红斑; B. 胸腹部淡红色环状红斑

Figure 11-4-1　A. Annular violaceous macules on the head and face; B. Annular slight red macules on the chest and abdomen

5. 抗磷脂抗体综合征
Antiphospholipid syndrome

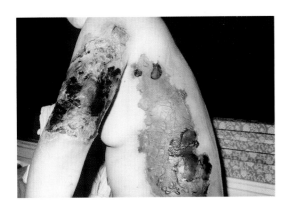

图 11-5-1 左上臂伸侧及左胁部大片浸润性红斑伴紫黑色厚痂和糜烂面

Figure 11-5-1 Infiltrate erythema and dark crusts and erosions on the extensor of the left upper arm and flank

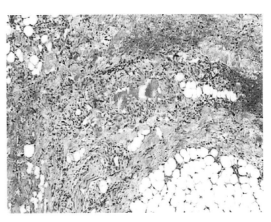

图 11-5-2 皮下小血管周围有炎症细胞浸润,小血管内有血栓形成(HE 染色, ×400)

Figure 11-5-2 Inflammatory infiltrate around small perivascular in subcutaneous, embolism in the small vascular (HE stain, ×400)

6. 结节性(假肉瘤性)筋膜炎
Nodular (pseudosarcomatous) fasciitis

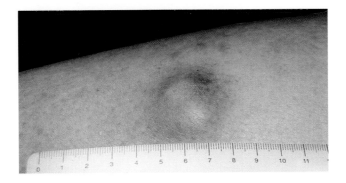

图 11-6-1 左小腿有一个皮下无疼痛和破溃的结节

Figure 11-6-1 A subcutaneous nodule without pain and ulcer on the left leg

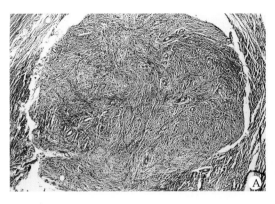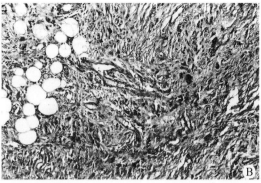

图 11-6-2　A. 真皮及皮下组织有大量梭形细胞增生(HE 染色,×50); B. 有些梭形细胞核外形不规则深染(HE 染色,×250)

Figure 11-6-2　A. Lots of fusiform cells in the dermis and hypodermis(HE stain,×50); B. Some of fusiform cells has hyperchromatic and irregularly shaped nuclei(HE stain,×250)

7. 对侧萎缩合并皮肤斑状萎缩
Crossed total hemiatrophy associated with atrophoderma of Pasini-Pierini

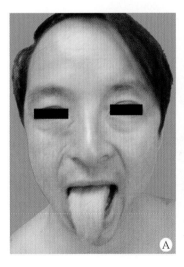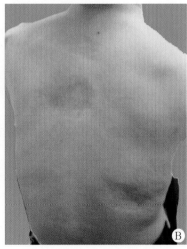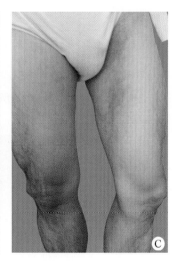

图 11-7-1　A. 舌右侧明显萎缩; B. 背部和腰部出现褐色斑片; C. 左大腿内侧褐色斑片,斑片中央浅静脉清晰可见,无炎症和硬结

Figure 11-7-1　A. Significant atrophy in right side of the tongue; B. A few brownish patches appeared on his back and lumbar; C. A few brownish patches appeared on the medial region of the left thigh. In the centers of these patches variciform superficial veins could be seen clearly without of redness or induration

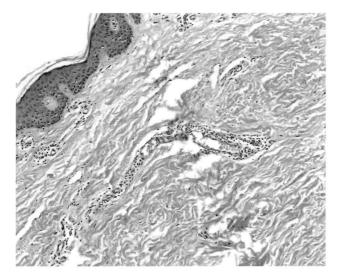

图 11-7-2　表皮正常,基底层黑素颗粒增加,真皮萎缩,真皮血管周围单核细胞浸润,皮下脂肪组织上移(HE 染色,×100)

Figure 11-7-2　Normal epidermis with increased pigment granules in the basal layer, perivascular mononuclear infiltration of the atrophic dermis, and subcutaneous adipose tissue moving up (HE stain, ×100)

8. 萎缩性肢端皮炎
Acrodermatitis atrophicans

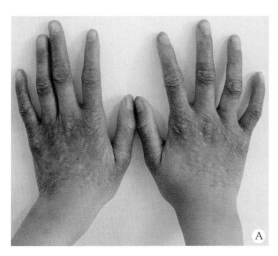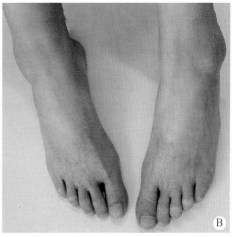

图 11-8-1　双手手背手指(A)和足背(B)褐色轻度萎缩性斑片,表面角化,皮疹以关节处明显

Figure 11-8-1　Brown plaques with keratotic and slightly atrophic appearance distributed on the back of hands(A), fingers and feet(B), especially on the joints

9. Moulin 线状皮肤萎缩
Linear atrophoderma of Moulin

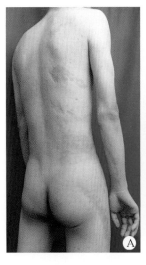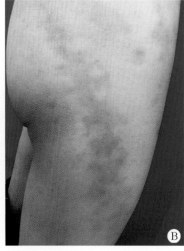

图 11-9-1　A. 右侧背部、前臂、臀部可见沿 Blaschko 线分布的暗褐色萎缩斑；B. 臀部暗褐色萎缩斑，未见毛细血管扩张

Figure 11-9-1　A. Dark-brown atrophic patches along Blaschko's lines on the right backside, right forearm, and buttock；B. Hyperpigmented atrophic patches without angiotelectasis on the right buttock

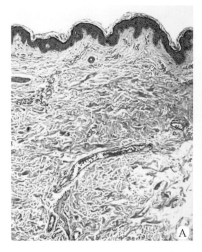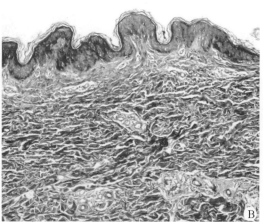

图 11-9-2　A. 表皮大致正常，基底层色素稍增多。真皮浅层血管扩张、充血，血管周围个别至少量单一核细胞浸润(HE 染色，×40)；B. 真皮层可见弹性纤维减少，弹性纤维未见断裂(弹性纤维染色，×100)

Figure 11-9-2　A. Normal epidermis with increased melanin in the basal layer；Telangiectasia and perivascular mononuclear cell infiltration in the upper dermis(HE stain，×40)；B. Reduced elastic fibers without fragmentation in upper dermis(Elastic fibers stain，×100)

10. 带状分布的皮肤萎缩

Atrophoderma of Pasini and Pierini in zosteriform distribution

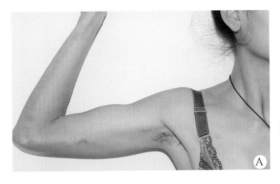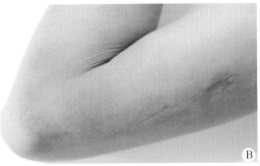

图 11-10-1 A. 右上肢内侧沿尺神经走向的紫色条带；B. 与周围皮肤相比,斑片凹陷,界限不清,边界无炎症

Figure 11-10-1 A. A violaceous band from the inner side of right arm extending along the ulnar nerve to the wrist; B. Numerous macules were depressed below the level of the surrounding skin, with ill-defined and non-inflamed borders

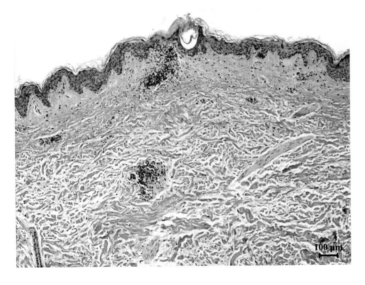

图 11-10-2 表皮轻度角化过度,基底层局灶性液化变性,胶原纤维增粗紊乱,真皮血管周围可见单核细胞浸润(HE 染色,× 40)

Figure 11-10-2 Mild hyperkeratosis of the epidermis, focal liquifaction degeneration of basal cells, slightly thickened, disorganized collagen fibrils, mononuclear cell infiltration around dermal vessels were seen (HE stain, × 40)

11. 巨大型和多发型斑状皮肤萎缩
Atrophoderma of Pasini and Pierini: multiple and giant

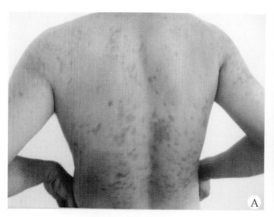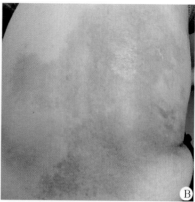

图 11-11-1　A. 背部、肩背和上肢伸侧多发性(超过 200 个)萎缩性红色斑块；B. 右腰背部 27 cm ×23cm 大小的萎缩性斑片

Figure 11-11-1　A. Multiple atrophic erythematous plaques on the back, shoulders and the extensor aspects of the proximal ends of the upper limbs; B. A single slightly depressed patch with normal texture, approximately a size of 27 cm × 23 cm, was present on the right back and lumbosacral region

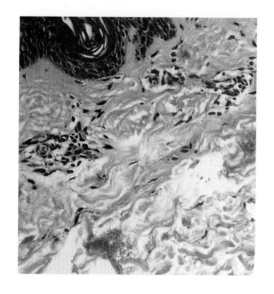

图 11-11-2　受累皮肤显示表皮萎缩,基底层黑素颗粒增加,真皮层胶原束增厚、致密(HE 染色,×200)

Figure 11-11-2　The involved skin showed atrophic epidermis, an increased amount of melanin in the basal cell layer and thickened, tightly packed collagen bundles in the dermis(HE stain, ×200)

12. 类风湿嗜中性皮炎
Rheumatoid neutrophilic dermatitis

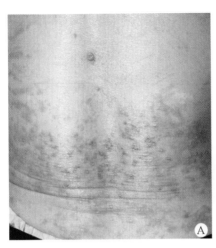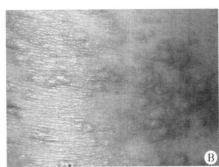

图 11-12-1　A. 患者腰背、腹部密集性红色或正常肤色丘疹、结节，大小 2～4mm 不等。未见糜烂、坏死及结痂；B. 局部放大后，可见风团样红斑和假性水疱样皮损

Figure 11-12-1　A. On the waist, back and abdomen, there were densely distributed red or skin colored papules and nodules, ranging from 2 to 4 mm in diameter. Erosions, crusts and ulcers were not discovered. B. urticarial erythema or pseudo-vesicles upon amplification of the lesions

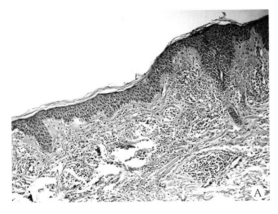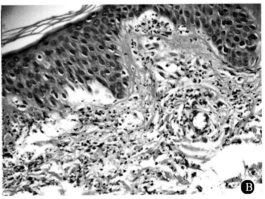

图 11-12-2　A. 真皮浅层水肿，并见带状中性粒细胞浸润(HE 染色，×100)；B. 白细胞碎裂明显，未见明显血管壁纤维素样坏死及血管栓塞，无红细胞外渗。真皮浅层可见局灶性胶原纤维碎裂。真皮乳头见中性粒细胞微脓肿(HE 染色，×400)

Figure 11-12-2　A. There was edema in the dermis, with neutrophilic cells infiltration in a band-like pattern(HE ×100)；B. Skin biopsy revealed leukocytoclasis without fibrinoid necrosis, thrombosis or extravasation of erythrocytes. There is collagen degeneration in the foci, as well as neutrophilic microabscess (HE stain, ×400)

13. 结节性皮肤狼疮性黏蛋白病
Nodular cutaneous lupus mucinosis

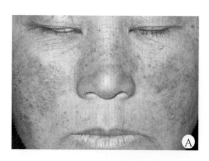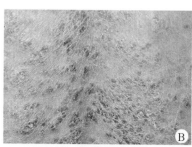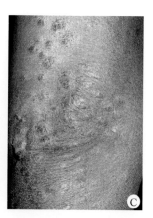

图 11-13-1　A. 两侧面颊部蝶形红斑,其表面有少许黏着性鳞屑;B. 背部许多暗紫红色丘疹和结节,表面有黏着性鳞屑,有的丘疹和结节互相融合;C. 左肘关节伸侧散在分布许多暗紫红色丘疹和结节,表面有黏着性鳞屑

Figure 11-13-1　A. Butterfly-like erythema covered with few adherent scales on the both of malar area; B. Multiple dark erythematous to violaceous papules or nodules covered with adherent scales on the back, part papules and nodules confluented; C. Multiple dark erythematous to violaceous papules and nodules covered with adherent scales on the extensor surface of left elbow joint

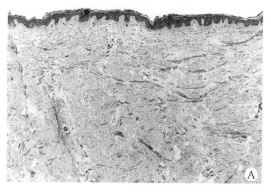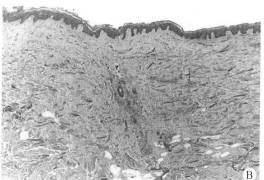

图 11-13-2　A. 表皮基本正常,真皮胶原纤维束有不同程度分离(HE 染色,×40);B. 真皮胶原纤维束有许多黏液样物质沉积(阿新蓝染色,×40)

Figure 11-13-2　A. The collagen bundles are seperated variously in the dermis (HE stain, ×40); B. A lot of mucin deposition between collagen bundles in the dermis (Alcian blue stain, ×40)

第 12 章
与皮肤有关的免疫缺陷病
Skin Related Immunodeficiency Disorder

1. 先天性胸腺发育不良
Congenital thymic dysplasia

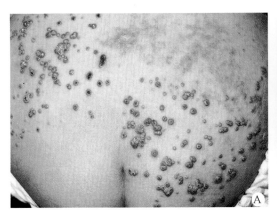
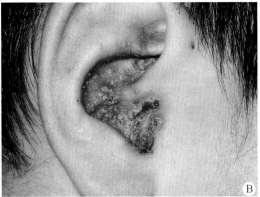

图 12-1-1　A. 臀部散在分布许多粟粒至绿豆大暗红色丘疹、水疱，部分表面结痂；B. 耳郭许多暗红色丘疹、水疱，部分表面结黄痂

Figure 12-1-1　A. Numerous millet to mung bean size, brownish red papules and vesicles partly with crust on the buttocks; B. Numerous papules and vesicles with crusts on the auricle

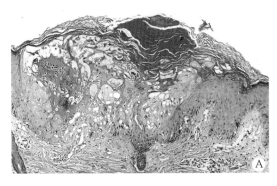
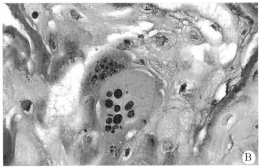

图 12-1-2　A. 表皮内可见角质形成细胞气球样变性形成的水疱(HE 染色, ×100)；B. 表皮内水疱中可见形态奇特的多核巨细胞(HE 染色, ×400)

Figure 12-1-2　A. Ballooning degeneration of epidermis forming vesicles(HE stain, ×100); B. Strange multi-nucleated giant cells in the vesicles (HE stain, ×400)

2. 移植物抗宿主病
Graft-versus-host disease

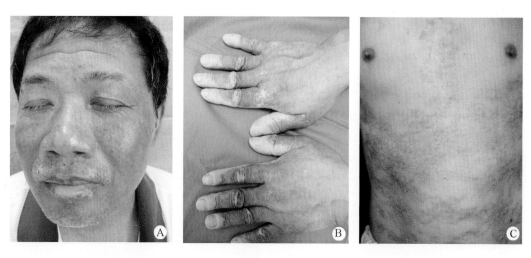

图 12-2-1　慢性移植物抗宿主病患者面部(A)、手(B)及躯干(C)弥漫性色素异常和色素沉着
Figure 12-2-1　Chronic GVHD with diffuse dyschromia and hyperpigmentation on the face(A), hands(B) and trunk(C)

第 13 章
角化性皮肤病 Keratoderma

1. 角化过度型汗孔角化症
Hyperkeratotic porokeratosis

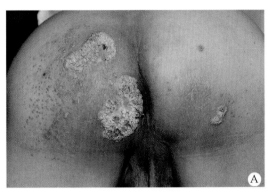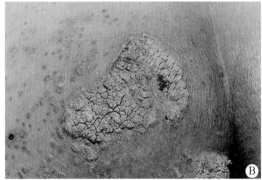

图 13-1-1　两侧臀部可见 3 片疣状增厚性斑块,表面粗糙为灰白色的角化物,其周围有许多粟粒至黄豆大疣状丘疹,似"卫星灶"

Figure 13-1-1　Three thick hyperpigmented and hyperkeratotic plaques with a verrucous surfaces on the both buttocks

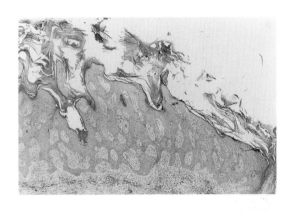

图 13-1-2　表皮显著角化过度,棘层肥厚,皮突延长,可见多个角化不全柱,嵌入表皮凹陷处,凹陷处底部颗粒层变薄消失,真皮浅层有少许慢性炎症细胞浸润(HE 染色,×40)

Figure 13-1-2　Marked hyperkeratosis with multiple parakeratotic column,a sparse,chronic inflammation infiltrate in the upper part of the dermis(HE stain,×40)

2. 偏侧性汗孔角化症
Porokeratosis localized on the left side of the body

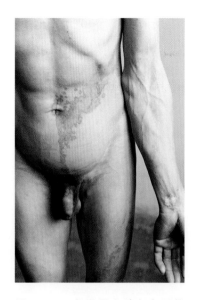

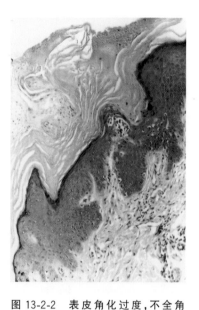

图 13-2-1 躯干及上肢多个环状和地图状淡褐色色素斑，边缘隆起

Figure 13-2-1 Multiple brown annular and atlas maculae on the trunk and upper arms

图 13-2-2 表皮角化过度，不全角化柱嵌入表皮浅层，血管周围淋巴细胞浸润（HE 染色，×100）

Figure 13-2-2 Hyperkeratosis, parakerototic column in superficial epidermis, perivascular lymphocyte infiltrate (HE stain, ×100)

3. 汗孔角化症合并假性阿洪病
Pseudoainhum with porokeratosis of Mibelli

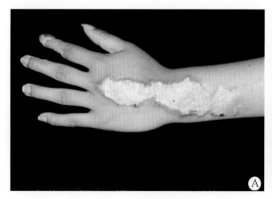

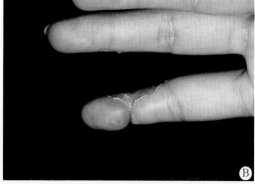

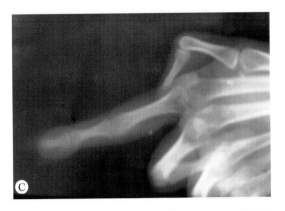

图 13-3-1 A. 左手背及左手示指伸侧不规则的环状红斑,边界清楚,周边呈堤状隆起,中央萎缩;B. 左手示指末端指关节屈侧横沟出现线性缩窄;C.X线:左手示指末端指关节处软组织萎缩、缩窄,骨质未见明显破坏

Figure 13-3-1 A. Well-circumscribed annular erythema with elevated margin and central atrophy on the left hand dorsal and extensor surface of left index finger; B. Transverse groove of first interphalangeal joint was constricted on the middle finger of left hand; C. Parenchyma atrophy and shrink on the terminal joint of left index finger

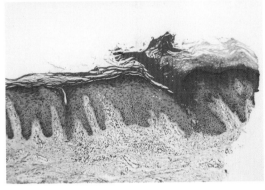

图 13-3-2 表皮角化过度,可见角化不全柱,棘层肥厚,真皮浅层可见少量慢性炎症细胞浸润(HE 染色,×100)

Figure 13-3-2 Hyperkeratosis, parakeratotic column, and a few chronic inflammation infiltrate in superficial dermis(HE stain,×100)

4. 播散性浅表性光线性汗孔角化症

Disseminated superficial actinic porokeratosis

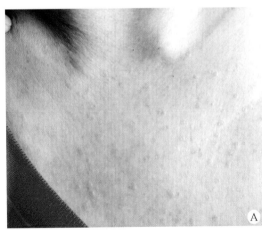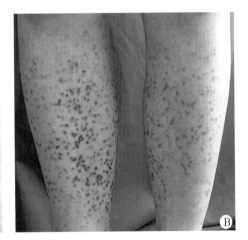

图 13-4-1 前胸部(A)、双下肢(B)泛发性环状淡红色或红褐色斑疹,皮损中央轻度萎缩,部分边缘轻微增厚隆起呈堤状

Figure 13-4-1 Multiple pink or red - brown annular macules distributed on the chest(A) and bilateral lower extremities(B). Close examination showed central atrophy and an elevated hyperkeratotic ridge

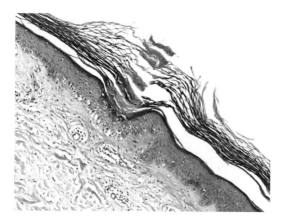

图 13-4-2　表皮见沟状凹窝,窝内充满角化不全柱,呈圆锥形板层状,其下方颗粒层减少,真皮浅层小血管周围少量淋巴细胞浸润(HE 染色,×40)

Figure 13-4-2　Characteristic cornoid lamella, as well as atrophy of the epidermis, flattening of the rete ridges, and absence of the granular layer. Perivascular lymphocytic infiltrate was present in the upper dermis (HE stain, ×40)

5. 点状掌跖角皮症
Punctate palmoplantar keratoderma

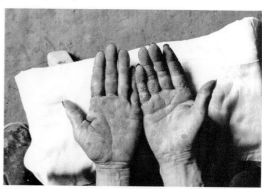

图 13-5-1　双手掌部角质丘疹

Figure 13-5-1　Keratotic punctuate papules on both palms

6. 条纹状掌跖角皮症
Striated palmoplantar keratoderma

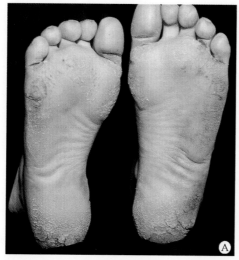
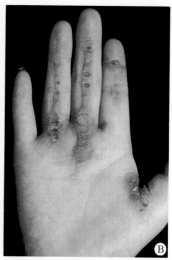

图 13-6-1　A. 双足跖受压部位明显角化、增厚,伴有皲裂;B. 右手示指、中指、环指的掌侧条带状角化增厚,右手虎口处明显角化、增厚、皲裂

Figure 13-6-1　A. Marked hyperkeratosis, thickened, and chaps on the pressed soles; B. Striated hyperkeratosis and thickened on the right index finger, middle finger and ring finger

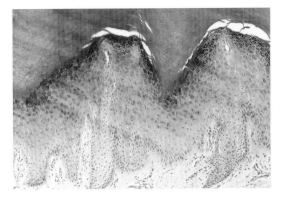

图 13-6-2　表皮明显角化过度,颗粒层增厚,轻度乳头瘤样增生,真皮浅层血管周围少量慢性炎性细胞浸润(HE 染色,×100)

Figure 13-6-2　Marked hyperkeratosis,thickened granular layer,slight papillomatosis and chronic inflammatory infiltrate pervascular in the superficial dermis(HE stain,×100)

7. 棘状角皮症
Spiny keratoderma

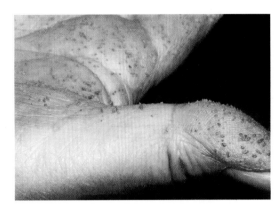

图 13-7-1　手掌似棘状角化性突起

Figure 13-7-1　Tiny spiked keratotic projection located at the palm

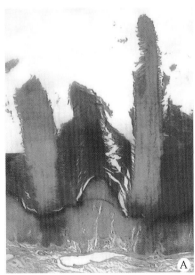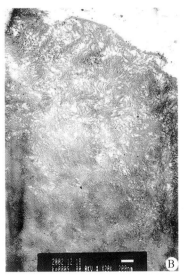

图 13-7-2　A. 表皮角化过度,可见界限清楚的角化不全柱,表皮凹陷,颗粒层变薄,棘层肥厚(HE 染色,×40);B. 电镜下表皮角质微丝排列疏松(×20 000)

Figure 13-7-2　A. Hyperkeratosis,columnar parakeratosis and acanthosis,the epidermis below parakeratotic column invaginated,granular layer thinned (HE stain,×40);B. Keratin filaments arranged rather loosely by transmission electron microscopy (×20 000)

8. 表皮松解性掌跖角化病
Epidermolytic palmoplantar keratoderma

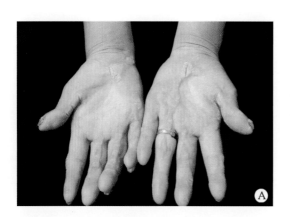
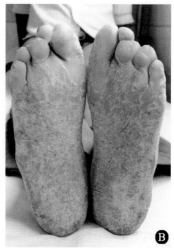

图 13-8-1 　显著的表皮角化过度,双手掌呈条状(A),双足跖为弥漫性(B)

Figure 13-8-1 　Marked epidermal hyperkeratosis in linear pattern in the both palms(A), in diffuse pattern in the both soles(B)

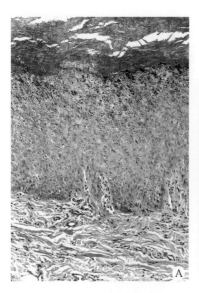
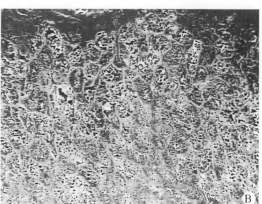

图 13-8-2 　表皮角化过度显著,中等度棘层肥厚和颗粒层增厚(A)(HE 染色,×100)颗粒层细胞肥大,透明角质颗粒密集成块(B)(HE 染色,×200)

Figure 13-8-2 　Pronounced hyperkeratosis, moderate acanthosis, and thick of granular layer(A)(HE stain, ×100), the granules in the swollen granular cells appear clumped (B)(HE stain, ×200)

9. 疣状肢端角化症
Acrokeratosis verruciformis

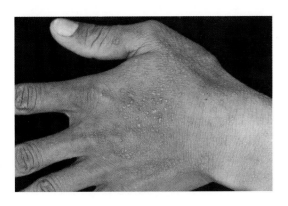

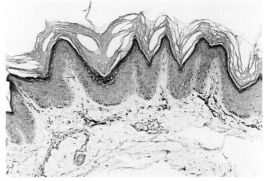

图 13-9-1 左手背可见肤色或灰白色多角形扁平丘疹,一至数毫米大,密集不融合,拇指甲部分变白
Figure 13-9-1 Skin-colored or greying flat papules on the left dorsa of hand, and thumb nail whitening

图 13-9-2 表皮高度角化过度,颗粒层及棘层肥厚,有明显乳头瘤样增生,部分表皮突起呈山峰样;表皮突轻度延长,但基底位于同一水平(HE 染色,×100)
Figure 13-9-2 Considerable hyperkeratosis, thickness of the granular layer and acanthosis, papillomatosis and the rete ridges slightly elongated (HE stain, ×100)

10. 疣状角化不良瘤
Warty dyskeratoma

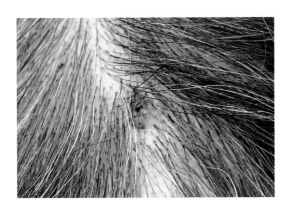

图 13-10-1 头皮有一个结节,中心呈脐凹状,有角化物质
Figure 13-10-1 An elevated nodule with umbilicated center on the scalp

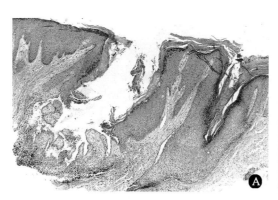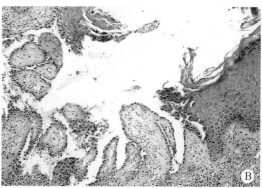

图 13-10-2　A. 表皮呈杯状凹隔,中含角化物质(HE 染色,×40);B. 大内隔中有多数绒毛,棘层松解细胞和角化不良细胞(HE 染色,×100)

Figure 13-10-2　A. A large invagination is connected with surface by a channel containing keratinous material (HE stain,×40); B. The large invagination contains numerous villi,acantholytic,dyskeratotic cells(HE stain,×100)

11. 进行性对称性红斑角皮症
Progressive symmetric erythrokeratodermia

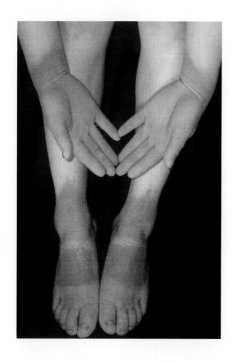

图 13-11-1　双手掌、足背对称性弥漫性红斑,边界清楚,浸润性肥厚、角化

Figure 13-11-1　Symmetric diffuse well-circumscribed erythema on the palms and the dorsa of feet

12. 砷角化病
Keratosis arsenica

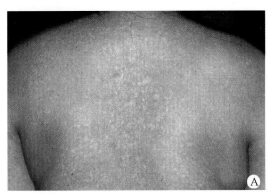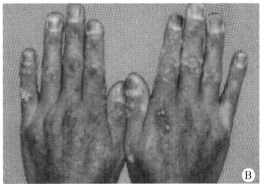

图 13-12-1　A. 背部皮肤呈灰黑色,其上可见"雨滴"样色素脱失斑; B. 双手背弥漫点状角化性丘疹
Figure 13-12-1　A. Grey-dark and raindrop-like depigmentation macule on the back; B. Diffuse punctate papules with keratosis on the dorsa of hands

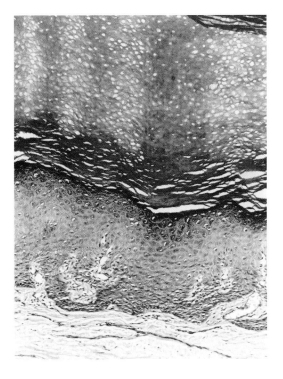

图 13-12-2　角化过度,表皮增生(HE 染色,×20)
Figure 13-12-2　Hyperkeratosis and epidermal hyperplasia(HE stain,×20)

13. 乳头乳晕角化过度症
Hyperkeratosis of the nipple and areola

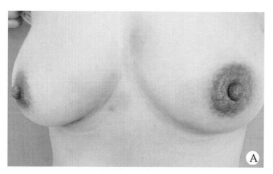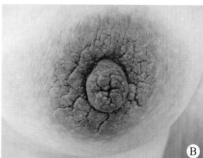

图 13-13-1　右侧乳头和乳晕(A、B)呈棕褐色疣状角化

Figure 13-13-1　Verrucous thickening and brownish discoloration on the right nipple and areola (A、B)

14. 光泽角化病
Waxy keratosis

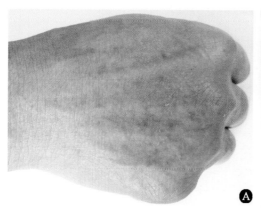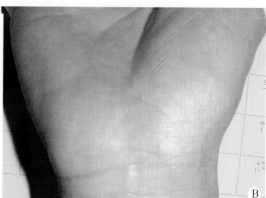

图 13-14-1　A. 手背多发性正常肤色或红色丘疹,稍微用力一刮,皮损整片分离;B. 手腕上见特征性发亮如蜡样光泽的丘疹(2~3mm)

Figure 13-14-1　A. Multiple skin-colored or red papules distributed on the dorsa of the hands. The lesions became flake-like and detached by a slight scratch;B. Primary shiny, "waxy" papules measuring 2-3 mm in diameter on the wrist

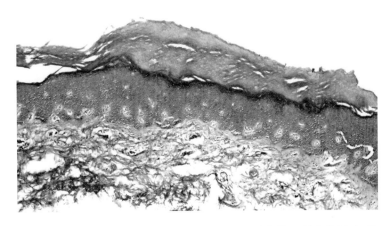

图 13-14-2　具有蜡样光泽原发性丘疹病理示：融合性正性角化过度，乳头瘤样增生和轻度颗粒层增厚。未见海绵水肿和其他炎症改变（HE染色，×100）

Figure 13-14-2　Skin biopsy of the primary shiny papules showed coalesced orthohyperkeratosis, papillomatosis and mild acanthosis without granular degeneration. No spongiosis or obvious inflammatory changes were apparent. (HE stain, ×100)

15. 肢端角化性类弹性纤维病
Acrokeratoelastoidosis

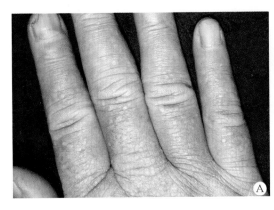
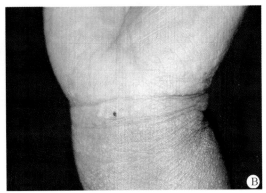

图 13-15-1　A. 双手背、大小鱼际外多发白色扁平角化丘疹，呈"铺路石"样，部分皮疹融合；B. 双手腕屈侧半透明丘疹，为半球形粟粒至绿豆大小，表面光滑

Figure 13-15-1　A. Numerous white firm papules on the dorsal of hands and hypothenar; B. Smooth translucent papules are the size of millet and mung bean on the flex of both wrists

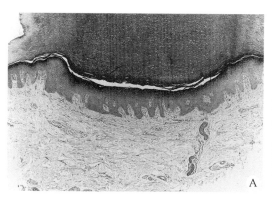
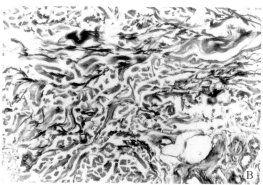

图 13-15-2　A. 表皮显著角化过度, 颗粒层增厚, 棘层肥厚, 皮突稍延长, 真皮浅层血管周围少量慢性炎性细胞浸润 (HE 染色, ×40); B. 真皮下部弹性纤维断裂、减少 (弹性纤维染色, ×100)

Figure 13-15-2　A. Marked hyperkeratosis, thickened granular layer and acanthosis, a few inflammatory cell perivascular infiltration in the upper of dermis (HE stain, ×40); B. Fragmentation and diminution of coarse elastic fibers in the reticular dermis (Verhalf-van Gieson stain, ×100)

16. 扁平苔藓样角化病
Lichen planus-like keratosis

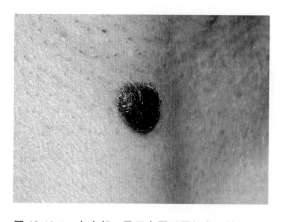

图 13-16-1　右肩部一蚕豆大圆形黑褐色斑块, 界限清楚, 表面粗糙, 轻度角化, 边缘有红晕

Figure 13-16-1　A solitary horsebean-sized, well-circumscribed, slight keratosis dark popular and plaques on the right shoulder

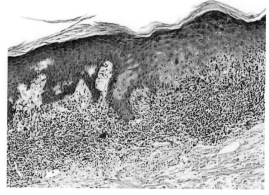

图 13-16-2　表皮角化过度, 颗粒层及棘层肥厚, 基底层可见灶性液化变性, 有胶样小体; 真皮浅层有致密的炎性细胞浸润, 并有较多噬色素细胞 (HE 染色, ×40)

Figure 13-16-2　Hyperkeratosis, hyperplasia of granular layer and liquefaction degeneration of basal cells in the epidermis with colloid body and band-shaped infiltration of lymphocytes, histiocytes, and melanophages in the superficial dermis (HE stain, ×40)

17. 水源性角化症
Aquagenic acrokeratoderma

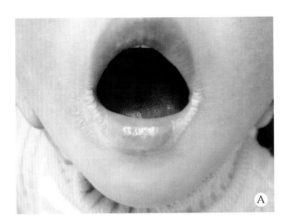
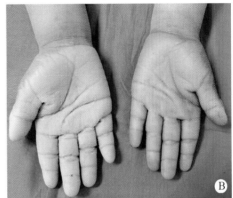
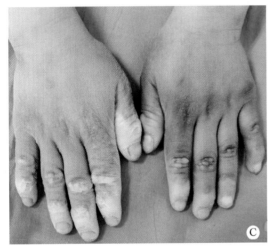

图 13-17-1　A. 由于唾液浸渍,口角发白;B. 右手浸水后,掌跖和手指发白、增厚;B、C. 左手正常

Figure 13-17-1　A. whitennig of corners of the mouth due to saliva dipping;B. Whitish discoloration of the palms and fingers with thickening of the palmar surface after immersion of the right hand in water;B、C. The left hand remains unaffected

第 14 章
红斑性皮肤病 Erythematous Disease

1. 匐形性回状红斑
Erythema gyratum repens

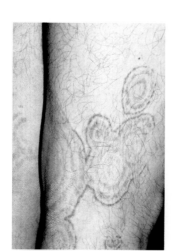

图 14-1-1　下肢散在排列成同心环形、半环形、扇形、弧形或水纹样的条形红斑，边缘略隆起

Figure 14-1-1　Concentric bands of flat-to-raised erythema on the lower limbs

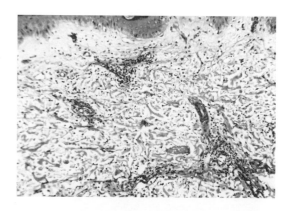

图 14-1-2　表皮角化过度，轻度萎缩，真皮浅中层可见中性粒细胞、淋巴细胞浸润（HE 染色，×200）

Figure 14-1-2　Hyperkeratosis, mild atrophied of the epidermis, and a superficial perivascular lymphocytes and neutrophils infiltrate in the dermis (HE stain, × 200)

2. 可触及游走性弧形红斑
Palpable archiform migratory erythema

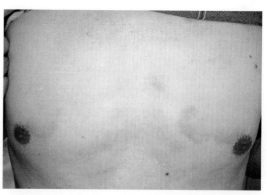

图 14-2-1　前胸部见二个 1/4 弧形红斑，长约 10cm，宽约 1cm，以手触之略高出皮面，但质地正常

Figure 14-2-1　There were two arciform erythemas on the chest which were approximate 10cm in length and 1cm in width, nomal texture with slightly elevated

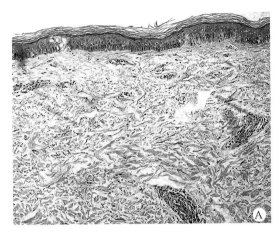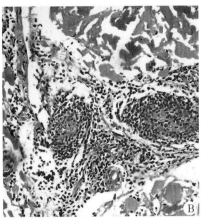

图 14-2-2　A. 表皮萎缩,基底层无液化变性;B. 真皮网状层血管周围致密单一核细胞袖口样浸润,浸润细胞无异形性

Figure 14-2-2　A. Epidermis was slight atrophied without liquefaction degeneration of basal cells; B. Mononuclear cells infiltrated densely around the blood vessels in the reticular layer of the dermis

3. 掌跖疼痛性红斑为首发表现的左心房黏液瘤

Left atrial myxoma presenting with painful erythematous macules on the palms and soles

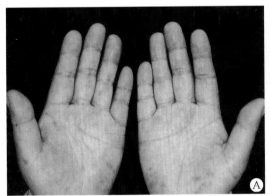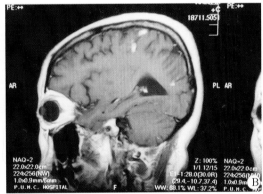

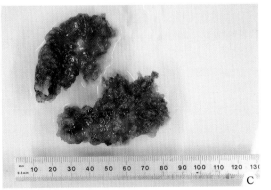

图 14-3-1　A. 双手掌散在粟粒大小的红色斑疹;B. 左心房黏液瘤患者头颅磁共振成像发现颅内多发性栓塞;C. 手术切除的黏液瘤

Figure 14-3-1　A. The painful erythematous macules on the palms; B. The MRI of the skull showed multiple cerebral infarctions; C. The appearance of excised tumor

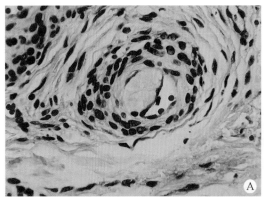

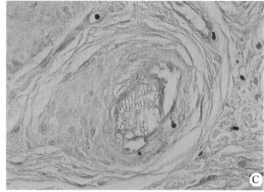

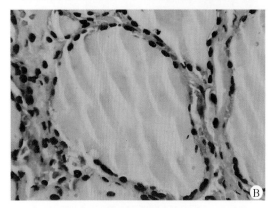

图 14-3-2　A. 真皮中部动脉血管内见折光性透明蛋白栓子(HE 染色,×400); B. 真皮血管内见阿新蓝染色阳性栓子(阿新蓝染色,×400); C. 肿瘤呈黏液性,瘤细胞排列成单层环状,周围有丰富的血管(HE 染色,×400)

Figure 14-3-2　A. An embolus within a vessel in the reticular dermis(HE stain,×400); B. Alcian blue staining positive embolus in blood vessel in the dermis (Alcian blue stain,×400); C. Scattered spindle cells with scant pink cytoplasm in a loose myxoid stroma(HE stain,×400)

4. 复发性疼痛性红斑
Recurrent painful erythema

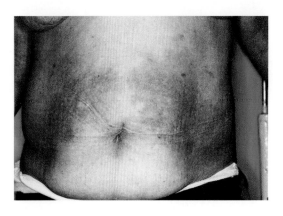

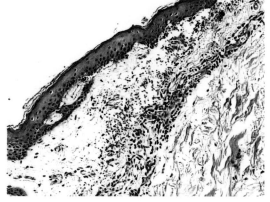

图 14-4-1　腹部红斑在脐周融合成片

Figure 14-4-1　Erythema on the abdomen, and confluent around the umbilicus

图 14-4-2　表皮角化过度,真皮浅层水肿,毛细血管扩张,血管周围有少许淋巴细胞浸润(HE 染色,×100)

Figure 14-4-2　Hyperkeratosis, edema in the upper dermis and capillaries dilated, a few lymphocytes infiltrated around the vessels (HE stain,×100)

5. 复发性半环状丘疹和红斑
Erythema papulosa semicircularis recidivans

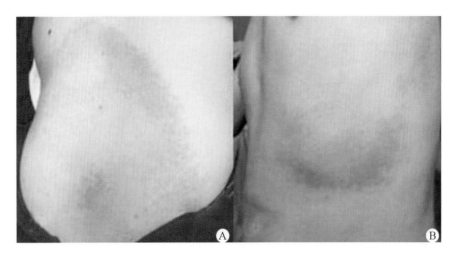

图 14-5-1 躯干部位的半环形排列的丘疹红斑性皮损(A、B)

Figure 14-5-1 Papuloerythematous lesions arranged in semicircles on the trunks(A、B)

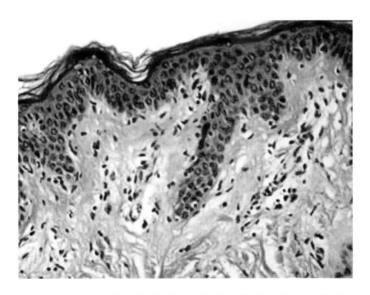

图 14-5-2 轻度角化过度,真皮乳头轻度水肿,浅层稀疏的管周淋巴细胞浸润(HE 染色,×100)

Figure 14-5-2 Mild hyperkeratosis, slight papillary dermal edema, and sparse superficial perivascular lymphocytic infiltrate (HE stain, ×100)

6. 红色阴囊综合征

Red scrotum syndrome

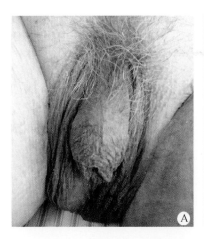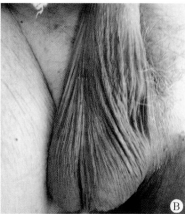

图 14-6-1　A. 边缘清楚的阴囊红斑；B. 阴茎根部红斑

Figure 14-6-1　A. Demarcated erythematous lesion on the scrotum；B. the skin at the root of penis

第 15 章
丘疹鳞屑性皮病
Papule and Scale Diseases

1. 掌跖银屑病
Palmoplantar psoriasis

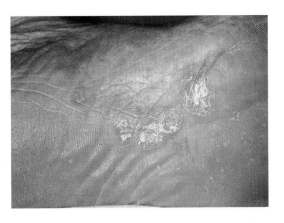

图 15-1-1　左足跖见境界清楚的角化性斑块，表面覆鳞屑

Figure 15-1-1　Demarcated, hyperkeratotic plaques covered with scales on the left soles

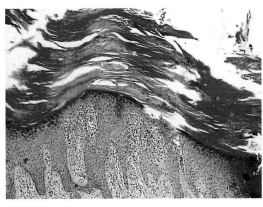

图 15-1-2　表皮角化不全，表皮突下延，真皮乳头上延，毛细血管扩张，真皮浅层血管周围淋巴细胞浸润液化变性(HE 染色，×40)

Figure 15-1-2　Parakeratosis, the rete ridges show regular elongation with thickening in the lower portion, the papillae are elongated and the capillaries dilated, lymphocytes infiltrated around the vessels in the upper dermis (HE stain, ×40)

2. 反向银屑病
Inverse psoriasis

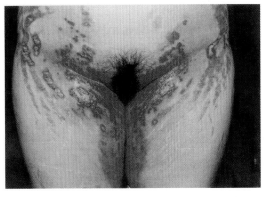

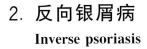

图 15-2-1　腹股沟大片境界清楚的鲜红斑

Figure 15-2-1　Circumscribed large erythematous patches in inguinal region

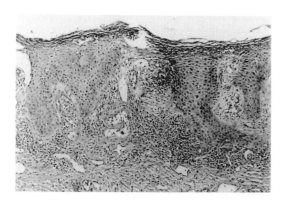

图 15-2-2 表皮角化过度,角化不全,棘层肥厚,皮突延长,见 Munro 微脓肿(HE 染色,×100)

Figure 15-2-2 Hyperkeratosis, parakeratosis, acanthosis and elongated rete ridges, a Munro microabscess presents in the stratum corneum (HE stain,×100)

3. 急性痘疮样苔藓状糠疹
Pityriasis lichenoides et varioliformis acuta

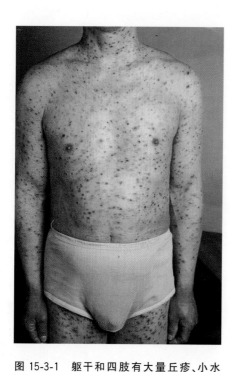

图 15-3-1 躯干和四肢有大量丘疹、小水疱,皮疹表面附鳞屑或黑痂

Figure 15-3-1 A large of papules and vesicles covered with scales and dark crests on the trunck and extremites

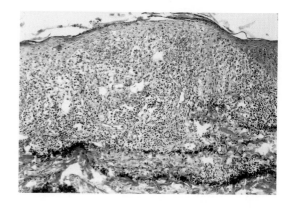

图 15-3-2 表皮内有明显的淋巴细胞浸润,角质形成细胞坏死和基底细胞液化变性(HE 染色,×100)

Figure 15-3-2 A predominantly lymphocytic infiltrate invades the epidermis. The necrotic keratinocytes and liquefaction degeneration of basal cells appear in the epidermis(HE stain,×100)

4. 紫癜型玫瑰糠疹
Purpuric pityriasis rosea

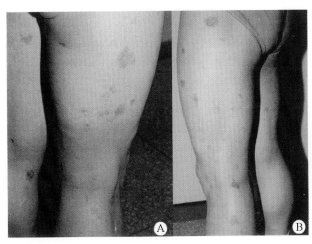

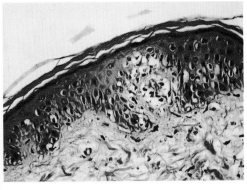

图 15-4-2 表皮细胞内及细胞间水肿,基底细胞灶性液化变性,真皮乳头水肿,血管扩张伴红细胞外渗(HE 染色,×400)

Figure 15-4-2 Intracelluar and intercellular edema, hydrophic degeneration of basal cells in the epidermis, edema and dilated vessels with extravasation of erythrocytes in the papillar dermis (HE stain, ×400)

图 15-4-1 A、B 下肢散在瘀点或瘀斑,部分瘀斑中央可见细小粉状鳞屑

Figure 15-4-1 Petechiae and ecchymoses covered with finely crinkled scaling on the lower limbs(A、B)

5. 泛发性丘疹型玫瑰糠疹
Pityriasis rosea

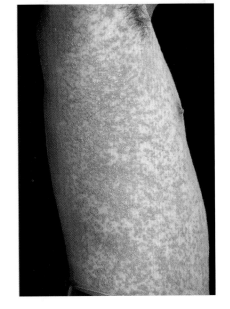

图 15-5-1 右胁和腰部密集红色丘疹,部分融合成不规则斑片,其上附有细薄鳞屑

Figure 15-5-1 Dense red scaly papules on the right flank and waist, part of them confluent macules

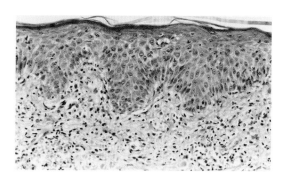

图 15-5-2　表皮角化不全，棘层轻度肥厚，细胞内和细胞间灶状水肿，真皮上部毛细血管扩张，红细胞外溢，围管性淋巴细胞浸润（HE 染色，×200）

Figure 15-5-2　Parakeratosis and slight acanthosis, spongiosis intracellular edema, and dilated capillaries, erythrocyte extravasate and perivascular lymphocytes infiltrate were present (HE stain, ×200)

6. 色素性玫瑰糠疹
Pigmentary pityriasis rosea

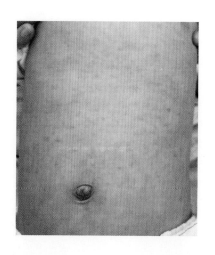

图 15-6-1　许多圆形和卵圆形色素斑沿躯干肋骨长轴排列

Figure 15-6-1　Many oval or circinate pigmented patches were arranged along the long axis of ribs

7. 鳞状毛囊角化症（土肥）
Keratosis follicularis squamosa（Dohi）

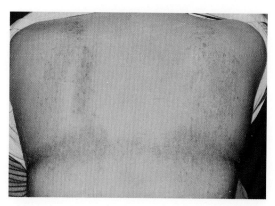

图 15-7-1　文胸下有褐色鳞屑斑，中心有黑色毛囊角栓

Figure 15-7-1　The brownish scales with black follicular horny plugs in the center were limited to the areabeneath cloth brassiere

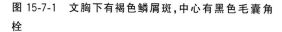

8. 面部鳞状毛囊角化病
Facial keratosis follicularis squamosa

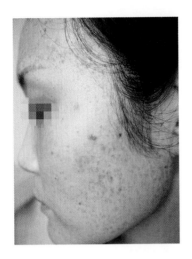

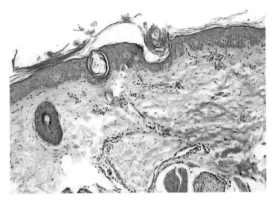

图 15-8-1 左侧面部萎缩性痤疮瘢痕样皮损,中央可见细小的褐色毛囊角栓

Figure 15-8-1 Atrophic acne scar like lesions, with a tiny brownish follicular plug in the center

图 15-8-2 表皮角化过度,毛囊扩大伴角质栓,鳞屑侧缘与颗粒层轻度分离(HE 染色,×40)

Figure 15-8-2 Dilated follicles with keratotic plugs and orthohyperkeratosis of epidermis. Lateral margins of the scales were slightly detached from the granular layer (HE stain, ×40)

9. 肥厚性扁平苔藓
Hypertrophic lichen planus

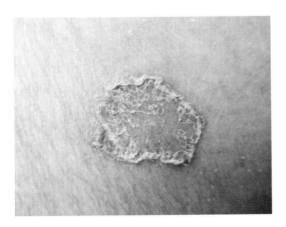

图 15-9-1 一个大疣状鳞屑性斑块,边缘隆起,中心色素沉着

Figure 15-9-1 A large verrucous plaque with a few scales had an elevated border and center pigmentation

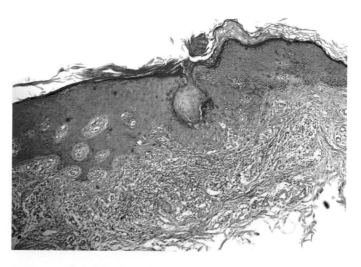

图 15-9-2　表皮角化过度和肥厚,基底细胞液化变性和真皮上部带状分布炎细肥浸润

Figure 15-9-2　Hyperkeratosis and epidermal hyperplasia, liquefaction of the basal cells and a band like infiltration of inflammatory cells in the upper dermis

10. 毛发扁平苔藓
Lichen planopilaris

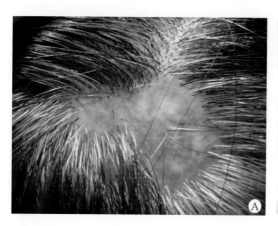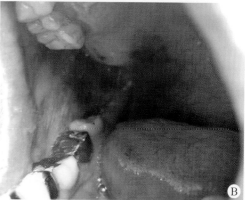

图 15-10-1　A. 头顶有象牙样不规则假性斑秃样脱发斑；B. 口腔颊黏膜见花纹状白斑

Figure 15-10-1　A. The ivory white irregular patches of pseudopelade on the vertex; B. The lacy white lesions were noted on the buccal mucosa

11. 色素性扁平苔藓
Lichen planus pigmentosus

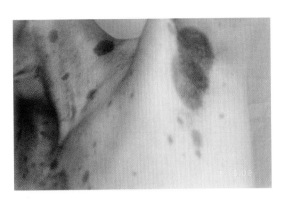 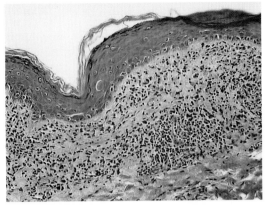

图 15-11-1　椭圆形褐色斑片，四周有大小不一的斑点

Figure 15-11-1　Oval brown patches and varying sized maculae

图 15-11-2　基底层色素增加，局灶性基底细胞液化变性，真皮上部带状浸润，红染的 Civatte 小体（HE 染色，×100）

Figure 15-11-2　Hyperpigmentation in the basal layer, focal liquefaction degeneration of basal cells, bandlike infiltrate in the upper dermis with Civatte bodies（HE stain, ×100）

12. 皱褶部色素性扁平苔藓
Lichen planus pigmentosus-inversus

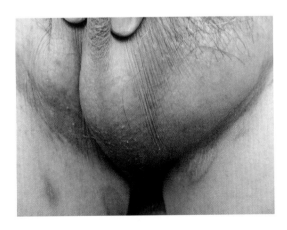

图 15-12-1　双侧腹股沟对称性褐灰色斑沿皮肤张力线分布

Figure 15-12-1　Brownish to grayish macules distributed along Langer's lines in the bilateral gluteal areas

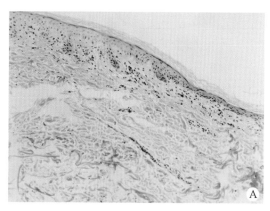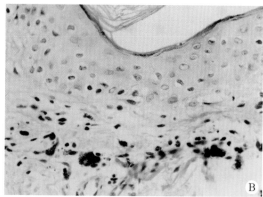

图 15-12-2　A. 角化过度，表皮萎缩，皮突消失，带状浸润不明显，真皮浅层淋巴细胞沿血管周围浸润（HE 染色，×100）；B. 基底细胞液化变性，真皮可见较多载色素细胞（HE 染色，×400）

Figure 15-12-2　A. Hyperkeratosis, epidermal atrophy and lymphocytic infiltration in the dermis(HE stain, ×100); B. Liquefaction degeneration of basal layer cells, melanophages can be noted in the dermis(HE stain, ×400)

13. 色素性扁平苔藓沿小腿静脉分布
Supravenous lichen planus pigmentosus on the leg

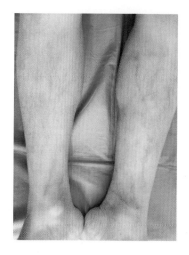

图 15-13-1　紫褐色丘疹性条纹沿表浅静脉网分布，主要见于小腿和内踝

Figure 15-13-1　Sable papular streaks were following the superficial venous network, predominately in the the lower leg and region medial malleolus

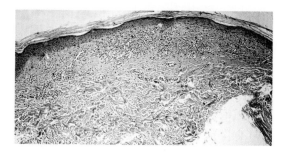

图 15-13-2　棘层轻度角化、萎缩，表皮嵴消失，基底层小灶状液化，血管周围轻微炎症浸润、色素失禁（HE 染色，×100）

Figure 15-13-2　Mild orthokeratosis, atrophy of spinous layer and disappearance of epidermal ridges, with focal basal liquefaction, sparse perivascular inflammatory infiltration and pigmentary incontinence (HE stain, ×100)

14. 线形色素性扁平苔藓
Linear lichen planus pigmentosus

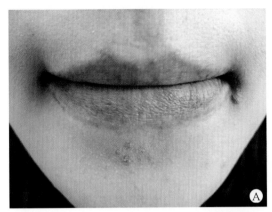
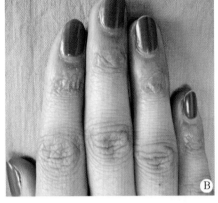
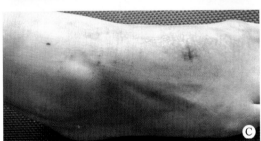

图 15-14-1　A. 下唇线下方边界清楚的深褐色条纹；B. 靠近指甲皱襞处簇集紫红色斑点，右手拇指除外；C. 右足背带状分布粟米大小、紫红色、扁平多角性丘疹

Figure 15-14-1　A. There was a well-defined dark brown streak paralleling near the lower lip line; B. A few dark porphyreous speckles clustered on the skin near to the nail fold of the right fingers except the thumb; C. On the dorsum of right foot, many flat-topped, shiny, purple and polygonal papules, showding a distribution of zosteriform pattern

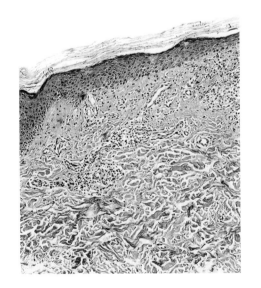

图 15-14-2　表皮角化过度、角化不全和萎缩，基细胞液化变性。血管周围淋巴细胞浸润，真皮色素失禁（HE 染色，×200）

Figure 15-14-2　Hyperkeratosis, parakeratosis and atrophy of the epidermis with liquescent degeneration of the basal cells. A perivascular lymphohistiocytic infiltration and pigmentary incontinence in the dermis were also noted (HE stain, ×200)

15.20 甲扁平苔藓
Lichen planus of nails

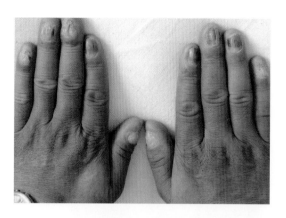

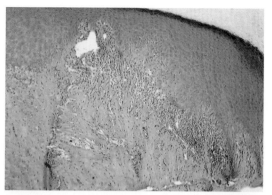

图 15-15-1 双手 10 指甲部分变薄、萎缩,呈翼状胬肉样改变,部分指甲肥厚、弯曲,呈棕褐色,上有纵行裂纹
Figure 15-15-1 Irregular longitudinal grooving and ridging of the nail plate,thinning of the nail plate,pterygium formation,shedding of the nail plate with atrophy of the nail bed

图 15-15-2 表皮棘层增生肥厚,基底细胞液化变性,真皮浅层淋巴细胞呈带状浸润(HE 染色,×100)
Figure 15-15-2 Acanthosis,liquefaction degeneration of basal layer cells,lymphocytes bandlike infiltrate in the upper dermis(HE stain,×100)

16. 扁平苔藓合并白癜风
Coincidence of lichen planus and vitiligo

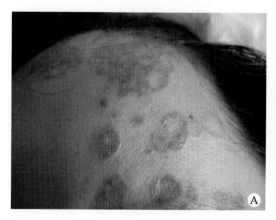

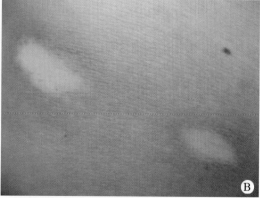

图 15-16-1 A. 左额部散在直径 0.3～3.0cm 暗红色或褐色、圆形或多角形斑或斑块,边缘稍隆起,中央色淡,轻度萎缩;B. 右下腹部不规则形色素脱失斑(2cm×2 cm～2cm×5cm)
Figure 15-16-1 A. Madder red or brown,round or polygonal,0.3～3.0cm in diameter maculae or patches, with an elevated borderline on left side of the frontal region;B. Irregular depigmented patches on right side of the waist(2cm×2cm～2cm×5cm)

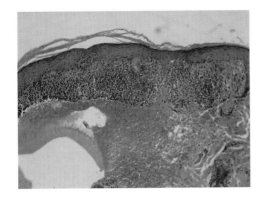

图 15-16-2　表皮角化过度,局灶性颗粒层增生,棘层不规则增厚(HE 染色,×40)

Figure 15-16-2　Hyperkeratosis, focal hypergranulosis and irregular acanthosis in the epidermis. (HE stain, × 40)

17. 急性泛发性扁平苔藓
Acute generalized lichen planus

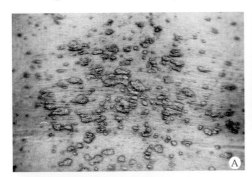

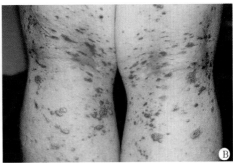

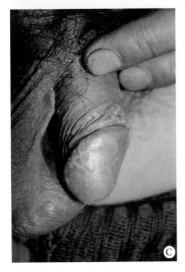

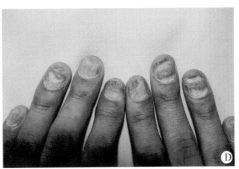

图 15-17-1　A. 腰部密集紫红色多角形丘疹,表面角化过度;B. 双下肢屈侧见较密集的紫红色丘疹;C. 龟头及包皮可见树枝状白斑;D. 指甲表面粗糙,覆有白屑

Figure 15-17-1　A. Thick, polygonal, violaceous, hyperkeratotic papules on the waist; B. A dense violaceous papules on the flexor surfaces of the both lower limbs; C. Dendritic whitish maculae on the glans penis and foreskin; D. Roughened nails with white scales on the fingers

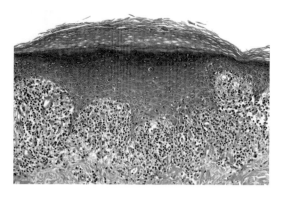

图 15-17-2 表皮角化过度,颗粒层、棘层增厚,基底细胞液化变性,真皮浅层淋巴细胞呈带状浸润(HE 染色,×100)

Figure 15-17-2 Hyperkeratosis, hypergranulosis and acanthosis, the basal cells liquefaction degeneration, a bandlike lymphocytes infiltrate in the upper dermis (HE stain, ×100)

18. 黑色丘疹性皮病
Dermatosis papulosa nigra

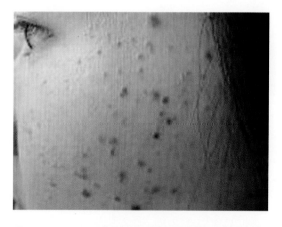

图 15-18-1 双颞颧对称散在分布米粒至绿豆大小棕色至深褐色扁平丘疹,直径为 1~5 mm,表面起皱,呈乳头瘤样,触之柔软,皮损间皮肤正常

Figure 15-18-1 Diffuse symmetric distribution of flat, round papules with papillamatus tops in sizes of 1-5 mm in diameter

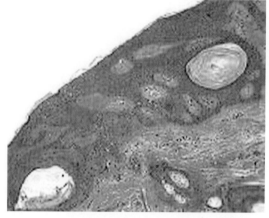

图 15-18-2 角质层轻度角化,颗粒层正常,棘层轻度肥厚,表皮突下伸,互连成网状。基底层色素颗粒增多,棘层内见 2 个角囊肿,真皮浅层小血管周围少量淋巴细胞浸润(HE 染色,×40)

Figure 15-18-2 Hyperkeratosis, mild acanthosis and normal granular layer; Elongation of rete ridge forming net-like structure; Two keratin cysts in spinous layer and increased melanin granules in basal layer; A few of lymphocytes arounded the small vessels in super dermis(HE stain, ×40)

19. 硬化性苔藓
Lichen sclerosus

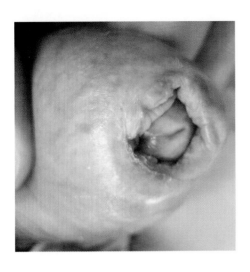

图 15-19-1　阴茎和龟头有白色硬化斑块

Figure 15-19-1　White and sclerosus plaques involved the penile shaft and the glans penis

20. 非生殖器部位特殊形态硬化性萎缩性苔藓
Lichen sclerosus in non-genital area with special shape

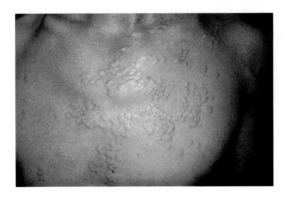

图 15-20-1　胸部许多黄豆大小群集分布之瓷白色扁平或蝶形丘疹,边缘略显红晕,中心可见毛孔扩大,毛囊性角栓

Figure 15-20-1　White flat-topped or discoid papules or plaques covered with horny plugs and surrounded by an erythematous halo on the chest

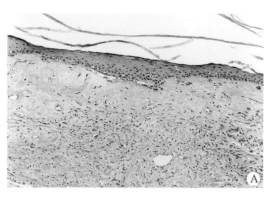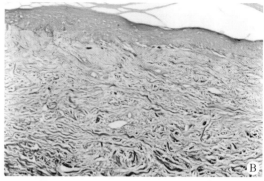

图 15-20-2　A. 表皮轻度角化过度,棘细胞层次减少,个别部位灶性萎缩,上皮脚变平,基底细胞灶性液化。真皮浅层胶原纤维水肿、纯一化、均质化,真皮中部弥漫性炎症细胞浸润(HE 染色,×20);B. 真皮上部网状纤维细疏,数量减少,淡染(网状纤维染色,×20)

Figure 15-20-2　A. Hyperkeratosis with follicular plugging, atrophy of stratum malpighii with hydropic degeneration of basal cells, pronounced edema and homogenization of the collagen in the upper dermis, and an inflammatory infiltrate in the middermis (HE stain, ×20); B. The diminution of elastic fibers sparse in the upper dermis (Verhoff stain, ×20)

21. 面颈部毛囊性红斑黑变病
Erythromelanosis follicularis faciei et colli

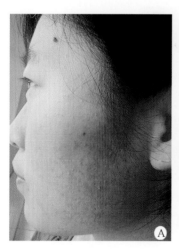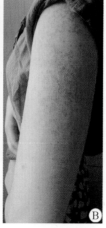

图 15-21-1　A. 颊部和颞部有毛囊性丘疹和淡红斑褐色斑;B. 上臂伸侧有毛囊角化丘疹,其母有类似病

Figure 15-21-1　A. Follicular papules and raddish-brown spots or pathes on the cheeks and temples; B. Follicular keratosis papules on the extenor aspect of arms. Her mother had similar condition

22. 金色苔藓

Lichen aureus

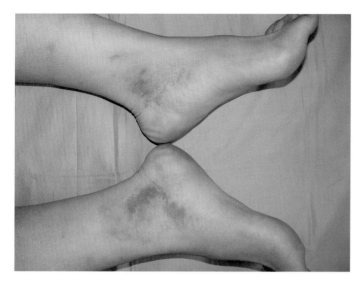

图 15-22-1　双内踝部金色斑疹融合成片状,皮损色素分布不均匀,表面无鳞屑

Figure 15-22-1　Golden pigmented maculae presented as "cayenne pepper" on the dorsum of both feet. The skin lesions are confluent on the inner malleolus

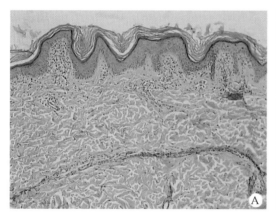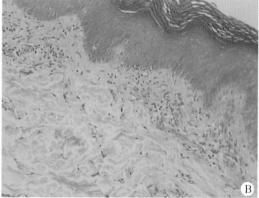

图 15-22-2　A. 真皮上部炎性细胞呈带状浸润(HE 染色,×100);B. 真皮上部大量染成蓝色的含铁血黄素(Perls 染色,×200)

Figure 15-22-2　A. A band-like infiltration of mononuclear and histiocytic cells in the upper dermis(HE stain, ×100); B. Perls staining showed the presence of massive haemosider in the upper dermis(Perls stain, ×200)

23. 泛发性光泽苔藓
Lichen nitidus

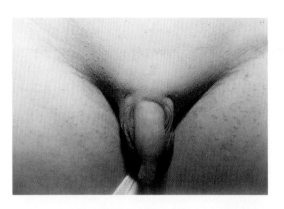

图 15-23-1　肤色圆形或多角形扁平小丘疹,累及阴茎包皮,孤立散在

Figure 15-23-1　Numerous flat-topped, skin-colored round or polygonal papules without coalesce on the penis and foreskin

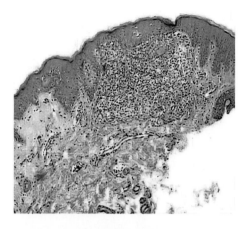

图 15-23-2　真皮乳头部有局限性细胞团,其顶部表皮突消失,两侧表皮突向内向下延伸,基底细胞灶性液化变性,细胞团内主要为淋巴细胞、上皮样细胞、组织细胞及个别多核巨细胞,未见干酪样坏死(HE 染色,×100)

Figure 15-23-2　A circumscribed nest of cells in the dermis papillary, the infiltrate consisted of lymphocytes, epithelioid cells, histiocytes and a few multinucleated giant cells (HE stain, ×100)

24. 连圈状秕糠疹
Pityriasis circinata

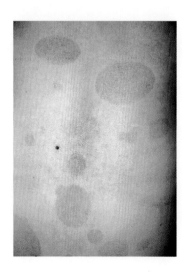

图 15-24-1　背部有多数大小不一圆形和卵圆形鳞屑斑

Figure 15-24-1　Muitiple, strikingly circular or oval scaly patches on the trunk

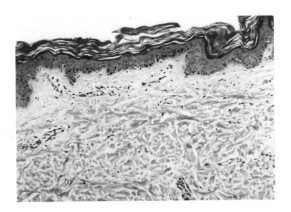

图 15-24-2 表皮角化过度,真皮小血管周围少量淋巴细胞和组织细胞浸润(HE 染色,×100)

Figure 15-24-2 Hyperkeratosis and infiltrate of a few lymphocytes and histocytes around blood vessels in the dermis(HE stain,×100)

第 16 章
大疱和无菌性脓疱性皮病
Chronic Blistering Dermatoses

1. 天疱疮患儿(新生儿)
Pemphigus neonatorum baby

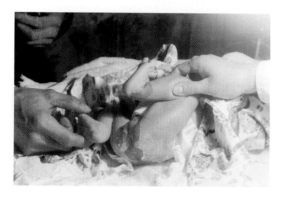

图 16-1-1　臀部、左下肢见散在大小不等的表皮剥蚀面

Figure 16-1-1　Varying size erosions on the buttocks and the left lower limb

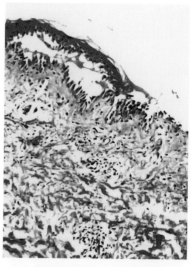

图 16-1-2　基底细胞层上方棘层松解,其上方部分表皮缺损,真皮见少量炎性细胞浸润(HE 染色,×100)

Figure 16-1-2　Acantholysis in the upper of basal layer,part epidermis absent,a few inflammatory infiltrate in the dermis(HE stain,×100)

2. 毛囊角化病样天疱疮
Follicularis kerotosoid pemphigus

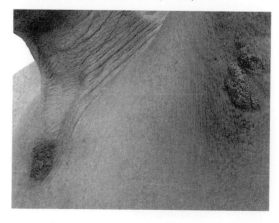

图 16-2-1　胸前及腋窝红棕色斑块,其上有小丘疹、小水疱及褐色结痂,周围有红晕

Figure 16-2-1　Red papules, vesicles, brownish-red eczematous plaques on the chest and axillae

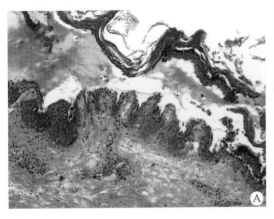
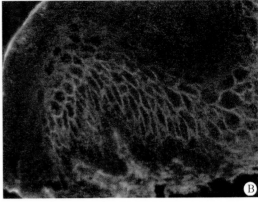

图 16-2-2 A. 基底层上棘层松解,可见棘突松解细胞及谷粒,有绒毛形成(HE 染色,×20);B. 表皮细胞间有 IgG 及 C3 沉积(直接免疫荧光,×200)

Figure 16-2-2 A. Acantholysis in the upper basal layer with acantholytic cells,grain and villi (HE stain,×20);B. Direct immunofluorescence examination showed a positive deposition of IgG and C3 among the keratinocytes(DIF,×200)

3. 伴局限性 Castleman 病的副肿瘤性天疱疮

Paraneoplastic pemphigus with Castleman's disease

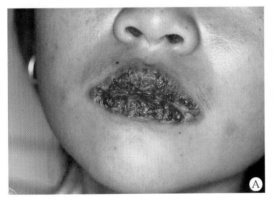
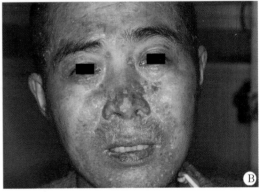

图 16-3-1 A. 口唇糜烂、结痂;B. 头面部红斑、结痂,口唇及眼糜烂

Figure 16-3-1 A. Erosions and crusting of the lips;B. Erythematous macules and crusting on the face,erosions of the lips and eyes

111

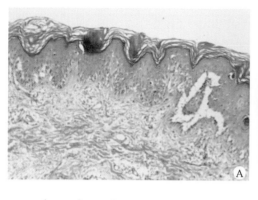
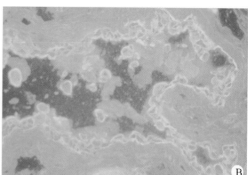

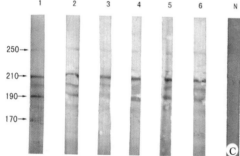

图 16-3-2　A. 表皮内散在坏死的角质形成细胞；B. 上皮细胞间免疫荧光抗体沉积（皮损直接免疫荧光）；C. 相对分子质量250ku,210ku,190ku处均有阳性条带,1～6为患者,N为正常人（免疫印迹结果）

Figure 16-3-2　A. Necrobiosis of keratinocytes in the epidermis；B. IgG and C3 deposition in the intercellular spaces of the epithelium（DIF）；C. Desmoplakin 1(250KD),envoplakin(210KD),and periplakin(190KD) were positive by western-blotting

4. 副肿瘤性天疱疮
Paraneoplastic pemphigus

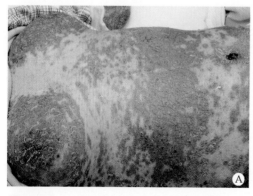
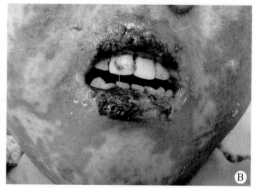

图 16-4-1　A. 躯干部有大片暗红色及褐色斑,部分皮疹表面有糜烂、渗出及结痂；B. 上下唇广泛糜烂,有血痂

Figure 16-4-1　A. Dark red or brown macules with erosion,effusion and crust on the trunk；B. Extensive erosion with blood crust on the bilabial

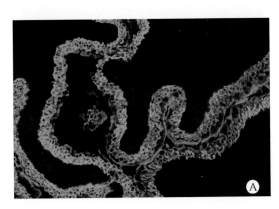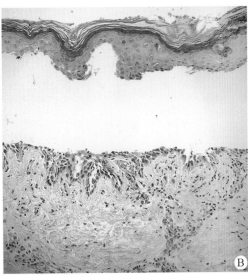

图 16-4-2　A. 血液间接免疫荧光检查大鼠膀胱作为底物,棘细胞间见 IgG 荧光阳性；B. 表皮基底层上大疱,棘细胞层可见散在红染的坏死角质形成细胞,基底细胞液化变性,真皮浅层血管周围淋巴细胞浸润(HE 染色,×100)

Figure 16-4-2　A. Squamous intercellular substance deposition of IgG (Indirect immunofluorescence testing); B. Bulla above the basal layer, necrosis of keratocytes in the stratum malpighii, liquefaction degeneration of basal cells, lymphocytes infiltrate perivascular in the superficial dermis(HE stain, ×100)

5. 结节性类天疱疮

Pemphigoid nodularis

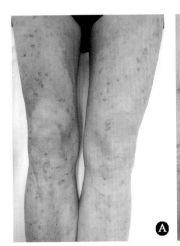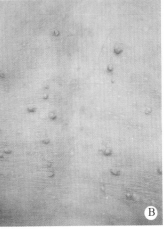

图 16-5-1　四肢(A)及躯干部(B)多散在丘疹、结节,孤立不相融合,绿豆大小,未见水疱

Figure 16-5-1　Multiple scaltered papules and nodules in the size of bean on the trunk (A) and extremities(B)

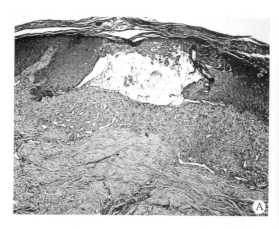
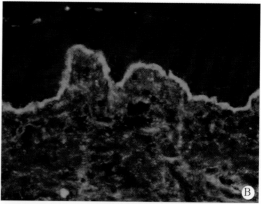

图 16-5-2　A. 表皮角化过度伴角化不全,棘层肥厚,表皮下一水疱,疱内及真皮浅层血管周围少量淋巴细胞、嗜酸性粒细胞及嗜中性粒细胞浸润(HE 染色,×200); B. (直接免疫荧光可见)表皮基膜带有 IgG 线状沉积(直接免疫荧光,×200)

Figure 16-5-2　A. Hyperkeratosis, parakeratosis, acanthosis and a subepidermal blister; lymphocytes, eosinophils and neutroplils in the blisters and around the blood vessels in the upper dermis(HE stain, ×200); B. A linear deposition of IgG and C3 at the basement membrane zone.(DIF, ×200)

6. 儿童线状 IgA 大疱性皮病
Linear IgA bullous dermatosis of childhood

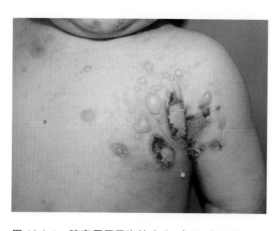

图 16-6-1　腋窝周围紧张性大疱,糜烂,表面结痂

Figure 16-6-1　Tensional blisters and erosion with crust around the axilla

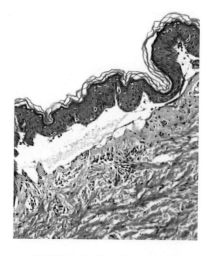

图 16-6-2　表皮下水疱,真皮有少许中性粒细胞等炎症细胞浸润(HE 染色,×100)

Figure 16-6-2　Subepidermal blister with mild neutrophil infiltration in the dermis(HE stain, ×100)

7. 成人线状 IgA 大疱性皮病
Linear IgA bullous dermatosis in adult

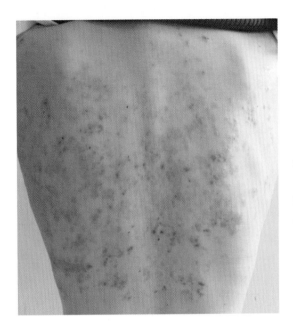

图 16-7-1 背部泛发水肿性红斑、丘疹,上有米粒至绿豆大小张力性水疱,可见环状或弧形排列,少许糜烂面、血痂和抓痕

Figure 16-7-1 Generalized erythemas, distributed in an annular form on the back

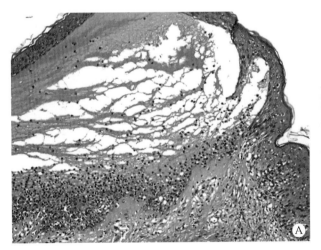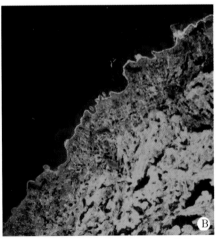

图 16-7-2 A. 表皮下水疱,疱内及真皮可见大量嗜酸性粒细胞浸润,真皮有少许中性粒细胞等炎性细胞浸润(HE 染色,×100);B. 直接免疫荧光示表皮基底膜带 IgA 呈亮绿色线状沉积(直接免疫荧光,×100)

Figure 16-7-2 A. A subepidermal blister contained with dermal eosinophils and a few neutrophils infiltration (HE stain,×100);B. Direct immunofluorescence showed continuous linear deposits of IgA along the basement membrane zone(DIF,×100)

8. 复发性线状棘层松解皮病
Relapsing linear acantholytic dermatosis

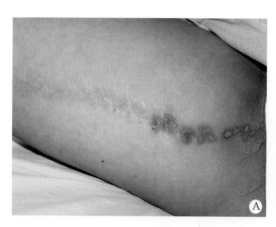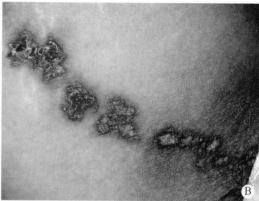

图 16-8-1　A. 右大腿内侧至屈侧沿 Blaschko 线分布的陈旧性暗红色斑块、色素沉着斑及新发红斑、水疱；B. 右大腿线状皮损上端新发红斑、水疱，部分水疱破溃后形成糜烂面及结痂

Figure 16-8-1　A. Erythema and vesicula eruption on the interior of right thigh and distributed along Blaschko's line；B. New erythema and vesicula on the upper of line eruption of right thigh，part broken vesicula forming erosion and scab

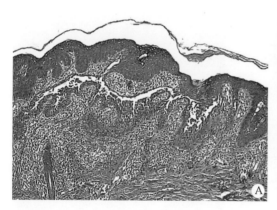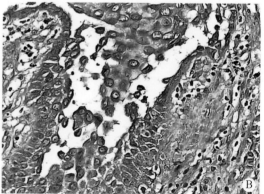

图 16-8-2　表皮基底细胞层上水疱形成，表皮见单个或倒塌砖墙样棘层松解细胞（HE 染色，A×40；B×200）

Figure 16-8-2　Epidermal acantholysis with multiple acantholytic keratinocytes and the appearance of a "dilapidated brick wall" in suprabasal cell layer（HE stain，A×40；B×200）

9. 具有掌跖损害的外生殖器部位的棘层松解性皮病
Acantholytic dermatosis of genitocrural area associated the lesions on the palms and soles

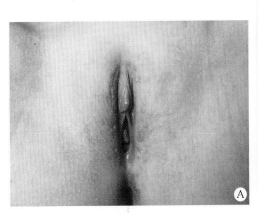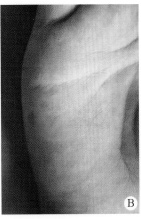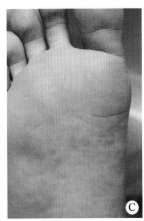

图 16-9-1　A. 双侧大阴唇多个肤色圆形丘疹；B、C. 掌、跖角化性丘疹和点状凹陷

Figure 16-9-1　A. Multiple skin-color round papules on both labia majora；B、C. Keratotic papules and pitting on the palms and soles

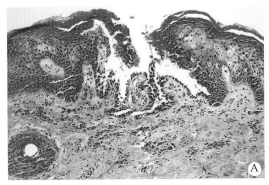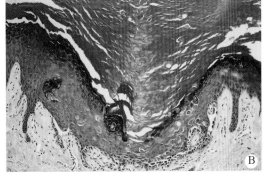

图 16-9-2　A. 大阴唇表皮角化过度，棘层增厚，基底层上裂隙形成，可见棘层松解细胞，真皮浅层散在的淋巴细胞浸润(HE 染色，×100)；B. 手掌明显角化过度，基底层上裂隙形成，颗粒层和棘层见圆体和谷粒，真皮浅层少许淋巴细胞浸润(HE 染色，×100)

Figure 16-9-2　A. (labium majus) Hyperkeratosis, acanthosis, cracks in the basal layer and acantholytic cells；Scattered lymphocyte infiltration in the upper dermis (HE stain, ×100)；B. (Palm) Significant hyperkeratosis, acanthosis, cracks in the basal layer, rounds and grains in the stratum granulosum and stratum spinosum；a few lymphocyte infiltration in the upper dermis (HE stain, ×100)

10. 获得性大疱性表皮松解症
Epidermolysis bullosa acquisita

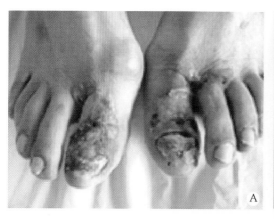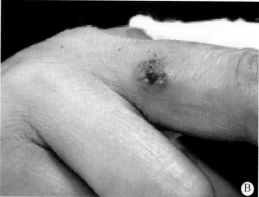

图 16-10-1　A. 双足跗趾伸侧、趾间水疱破裂后形成结痂；B. 指间皮肤上水疱破裂，表面结痂

Figure 16-10-1　A. The blister and scarring on the extensor surface of thumb and between toe；B. The blister and scarring between the fingers

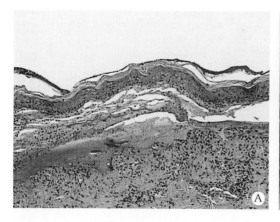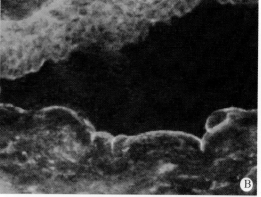

图 16-10-2　A. 表皮下水疱，疱内有大量中性粒细胞，真皮浅层中性粒细胞、单核细胞浸润（HE 染色，×40）；B. IgG、C3 沉积于真皮乳头侧（直接免疫荧光，×40）

Figure 16-10-2　A. Bullae in the subepidermis，numerous neutrophils in the bullae，neutrophils and monocytes infiltrate in the superficial dermis（HE stain，×40）；B. Deposition of IgG and C3 in the dermis papillary （DIF，×40）

11. 疱疹样脓疱病并发妊娠期肝内胆汁淤积症
Impetigo herpetiformis and gestational intrahepatic cholestasis

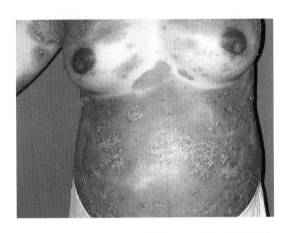

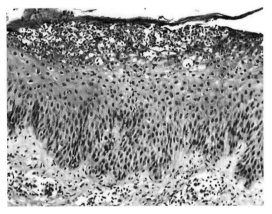

图 16-11-1　胸腹部可见大片红斑、脓疱，部分脓疱融合

Figure 16-11-1　Erythema and pustulae on the trunk

图 16-11-2　表皮内可见 Kogoj 样脓肿（HE 染色，×400）

Figure 16-11-2　The spongiform pustule of Kogoj in the epidermis（HE stain,×400）

12. 掌跖脓疱病合并前胸壁综合征
Pustulosis palmoplantaris accompanied with anterior chest wall syndromes

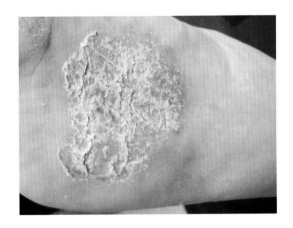

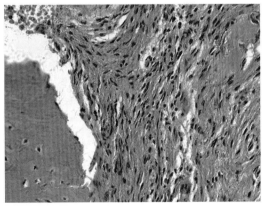

图 16-12-1　双足和手掌有多数脓疱

Figure 16-12-1　Multiple pustules on the both sole and palmar

图 16-12-2　左侧第 1 肋胸关节处在软骨间有单一核细胞和纤维细胞浸润（HE 染色，×200）

Figure 16-12-2　There are monocycle and fibroblast infiltrate among the articular cartilage of the first left sternocostal joint（HE stain,×200）

13. 嗜酸性脓疱性毛囊炎
Eosinophilic pustular folliculitis

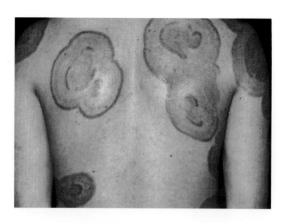

图 16-13-1 肩背部有多数大小不一的环形红斑，部分红斑边缘有脓疱

Figure 16-13-1 Neumerous and various size circle erythema, some of them have pustules at peripheral on the back

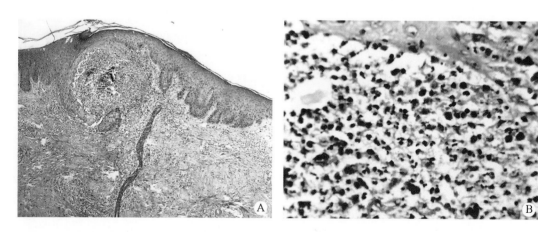

图 16-13-2 毛囊内微脓肿，含较多嗜酸性粒细胞和嗜中性粒细胞(HE 染色 A：×100；B：×400)

Figure 16-13-2 Microabscess formation contained numerous eosinophilis and neutrophilis in the hair follicular (HE stain A：×100；B：×400)

14. 婴儿肢端脓疱病
Infantile acropustulosis

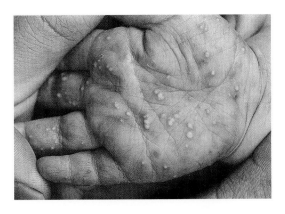

图 16-14-1   手掌、手指屈侧小米粒大脓疱,疱壁紧张,尼氏征阴性,疱液呈淡黄色

Figure 16-14-1   The pustules with intense wall and pale yellow fluid in size from 1 to 2 mm on the palms and flexor surface of the finger, intense wall and pale yellow fluid in the pustules

15. 泛发性连续性肢端皮炎
Generalized acrodermatitis continua

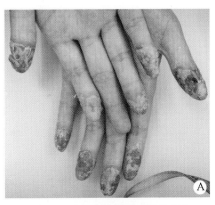

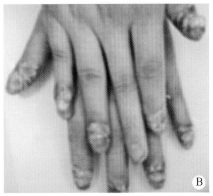

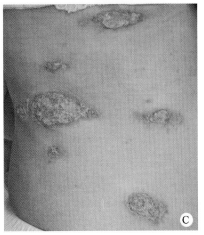

图 16-15-1   A. 十指皆有不同程度的红斑,其上散布芝麻大小的脓疱,部分脓疱融合、部分干枯结痂;B. 甲变形、部分变薄或缺失,部分增厚、甲下脓疱;C. 胸、腹部也见红斑基础上脓疱、部分融合成脓湖。部分趋于干枯、结痂

Figure 16-15-1   A. Different degree of erythema on ten fingers, which the size of sesame seeds scattered pustules on erythema, the pustules integration or dry scab; B. Nails deformed, some of them thin or missing, others thickened and pustules under them; C. Some pustules on erythema of chest and abdomen integrat into lake, others dry or crusted

第 17 章
真皮弹性纤维疾病
Dermal Elastic Tissue Diseases

1. 播散型匐行性穿通性弹性纤维病
Disseminated elastosis perforans serpiginosum

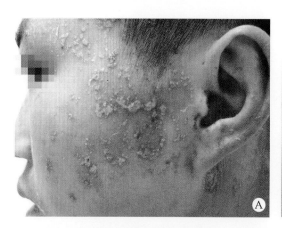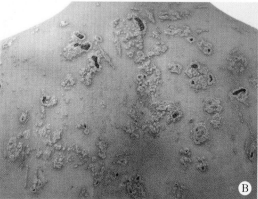

图 1/-1-1　群集丘疹排列成弓形或匐行状十面部(A)和背部(B)

Figure 17-1-1　These papules are arranged in arcuate or serpiginous groups on the face(A) and on the back(B)

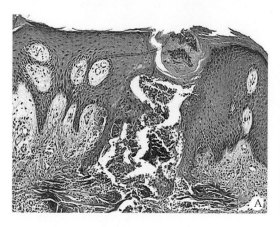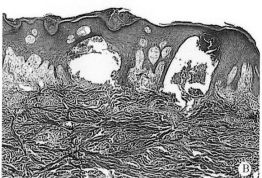

图 17-1-2　A. 棘层肥厚的表皮内有一个窄而弯曲管道穿通,中含嗜碱性坏死物质和炎症(HE stain, ×200); B. 变性的弹力纤维增多增粗(Verhoeff 染色, ×100)

Figure 17-1-2　A. A narrow, curved channel contained basophilic necrotic material and inflamate cells through an acanthotic epidermis is shown(HE stain, ×200); B. There are increased and thickened of degenerated elastic fibers(Verhoeff stain, ×100)

2. 先天性皮肤松弛症
Congenital cutis laxa

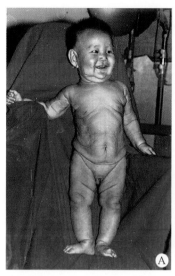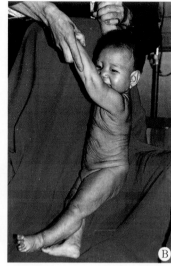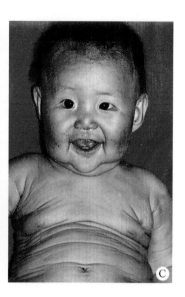

图 17-2-1　面、颌、颈、胸、腰部皮肤及双乳房松弛、下垂,多皱褶,呈早老貌

Figure 17-2-1　Loose, redundant skin, hanging in folds around the face, jaw, neck, chest and waist and breasts

3. 全身性皮肤松弛症
Generalized elastorrhexis

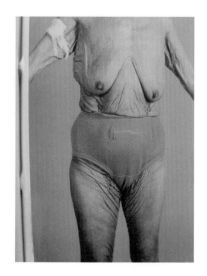

图 17-3-1　妇女皮肤松弛和悬垂

Figure 17-3-1　A woman with loose and pendulous skin

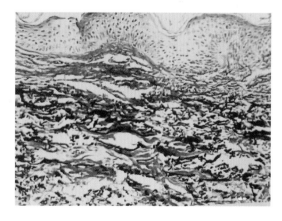

图 17-3-2　真皮弹性纤维数目减少断裂,呈颗粒样
(弹性纤维染色,×100)

Figure 17-3-2　Fragmentation, granular appearance and diminution of elastic fibers in the dermis(Verhoff stain, ×100)

4. 局限性皮肤松弛症
Circumscribed cutis laxa

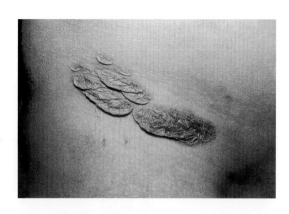

图 17-4-1　腹股沟中外段 3 片类椭圆形的松弛斑,边界清楚

Figure 17-4-1　Three oval, circumscribed loose maculae on the inguinal

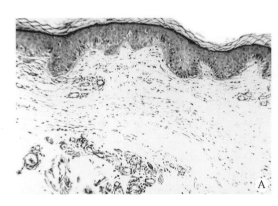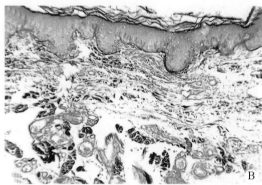

图 17-4-2　A. 表皮基底层色素增加,真皮结缔组织疏松排列,血管周围少量慢性炎性细胞浸润(HE 染色,×100);B. 真皮弹性纤维明显减少,形态异常,纤维变短、增粗,且粗细不一(双联染色,×100)

Figure 17-4-2　A. Hyperpigmentation in the basal layer, and connective tissue lined loosenly, a few chronic inflammatory cells infiltrated around blood vessels (HE stain, × 100); B. The elastic fibers diminished in the dermis, the shape of elastic fiber is abnormal (Combind stain, × 100)

5. 眼睑松弛症
Blepharochalasis

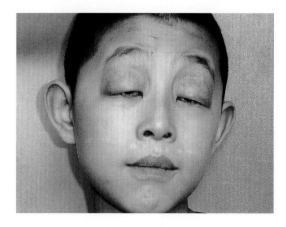

图 17-5-1　双上眼睑皮肤松软、下垂、水肿,表面菲薄呈浅橙色,皮下血管清晰可见

Figure 17-5-1　Swelling of the upper lids leading to thinning of the skin and excessive upper lid skin clear vein being seen

6. 弹性纤维性假黄瘤
Pseudoxanthoma elasticum

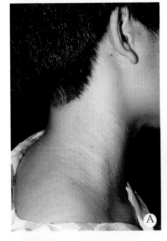
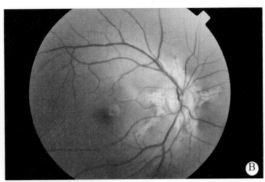
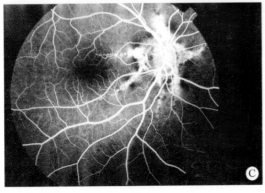

图 17-6-1　A. 颈部线状排列的淡黄色扁平小丘疹，皮肤柔软、轻度皱缩，呈鸡皮样外观；B. 眼底检查显示右眼有 6 条血管样条纹；C. 眼底荧光血管造影显示血管样条纹呈荧光

Figure 17-6-1　A. The soft yellowish flat papules in linear arrangement on the neck to appear loose and wrinkled; B. Six angioid streaks of the fundi in the right eye; C. The fluorescence of angioid streaks by fundus angiography

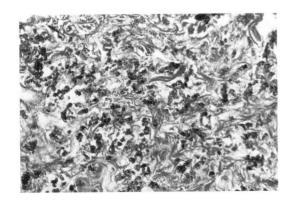

图 17-6-2　真皮内深蓝黑色弹性纤维增多、增粗、断裂，呈破毛线团状（弹性纤维染色，×400）

Figure 17-6-2　The dark black elastic fibers are increased in number and showed fragmentation and clamping in the dermis（Verhoeff staining, ×400）

7. 皮肤弹性过度伴免疫学检查异常
Cutis hyperelastica complicated by the abnormity in immunoassay

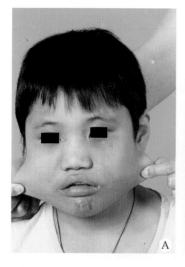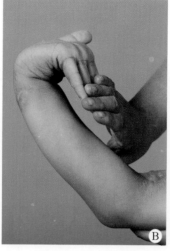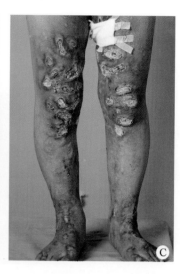

图 17-7-1　A. 皮肤弹性过度,面部皮肤可过度牵拉;B. 手腕关节伸展过度;C. 双下肢有较多蚕豆至核桃大的溃疡,表面有脓性分泌物,愈合处可见增生性瘢痕、色素沉着及色素脱失斑

Figure 17-7-1　A. Cutis hyperrelastica, stretched skin at face; B. Hyperextensibility of the wrist; C. Neumerous varying size ulcers with pus secretion, hyperplastic scar, hyperpigmentation and hypopigmentation macules in the scar

8. 巨大结缔组织痣
Giant connective tissue nevus

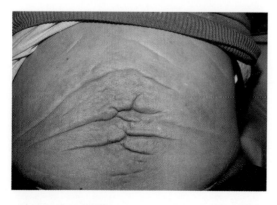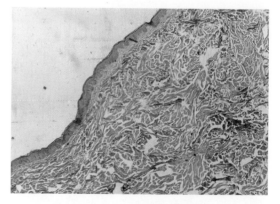

图 17-8-1　在腰骶部有 19 cm×22 cm 大轻微隆起和发硬的斑块

Figure 17-8-1　Slightly elevated and indurated plaques in 19 cm×22 cm size on the waist

图 17-8-2　真皮中胶原纤维束增厚和均质化(HE 染色,×100)

Figure 17-8-2　The collagen bundles are thickened and homogenized in the dermis(HE stain,×100)

9. 发疹性皮肤胶原瘤
Eruptive collagenoma of the skin

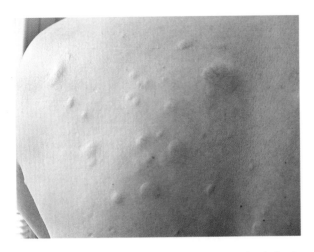

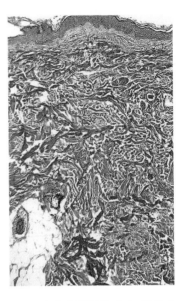

图 17-9-1　背部、肩部多发性肤色的扁平丘疹、结节、斑块

Figure 17-9-1　Multiple skin-colored flat papules, nodules and plaques on the shoulders and back

图 17-9-2　真皮胶原纤维增生、致密(HE 染色，×200)

Figure 17-9-2　Collagen fibers are coarse and increased in the dermis(HE stain, ×200)

10. 颈部白色纤维丘疹病
White fibrous papulosis of the neck

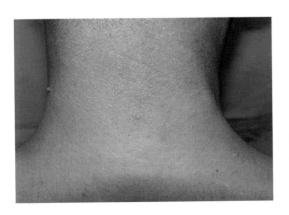

图 17-10-1　项部有多数圆形到椭圆形白色坚实丘疹

Figure 17-10-1　Maltiple round-to-oval, whitish, firm papules on the nape

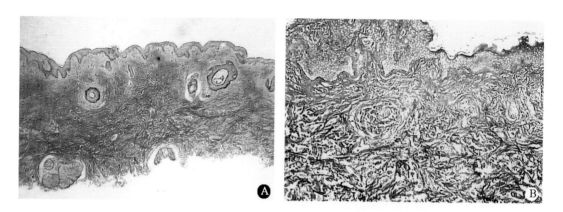

图 17-10-2　A. 真皮中胶原纤维束局限性增厚（HE 染色，×40）；B. 真皮内弹力纤维未发现异常（Verhoeff 染色，×100）

Figure 17-10-2　A. Circumscribed thickening collagen bundles in the dermis（HE stain，×40）；B. No abnormality of elastic fibers could be found in the dermis（Verhoeff stain，×100）

第 18 章
萎缩性皮肤病 Atrophy Diseases

1. 膨胀纹和局限性萎缩
Striae distensae and localized atrophy

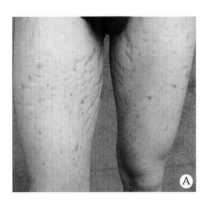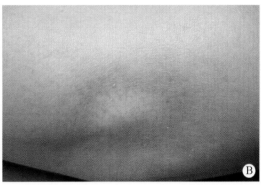

图 18-1-1　A. 0.1% 曲安奈德霜应用 3 个月后双大腿内侧有明显膨胀纹；B. 局部注射曲安奈德 5mg 2 次后，在注射部位发生皮下脂肪萎缩

Figure 18-1-1　A. The striae distensae widely distributed over both thighs after application of 0.1% tramicinolone cream for three months；B. Subcutaneous atrophy at the site injection of 5mg tramicinolone for two times

2. 原发性斑状萎缩
Macular atrophy

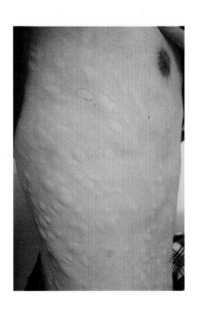

图 18-2-1　躯干泛发孤立约黄豆至蚕豆大小类圆形肤色柔软萎缩性斑，触之有轻度落空感

Figure 18-2-1　General lined isolated rounded and atrophic cuticolour patches with mild frustration feeling by touch distributed on the trunk

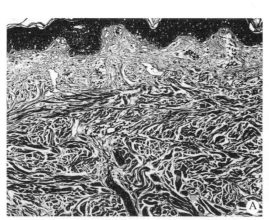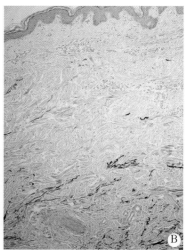

图 18-2-2　A. 表皮大致正常，真皮内血管及附件周围少量淋巴细胞浸润，乳头层及网状层弹力纤维稀疏，局限性胶原纤维呈结节状增生（HE 染色，×100）；B. 真皮内弹力纤维明显减少、断裂、消失（弹力纤维染色，×100）

Figure 18-2-2　A. Epidermis was normal, some lymphocytes infiltrated around the vessel and skin appendages in the dermi. The collagenous fibers proliferated at papillary layer（HE stain, ×100）; B. Elastin fibers fractured, decreased and even disappeared in the dermis（Elastic tissue stain, ×100）

3. 包皮假性阿洪病
Pseudoainhun of the penis

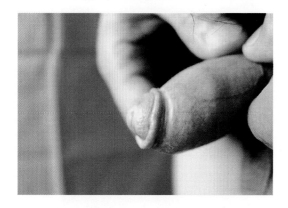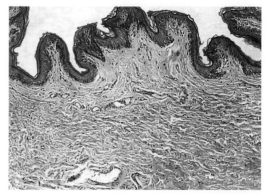

图 18-3-1　包皮前端有一个完整的环形缩窄带

Figure 18-3-1　Intact constricting band around the penis

图 18-3-2　表皮正常，真皮轻度胶原纤维增生（HE 染色，×100）

Figure 18-3-2　There is slight increase of collagen fibers in the dermis without epidermal charge（HE stain, ×100）

第 19 章
皮肤血管炎 Cutaneous Vasculitis

1. 持久性隆起红斑
Erythema elevatum diutinum

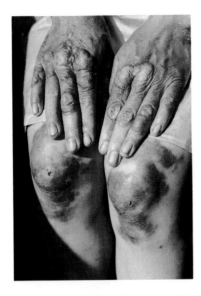

图 19-1-1 双手指间关节、掌指关节、膝关节伸侧见玉米至核桃大紫红色或棕红色隆起皮面的结节、斑块

Figure 19-1-1 Brownish red to purple nodules and plaques on the extensor surfaces of the joint of knees and hands

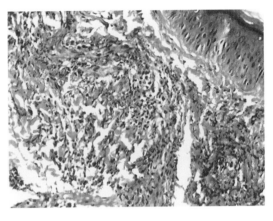

图 19-1-2 真皮浅层及血管周围弥漫致密的以中性粒细胞为主的浸润，间有少量淋巴细胞及组织细胞（HE 染色，×100）

Figure 19-1-2 Dense neutrophils intermingled with varying numbers of lymphocytes and histiocytes infiltrate in the superficial dermis and perivascular（HE stain，×100）

2. 急性发热性嗜中性皮病
Sweet's syndrome

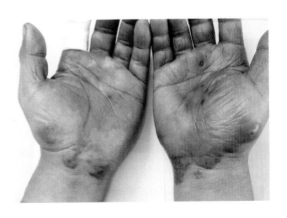

图 19-2-1 双手掌紫红色水肿性红斑，边缘清楚，略呈环状

Figure 19-2-1 Well-circumscribed annular-like violaceous plaques on both palms

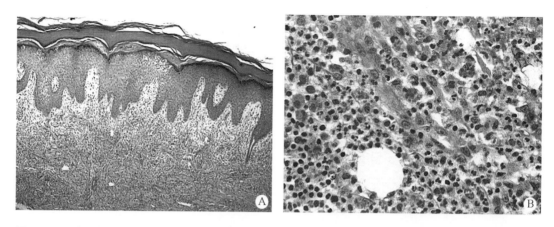

图 19-2-2　表皮灶性细胞间水肿,真皮血管周围弥漫性中性粒细胞、组织细胞及淋巴细胞浸润(HE 染色,A ×40,B×200)

Figure 19-2-2　Focal spongiosis in the epidermis and diffuse perivascular neutrophils,histocytes and lympho-cytes infiltrate in the dermis (HE stain,A×40,B×200)

3. 皮下型急性发热性嗜中性皮肤病
Subcutaneous acute febrile neutrophilic dermatosis

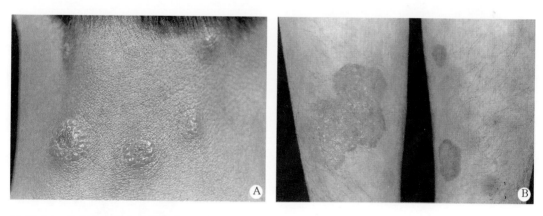

图 19-3-1　有红色斑块和结节发生于项部(A)和小腿(B)

Figure 19-3-1　Erythematous plagues and nodules on the nape(A) and the leg(B)

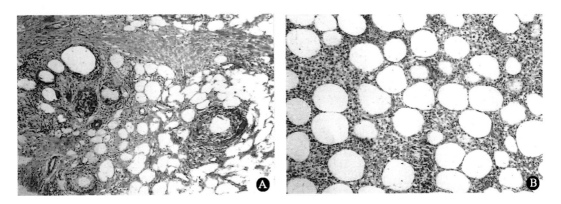

图 19-3-2　A. 真皮内围绕血管周围有显著的中性粒细胞浸润(HE 染色,×100);B. 在皮下脂肪组织中有致密的淋巴细胞浸润合并核分裂(HE 染色,×160)

Figure 19-3-2　A. Prominent infiltrate composed of neutrophils around the vascular in the dermis(HE stain,×100);B. There is a dense infiltrate composed of neutrophils associated with neuclear fragmentation in subcutaneous tissue(HE stain,×160)

4. Wegener 肉芽肿
Wegener's granulomatosis

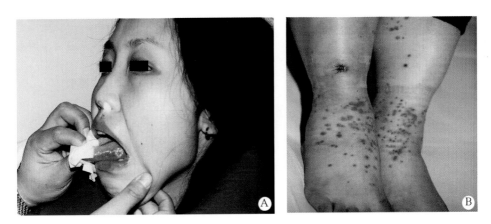

图 19-4-1　A. 左侧舌缘有一黄豆大肉芽肿性溃疡;B. 两足背和小腿散在米粒大红色丘疹,压之不退色,部分丘疹中央有水疱、脓疱和坏死性痂

Figure 19-4-1　A. A soybean-sized ulcer on the left aspect of tongue;B. Millet sized red papules with central vesicles,pustule and necrosis crust on the back of feet and calves

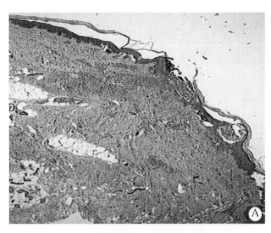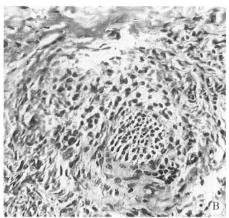

图 19-4-2　A. 血管周围肉芽肿性炎性浸润,以组织细胞为主,伴有淋巴细胞、少量多核巨细胞(HE染色,×10); B. 肉芽肿性血管炎(HE 染色,×40)

Figure 19-4-2　A. Leukocytoclastic vasculitis with granulomatous inflammation, and majority histocytes (HE stain, ×10); B. Granulomatous vasculitis (HE stain, ×40)

5. 坏疽性脓皮病
Pyoderma gangrenosum

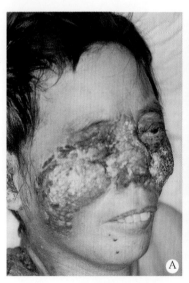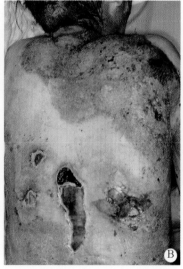

图 19-5-1　A. 面部蝶形溃疡性斑块; B. 肩背部大小不等的溃疡、瘢痕
Figure 19-5-1　A. Butterfly ulcerative plaques on the face; B. Varying size ulcers and scars on the shoulder and back

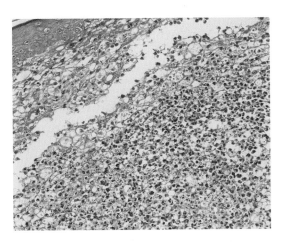

图 19-5-2　真皮层见大量中性粒细胞及嗜酸粒细胞浸润(HE 染色,×400)

Figure 19-5-2　A dense infiltrate of neutrophils and eosinophils in the dermis (HE stain,×400)

6. 恶性萎缩性丘疹病伴肠穿孔
Malignant atrophic papulosis accompanying intestinal perforation

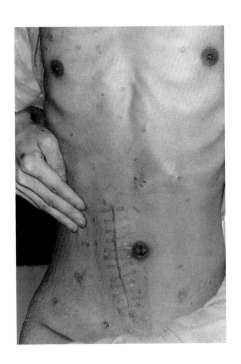

图 19-6-1　散在米粒至黄豆大淡红色、暗红色半球形丘疹,中央微凹,呈瓷白色,丘疹周围有红晕,部分丘疹表面有细小鳞屑

Figure 19-6-1　The size of millet to soybean pale red or yellowish red papules with atrophic porcelain-white center,partly with fine scales on the surface

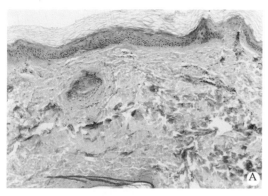
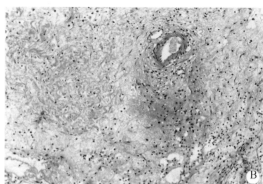
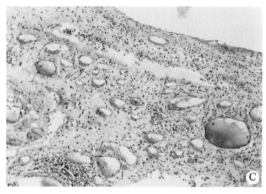

图 19-6-2 A. 表皮变薄,角化过度,表皮突消失(HE 染色,×100);B. 真皮灶性坏死,皮肤附属器减少,纤维组织增生伴胶原化,小血管周围可见灶状淋巴细胞浸润(HE 染色,×100);C. 肠黏膜散在中性粒细胞浸润,固有层及黏膜下血管淤血,血管内皮增生,血管炎及血管周围炎,部分血管血栓性闭塞(HE 染色,×100)

Figure 19-6-2   A. Marked atrophy of the stratum malpighii associated with slight hyperkeratosis and rete ridge vanishing (HE stain, ×100); B. Focal necrobiosis in the dermis, appendages decrease, collagen fibrous tissue hyperplasia and focal lymphocyte infiltrate in the perivascular (HE stain, ×100); C. Scattered neutrocyte infiltrate in the intestinal, with subserosal arterioles endothelial cell hyperplasia occluded by thrombosis (HE stain, ×100)

7. 青斑样血管炎
Livedoid vasculitis

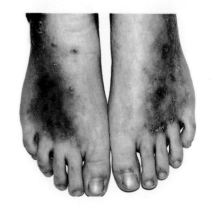

图 19-7-1 双足背部溃疡及色素沉着
Figure 19-7-1   Ulcer and hyperpigmentation on the dorsal of feet

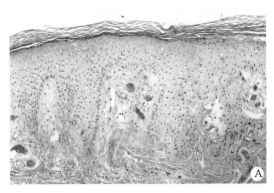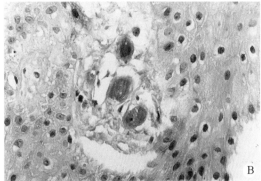

图 19-7-2　A. 真皮上部水肿,多处小血管血栓形成(HE 染色,×100);B. 真皮乳头小血管内血栓(HE 染色,×200)

Figue 19-7-2　A. Edema and multiple small vessels thrombogenesis in the upper dermis (HE stain,×100); B. Multiple thrombogenesis in small vessels in the dermis papilla (HE stain,×200)

8. 血小板增多性紫癜

Thrombocythemia purpura

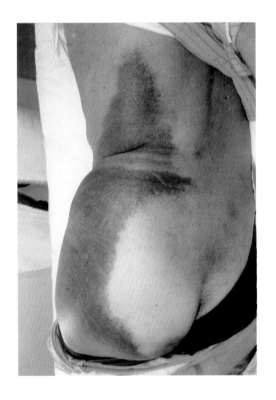

图 19-8-1　左侧腰部、臀部及大腿伸侧大片紫红色斑片,边界欠清

Figure 19-8-1　Uncircumscribed violaceous maculae on the left waist,buttocks and the extensor surface of thigh

9. 播散性瘙痒性血管性皮炎
Disseminnate pruriginous angiodermatitis

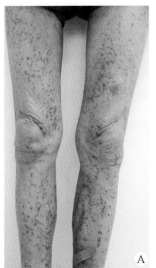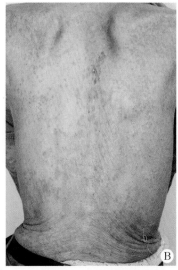

图 19-9-1　双下肢(A)和后背(B)散在或融合成片的紫癜性斑疹，部分表面有少许鳞屑

Figure 19-9-1　Irregular pink papules, plaques, petechias and ecchymosis distributed on the lower limbs(A) and back(B) of the patient, some lesions were covered with a few scales

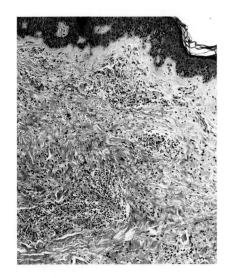

图 19-9-2　真皮上部小血管内皮细胞肿胀，血管周围以淋巴细胞和单核细胞浸润为主，可见嗜酸性粒细胞浸润，少量红细胞外渗(HE 染色，×200)

Figure 19-9-2　The dermal microvescular endothelia cells swelling, mainly lymphocyte and mononuclear cells around blood vessels, meanwhile a few erythrocytes leakage(HE stain, ×200)

第 20 章
皮肤脉管性疾病
Cutaneous Vascular Diseases

1. 发疹性复发性色素性沉着性毛细血管扩张症
Eruptive recurrent pigmented telangiectasia

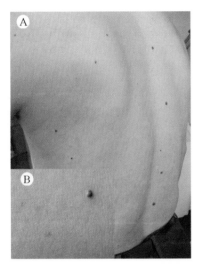

图 20-1-1　躯干部散在性分布红色、半球形丘疹,近距离可见在红色丘疹周围夹有大小类似的色素沉着斑(左下角图)

Figure 20-1-1　Bright red, dome-shaped papules measuring 1-4 mm on the trunk. Similar sized oval or guttate pigmented macules distributed around the red papules(left low)

2. 持久性发疹性斑状毛细血管扩张症
Telangiectasia macularis eruptive perstans

图 20-2-1　腹部及双下肢近端可见密集红斑及 0.3～0.5 cm 大小红色丘疹

Figure 20-2-1　Numerous red-tan macules and papules 0.3～0.5cm in diameter are scattered on the abdomen and lower limbs

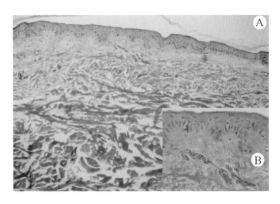

图 20-1-2　真皮乳头层及浅层毛细血管高度扩张,血管内皮细胞正常,血管周围淋巴细胞浸润不明显(A,HE stain,×100),扩张的血管腔隙内充满红细胞,基底层色素轻度增加(B,HE 染色,×400)

Figure 20-1-2　Superficial plexus are prominently dilated. There is no vessel proliferation, and perivascular lymphocytic infiltration is unremarkable (A, HE stain, ×100). Dilated superficial blood vessels laden with red blood cells. The basement layer is slightly hyperpigmented (B,HE stain,×400)

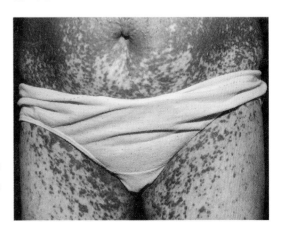

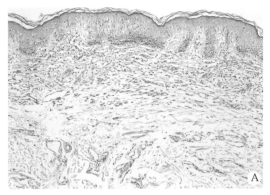

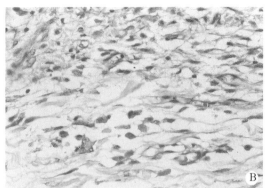

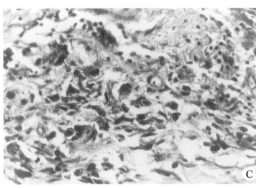

图 20-2-2　A. 表皮角化过度,基底层色素增加,真皮内多数肥大细胞浸润(HE 染色,×100); B. 真皮内多数肥大细胞浸润(HE 染色,×400); C. 肥大细胞内明显异染颗粒(Giemsa 染色,×400)

Figure 20-2-2　A. Hyperkeratosis and hyperpigmentation of the epidermal basal layer, an increased number of mast cells in the papillary dermis (HE stain, ×100); B. Numerous mast cells infiltrate in the dermis (HE stain, ×400); C. The metachromatic granules are found in mast cells (Giemsa stain, ×400)

3. 单侧性皮肤浅表毛细血管扩张症
Unilateral dermatomal telangiectasia

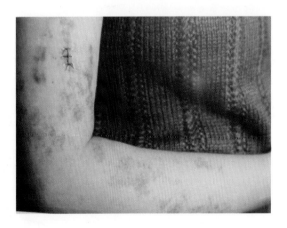

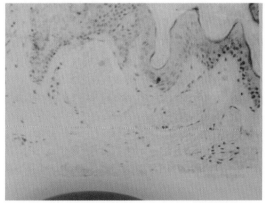

图 20-3-1　右前臂和上臂有带状分布的暗红斑和斑片近 25 片

Figure 20-3-1　About 25 erythematous macules in the band-like distribution on her right foream and arm

图 20-3-2　真皮浅层有很多高度扩张的毛细血管

Figure 20-3-2　Many marked dilated capilaries in the upper dermis

4. 单侧痣样毛细血管扩张症和 Bier 斑
Unilateral nevoid telangiectasia superimposed on the Bier spots

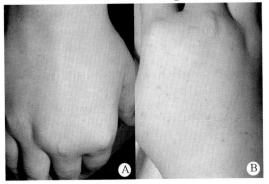

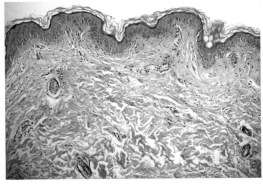

图 20-4-1　右上肢多发性针尖大小卷曲或蜘蛛样毛细血管扩张,周围有苍白圈

Figure 20-4-1　Multiple pin-sized wiry and spider-like telangiectases with peripheral pale macule unilaterally distributed on her right hand

图 20-4-2　皮肤病理示表皮正常。真皮乳头毛细血管扩张,周围有少量单一核细胞浸润,无血管增生(HE 染色,×100)

Figure 20-4-2　Skin biopsy revealed vascular dilation with mild perivascular infiltration of mononuclear cells in the papillary dermis. (HE stain,×100)

5. 胸腹壁血栓性静脉炎
Mondor's disease (Superficial thrombophlebitis of the chest)

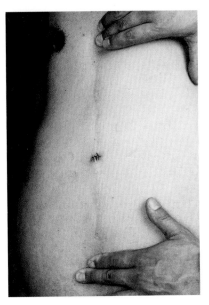

图 20-5-1　左侧胸腹壁有条状微凹陷,牵拉皮损走行区皮肤,凹陷更明显

Figure 20-5-1　Strip hollow on the left breast

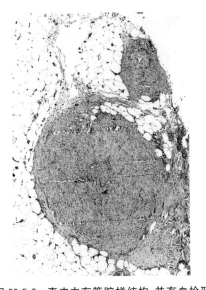

图 20-5-2　真皮内有管腔样结构,并有血栓形成,静脉壁增厚和纤维化(HE 染色,×100)

Figure 20-5-2　Tube structures with thrombosis in the dermis,and vein wall increment and fibrosis (HE stain,×100)

6. 闭塞性动脉硬化症
Arteriosclerosis obliterans

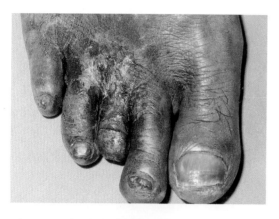

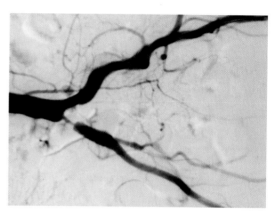

图 20-6-1　右足趾呈青紫色,其中第 3 趾已坏死、缩短

Figure 20-6-1　The toe of right foot being purple, the third toe is necrosis and shorten

图 20-6-2　双下肢动脉造影示右髂总动脉在腹主动脉分支处明显狭窄

Figure 20-6-2　The narrow of hypogastric arteria from arteria femoralis

7. 发疹性假性血管瘤病
Eruptive pseudoangiomatosis

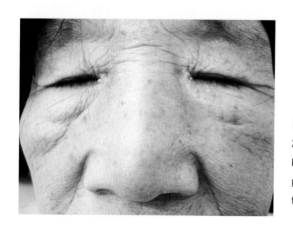

图 20-7-1　颜面见散在性血管瘤样丘疹,表面光滑,2～5mm 大小。皮疹分布区域无鳞屑、结痂和溃疡

Figure 20-7-1　Disseminated, smooth and angioma-like papules with diameters up to 2-5 mm mainly located on the face

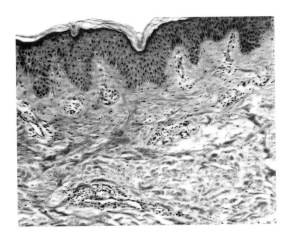

图 20-7-2　表皮正常。真皮血管无增生,毛细血管扩张、充血。真皮浅、中层血管周围主要以淋巴细胞及少量嗜酸性粒细胞浸润(HE 染色,×100)

Figure 20-7-2　The epidermis was normal. The blood vessels in the superficial dermis were dilated and surrounded mainly by a lymphocytes infiltration. (HE stain,×100)

第 21 章
皮下脂肪组织疾病
Subcutaneous Adipose Tissue Diseases

1. 组织细胞吞噬性脂膜炎
Cytophagic histiocytic panniculitis

图 21-1-1 双小腿胫前数个大小不等的红色斑块及瘀斑

Figure 21-1-1 Several violaceous plaques and petechia on the both pretibial

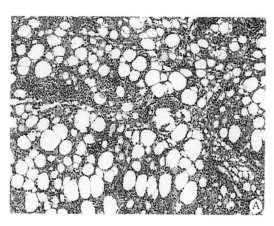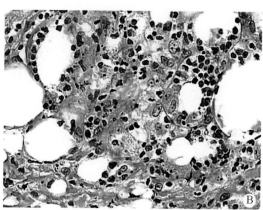

图 21-1-2 A. 皮下脂及小叶部分坏死,伴密集的淋巴细胞及组织细胞浸润(GE 染色,×40);B. 可见组织细胞吞噬白细胞及核碎块,形成"豆袋细胞"(HE 染色,×200)

Figure 21-1-2 A. Subcutaneous part fat lobes necrosis and a massive infiltration of lymphocytes and histiocytes phagocytosing nuclear debris in the subcutaneous (GE stain, ×40); B. Histiocytes phagocytosing leukocyte and nuclear debris, forming "bean bag cells" (HE stain, ×200)

144

2. 硬化性脂膜炎
Sclerosing Panniculitis

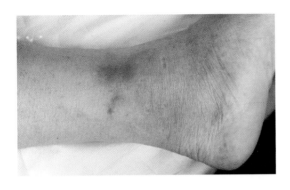

图 21-2-1　右小腿外踝上出现一持续性暗红色质硬结节,局部有色素沉着,边界清

Figure 21-2-1　A Well-circumscribed, indurated, erythematous plaque and hyperpigmentation on the lateral malleous of right leg

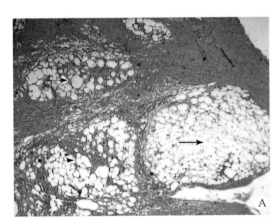

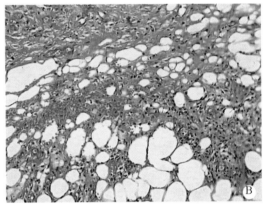

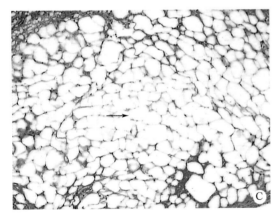

图 21-2-2　A. 小叶中央缺血性坏死,大小不等脂囊肿的形成,间隔纤维化(HE 染色,×40);B. 脂肪小叶中央缺血性坏死,呈苍白色,少见炎症细胞浸润(HE 染色,×100);C. 脂肪小叶内膜样脂肪坏死,坏死组织呈羽毛样外观(HE 染色,×400)

Figure 21-2-2　A. Centrilobular ischemic necrosis (arrows), fat microcysts (arrowheads) and septal fibrosis (HE stain, ×40); B. Pale Centrilobular ischemic necrosis with inflammatory infiltration (arrows) (HE stain, ×100); C. Centrilobular membranous fat necrosis (arrows) and feather-like appearance of necrotic tissue (HE stain, ×400)

3. 嗜酸细胞性脂膜炎
Eosinophilic panniculitis

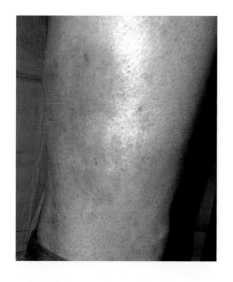

图 21-3-1　右大腿有红色硬化的斑

Figure 21-3-1　A red indurate patch on the right leg

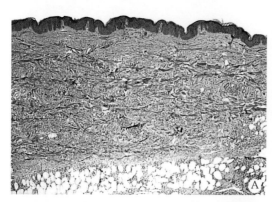

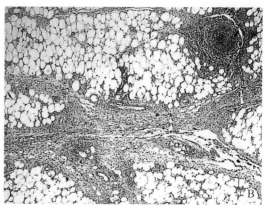

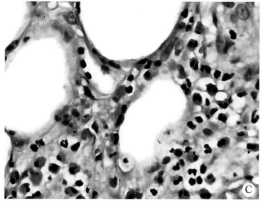

图 21-3-2　A. 表皮和真皮基本正常（HE 染色，×20）；
B、C. 脂肪小叶和间隔内丰富的嗜酸性细胞和单一核
细胞浸润（HE 染色，×20；×400）

Figure 21-3-2　A. The epidermis and dermis are normal
（HE stain, ×20）；B, C. Eosinophils and mononuclear
cells are very abundant in both septa and lobules（HE
stain, B, ×20；C, ×400）

4. 全身性脂肪萎缩
Total lipoatrophy

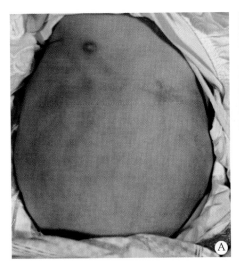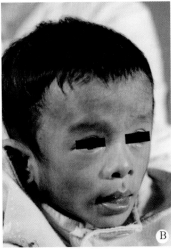

图 21-4-1　A. 腹部大片皮肤萎缩下陷,静脉清晰可见; B. 面部皮下脂肪大面积萎缩,前额有 4 个黄色瘤损害

Figure 21-4-1　A. A large depressed area on the abdomen associated clear veins；B. The loss of large areas of subcutaneous fat on the face, four lesions of xanthoma on the forehead

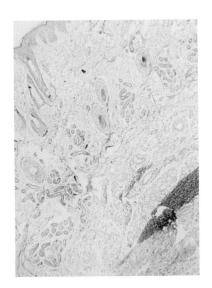

图 21-4-2　整个皮下脂肪的萎缩使真皮紧贴筋膜(HE 染色,×40)

Figure 21-4-2　Total loss of the subcutaneous fat producing dermis adjacent to fascia(HE stain,×40)

5. 幼儿腹部离心性脂肪营养不良
Lipodystrophia centrifugalis abdominalis infantilis

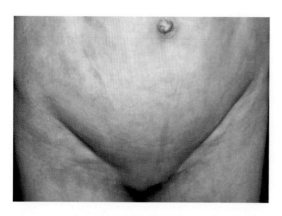

图 21-5-1 下腹部、腹股沟及外阴皮肤见大片凹陷性斑片,呈其浅褐色,边缘有轻度红斑,皮下静脉显露

Figure 21-5-1 Large depressed spadiceous patches with reddish edge on the lower abdomen, bilateral groin, from which could see subcutaneous veins

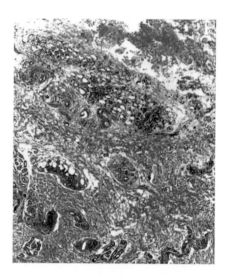

图 21-5-2 真皮下部及皮下脂肪周围可见中等量淋巴细胞浸润,皮下脂肪浸润细胞中可见较多浆细胞(HE 染色,×40)

Figure 21-5-2 Histopatholytic changes showed that a decrease or absence of subcutaneous fat and mild inflammatory infiltrate of lymphocytes and histiocytes in the lower dermis and subcutis. (HE stain, ×40)

第 22 章
非感染性肉芽肿
Noinfectious Granuloma

1. 环状肉芽肿
Granuloma annulare

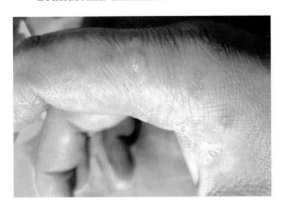

图 22-1-1　右手示指见淡红色丘疹,顶部稍扁平且光滑

Figure 22-1-1　A small papule presented on the lateral surface of index finger,with a flatt and smooth top

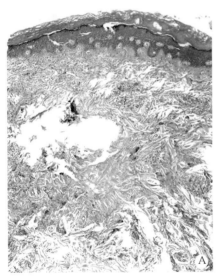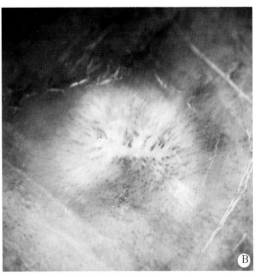

图 22-1-2　A. 病理真皮浅层及中层中央纤维素样坏死,边沿淋巴细胞呈栅栏样排列,偶见巨噬细胞(HE 染色,×40); B. 皮肤镜下,见白色条纹,如横出平行叶脉

Figure 22-1-2　A. Skin biopsy showed areas of fibronoid necrosis were surrounded by histiocytes and lymphocytes which showed palisading arrangement in the superficial and mid dermis(HE stain, ×40); B. Dermatoscopically,there were numerous,parrallel crystal-white striae interspersed with fine red dots at their roots,which were characterized by the pattern of transverse parallel venation

2. 儿童播散型环状肉芽肿

Generalized granuloma annularein in a boy

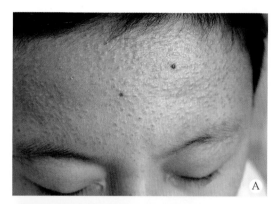
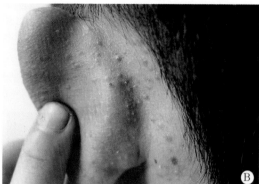

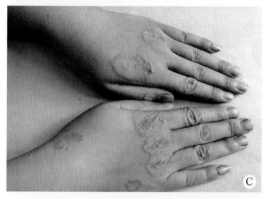

图 22-2-1 　A. 前额黄白色和淡红色坚实丘疹,表面光滑,密集而不融合;B. 耳后淡红色坚实丘疹;C. 双手背淡紫色环状斑疹,边缘隆起

Figure 22-2-1 　A. White yellow or pale red firm papules with smooth surface on the forehead; B. Pale red firm papules on the back of ear; C. Pale purple circinate macula on the dorsal of both hands with elevated edge

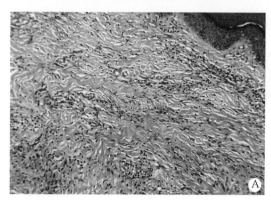
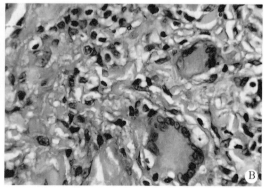

图 22-2-2 　A. 表皮角化过度,真皮浅层胶原纤维变性,周围上皮样细胞排列成栅栏状(HE 染色,×100);B. 真皮内可见多核巨细胞(HE 染色,×100)

Figure 22-2-2 　A. Hyperkeratosis, degeneration of collagen in the upper dermis, epithelioid cells in a palisading arrangement (HE stain, ×100); B. Multinuclear giant cells in the dermis (HE stain, ×100)

3. 穿通性环状肉芽肿
Perforating granuloma annulare

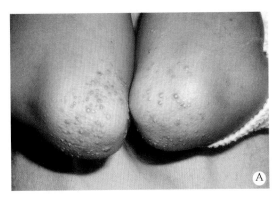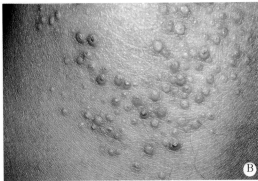

图 22-3-1　A. 双肘部有群集肤色和淡红色丘疹；B. 多数丘疹中心有角质栓

Figure 22-3-1　A. The flesh-colored or red-pale papules are grouped on the both elbows；B. Most of papules have a keratic plug at center

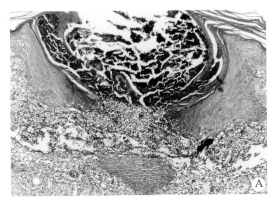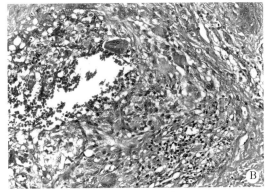

图 22-3-2　A. 表皮内有一个窄管道穿过,内含坏死组织和变性的胶原纤维(HE 染色,×100)；B. 在真皮上层坏死区周围有栅栏状分布组织细胞(HE 染色,×200)

Figure 22-3-2　A. A narrow channel contained necrotic tissues and degenerated collogen fibers throw the epidermis(HE stain,×100)；B. A palisade of histiocytes around the necrobiosis area in the upper dermis(HE stain,×200)

4. 播散性环状肉芽肿合并乙型肝炎病毒感染

Generalized granuloma annulare associated with the infection of chronic hepatitis B virus

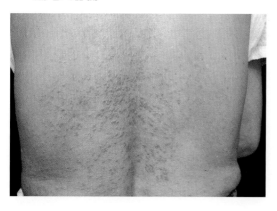

图 22-4-1　背部群集绿豆大坚实丘疹,正常皮色,表面光滑,皮损互不融合,中心未见明显凹陷

Figure 22-4-1　The skin-color firm papules with smooth surface grouped on the back

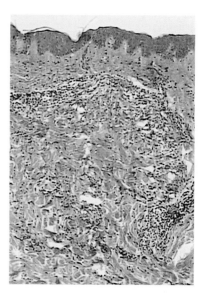

图 22-4-2　表皮大致正常,真皮浅中层变性的胶原束间较多的上皮样细胞和淋巴细胞成栅栏状排列(HE 染色,×200)

Figure 22-4-2　Considerable epithelioid cells and lymphocytes in a palisading arrangement between degeneration of collagen bundles in the middle of dermis (HE stain,×200)

5. 多形性肉芽肿

Granuloma multiforme

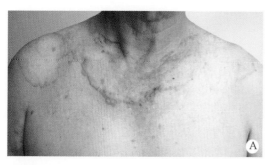
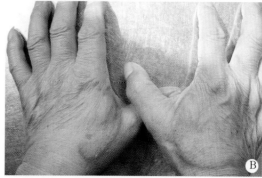

图 22-5-1　A. 颈部、胸部上 1/4 处可见丘疹融合成环形或地图状,皮损表面光滑无鳞屑,未见溃疡或瘢痕,皮损中央为正常皮肤、无色素改变;B. 双手背各见 1 个半弧形坚实、边沿隆起的皮损

Figure 22-5-1　A. Papules on the neck and upper quarter of the trunk coalesce to be reticular or irregular shape with a smooth surface. There were no ulcerations, scars or abno rmal pigmentary changes; B. On the dorsal hands, there were lesions with an elevated serpiginous border

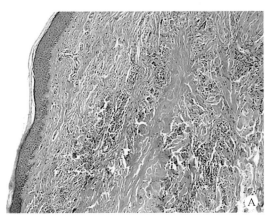
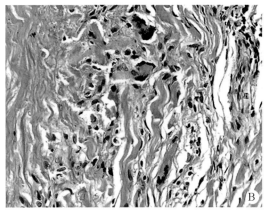

图 22-5-2　A. 真皮浅、中层见局灶性渐进性坏死及明显栅栏状肉芽肿(HE 染色,×40); B. 典型的栅栏状肉芽肿,可见较多多核巨细胞,星状小体偶见(HE 染色,×200)

Figure 22-5-2　A. Areas of necrobiosis surrounded by palisaded rim of histiocytes in the mid and upper dermis (HE stain,×40); B. Palisading granuloma were shown typically with multinucleated giant cells and occasional asteroid bodies(HE stain,×200)

6. 环状弹力纤维溶解性巨细胞肉芽肿
Annular elastolytic giant cell granuloma

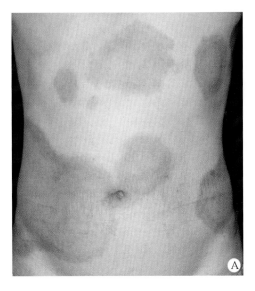
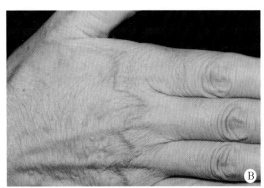

图 22-6-1　手背(A)及躯干(B)多发环形,边界清楚的红斑,边缘隆起,中心红斑消退,萎缩

Figure 22-6-1　Multiple annular,demarcated erythemas with elevated borders and a less erythematous, atrophic center on the trunk(A) and the dorsal of hands(B)

153

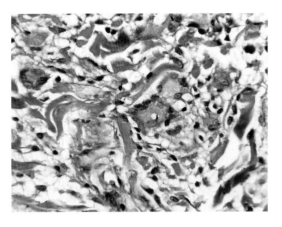

图 22-6-2　真皮内巨噬细胞和多核巨细胞浸润,损害中心无渐进性坏死(HE 染色,×100)
Figure 22-6-2　Dermal infiltrate of macrophages and multinucleated giant cells, and absence of necrobiosis in the center of the lesion (HE stain, ×100)

7. 皮肤硅石肉芽肿
Cutaneous silica granuloma

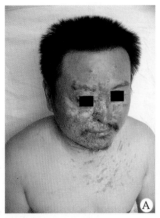
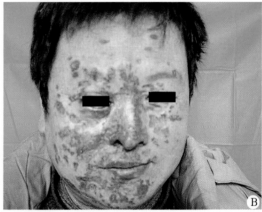

图 22-7-1　面、颈部满布大小不等的红色斑块、结节,部分破溃,覆白色鳞屑,中间呈环状、下陷,轻度萎缩(A. 治疗前;B. 治疗后)
Figure 22-7-1　Erythematous, nodues on his face, around the lips, left eye, submaxillary mentoniane furrow, chin and prothorax(A. before treatment; B. after treatmen)

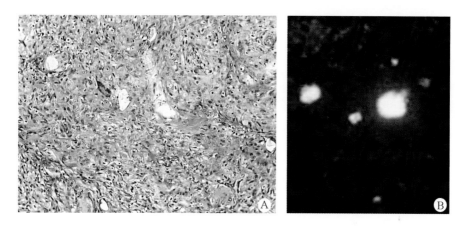

图 22-7-2　A. 真皮乳头层和网状层境界清楚的无干酪样坏死肉芽肿,由组织细胞、巨细胞及少量淋巴细胞组成;肉芽肿内可见明亮的折光结构(HE 染色,×200);B. 偏振光显微镜下可见灰白色晶体颗粒(×200)

Figure 22-7-2　A. Circumscribed granulomas of epithelioid cells tubercles showing no necrosis in dermis, giant cell with a foreign body in the cytoplasm (HE stain, ×200); B. Birefringent foreign body under polarized light in the cytoplasm of a giant cell. (×200)

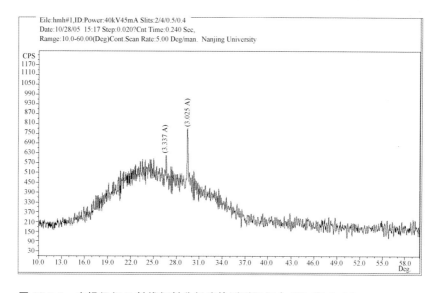

图 22-7-3　皮损组织 X 射线衍射分析法检测到组织中 SiO$_2$ 和 CaCO$_3$

Figure 22-7-3　X-ray spectrum of one of the crystalline structures shoused major constituents of silica, oxygen, and aluminum

8. 反应性结节性增生
Reactive nodular hyperplasia

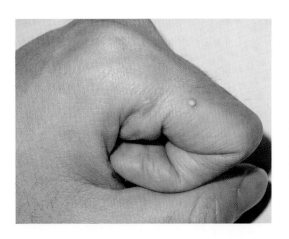

图 22-8-1　左手示指伸侧近端可见一绿豆大小的结节，正常肤色，表面角化明显，基底略窄

Figure 22-8-1　A solitary green bean sized hyperkeratotic nodule with narrow base on the extensor of left index finger

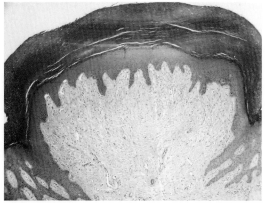

图 22-8-2　表皮角化过度，表皮增生形成衣领样外观，真皮成纤维细胞以及胶原纤维增生(HE 染色，×40)

Figure 22-8-2　Epidermal hyperkeratosis and the collar-like hyperplasia; Dermal fibroblast and collagen fiber hyperplasia were present. (HE stain,×40)

第 23 章
皮肤附属器疾病
Diseases of the Skin Appendages

1. 鼻红粒病
Granulosis rubra nasi

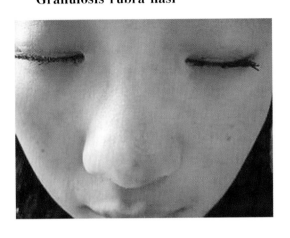

图 23-1-1　鼻尖部,双颊淡红斑,鼻尖表面可见串珠样汗滴

Figure 23-1-1　Erythema on the nose and cheeks. Beads of sweat on the nasal tip

2. Fox-Fordyce 病
Fox-Fordyce disease

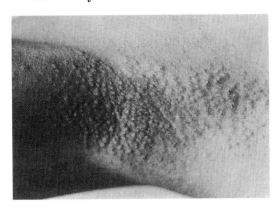

图 23-2-1　腋窝密集圆形粟粒大光滑毛囊性坚实丘疹,肤色或灰褐色,不融合

Figure 23-2-1　Dense, round, smooth, millet-sized, firm, follicular, skin-colored or dust color papules on the axillae

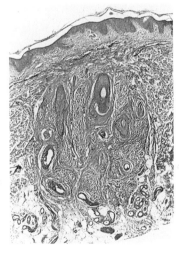

图 23-2-2　真皮内大汗腺导管扩张,慢性炎性细胞浸润(HE 染色,×20)

Figure 23-2-2　Dilated apocrine duct and chronic inflammatory infiltrate in the dermis(HE stain,×20)

3. 蛇形斑秃
Alopecia areata called ophiasis

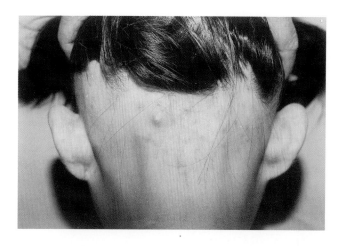

图 23-3-1　沿枕下、双耳后发际线见弯曲呈蛇形非瘢痕性脱发,宽 2～3cm

Figure 23-3-1　A bilateral serpentine extension of alopecia from the occiput to the temple regions in size from 2 to 3 cm in width

4. 全秃再生发呈马蹄形、蛇形嵌合型分布
Mosaic hair regrowth pattern of ophiasis and sisaipho in a patient with alopecia totalis

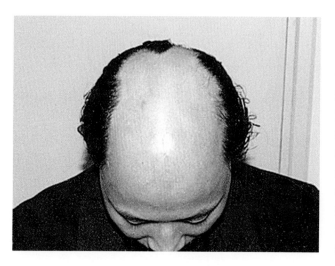

图 23-4-1　前额直到枕部头发成片缺失,距离发际线 3～5cm,酷似雄激素性脱发(Hamilton 分级 Ⅵ 级),右颞部有 3 cm 宽的脱发区

Figure 23-4-1　A circumscribed U-shaped display of hair loss over the center of the scalp, with persistence of hair only at the hair margin, mimicking grade Ⅵ male-pattern baldness in the Hamilton's scale, another affected hair margin of the right temple, with a area ranging 3 cm in diameter

5. Brocq 假性斑秃
Brocq pseudopelade

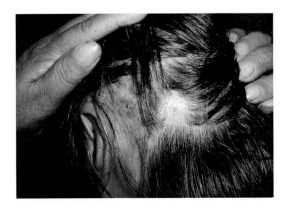

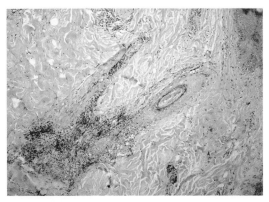

图 23-5-1　头皮有淡红色斑片,中央萎缩凹陷,上覆褐色结痂

Figure 23-5-1　Pale red macules with central atrophy and brown crusts on the scalp

图 23-5-2　真皮内多处毛囊受累,完整结构破坏,仅存少量残余毛囊(HE 染色,×100)

Figure 23-5-2　Numerous hair folliculars are destroyed in the dermis (HE stain,×100)

6. 蛇形脱发和 W 形脱发嵌合分布
Mosaic distribution of ophiasis and W-shaped alopecia areata

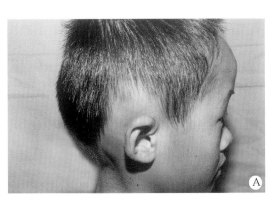

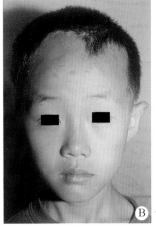

图 23-6-1　A. 耳上至枕部发际带状脱发,表面光滑,无红斑、鳞屑;B. 前额发际呈 W 形脱发

Figure 23-6-1　A. An ophiasis type of alopecia areata at the hair margin of both temples; B. W-shape pattern alopecia at frontal implantation line

7. 未累及皮损内白发的斑秃
Alopecia areata sparing white hairs within lesion

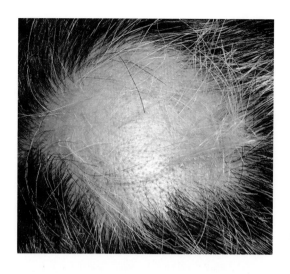

图 23-7-1　头顶可见直径约 5 cm 圆形脱发区,其中散在白发,其发干直径和长度与其他尚未脱落的黑发相同

Figure 23-7-1　A round, well-defined alopecic patch presented on the vertex of the scalp with a diameter of about 5 cm. Some graying hairs were randomly distributed among the balding patch, which showed similar diameters and lengths with neighboring unshedding pigmented hairs

8. 浸润性导管癌患者出现多毛和斑秃
Coexistence of acquired hypertrichosis and scalp alopecia in a patient with infiltrating ductal carcinoma

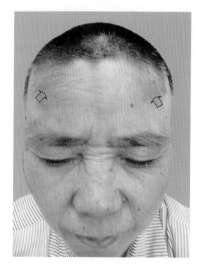

图 23-8-1　面部多毛,眉毛浓密,睫毛增长

Figure 23-8-1　Facial hypertrichosis, bushy eyebrows and trichomegaly

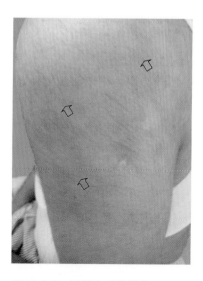

图 23-8-2　手臂上毛发增多

Figure 23-8-2　Hypertrichosis over the arms

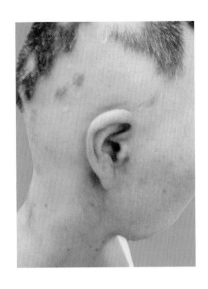

图 23-8-3　头皮局限性脱发,头皮光滑无炎症,毛囊口完整

Figure 23-8-3　Scalp alopecia with smooth noninflamed scalp and intact follicular openings

9. 羊毛状发
Woolly hair

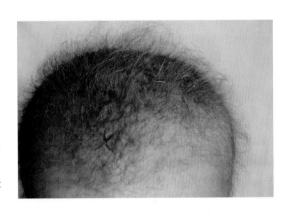

图 23-9-1　毛发稀疏,呈螺旋状卷曲,淡灰黄色,无光泽

Figure 23-9-1　Curled, light grey sparse hair without sheen

10. 念珠形发
Monilethrix

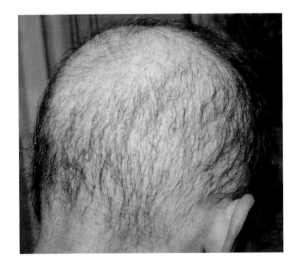

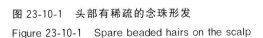

图 23-10-1　头部有稀疏的念珠形发

Figure 23-10-1　Spare beaded hairs on the scalp

11. 环状发
Pili annulati

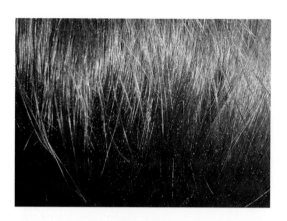

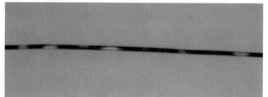

图 23-11-1　毛发正常颜色与白色交替,使毛发呈环纹状

Figure 23-11-1　Alternating segments of light and dark color annulated hairs

图 23-11-2　光镜下见毛干黑白带交替(×40)

Figure 23-11-2　Light microscopy revealed alternating light and dark bands at various lengths along the hair shaft(×40)

12. 结毛症
Trichonodosis(Knotted hair)

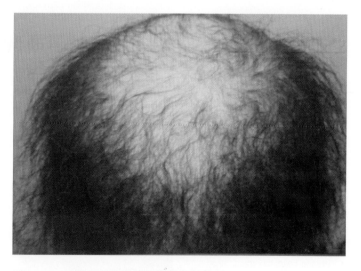

图 23-12-1　额上和头顶弥漫性脱发伴多汗

Figure 23-12-1　Diffuse alopecia of the frontal region and on the vertex with hyperhydrosis

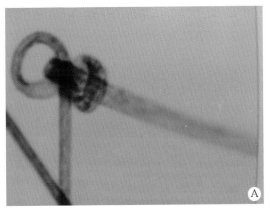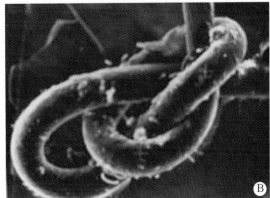

图 23-12-2　有 2 个毛干结节

Figure 23-12-2　Double knot in hair shaft

13. 管状发鞘

Hair cast

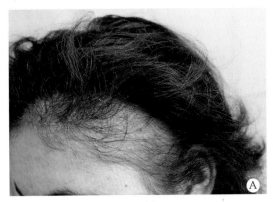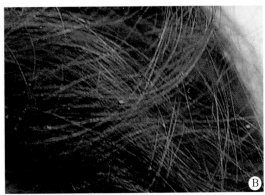

图 23-13-1　前额和颞部发稀疏(A),毛干上有白色结节(B)

Figure 23-13-1　Alopecia located in frontal and temporal areas of the scalp(A),white nodules on hair shafts (B)

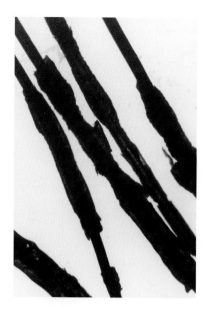

图 23-13-2　镜下管状发鞘（×100）

Figure 23-13-2　Close view of hair cast under microscope（×100）

14. 小棘毛壅症
Trichostasis spinulosa

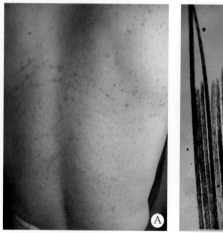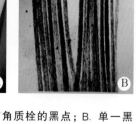

图 23-14-1　A. 背部有许多嵌有角质栓的黑点；B. 单一黑点中含有 16 根毳毛

Figure 23-14-1　A. Many black heads filled with horny plugs occur on the trunk；B. Bundle of sixteen vellus hairs within a single blackhead

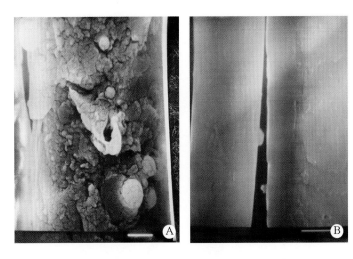

图 23-14-2 霾毛表面毛小皮消失或堆积许多角朊细胞碎片

Figure 23-14-2 Hair cuticle disappeared or many fragments of keratinocytes on the surface of lanugo

15. 皮肤匐行毛发

Cutaneous pili migrans

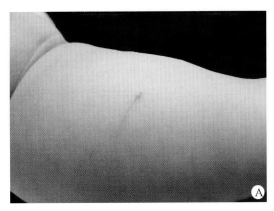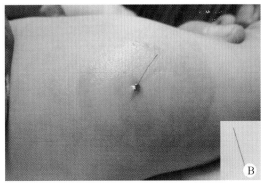

图 23-15-1 A. 左下肢后侧可见表皮下黑线,四周无炎症;B. 从表皮中拔出黑发,微量出血,拔出的毛发,长约 2.5cm

Figure 23-15-1 A. Fine, very superficial, black line was clearly visible through the skin surface, without any sign of inflammation on the surrounding skin; B. A dark hair was extracted from its epidermal bed with little bleeding. The insert was showing the extracted hair, measuring 2.5 cm in length

16. 黄发
Yellow hair

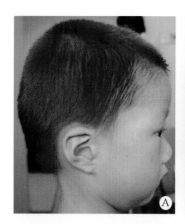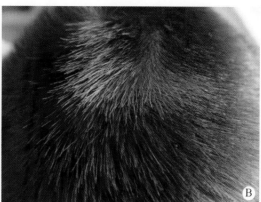

图 23-16-1　A. 头部全部黄发；B. 头顶有局灶黄发

Figure 23-16-1　A. Total yellow hair of the scalp；B. Local yellow hairs on the top of scalp

17. 拔须后永久性白须
Permanent poliosis after plucking

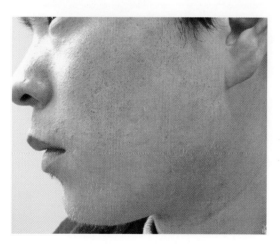

图 23-17-1　长期拔须后下颌部永久性白须，而其最外围黑须无变化，口周胡须正常着色，下颌部肤色也正常

Figure 23-17-1　Permanent poliosis affecting the submaxilla area after repetitive plucking, The pigment of several peripheral rows of beard hairs was unchanged, Perioral beard hairs were untouched, The color of the submaxilla skin was normal

18. 先天性厚甲症
Pachyonychia congenita

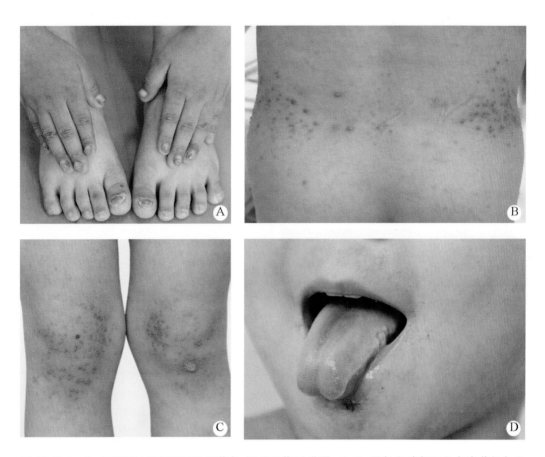

图 23-18-1　A. 手指和足趾指(趾)甲呈黄色,远端呈楔形增厚;B、C. 腰部和膝部可见多发黄褐色丘疹;D. 舌苔增厚呈黄黑色

Figure 23-18-1　A. Thick yellow keratoses are wedge-like thickening of distal finger and toenails;B、C. Many brown papules on the waist and knees;D. The thickening of tongue coating was yellow and black

19. 先天性全白甲
Congenital leukonychia totalis

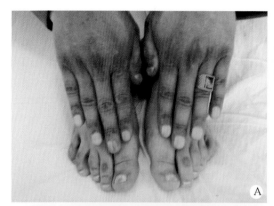
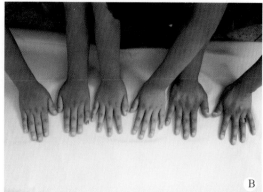
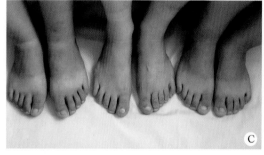

图 23-19-1　A. 20 甲呈奶白色；B、C. 患先天性全白甲的家族成员的手足皮损

Figure 23-19-1　A. Twenty nails with milk-white color in both hands and feet; B, C. Hands and feet of members suffered from congenital leukonychia totalis in his family

20. 铅沉积黑甲
Hyperpigmentation of the nail from lead deposition

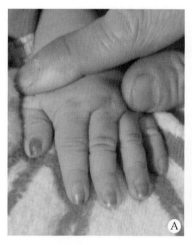
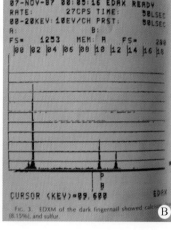

图 23-20-1　A. 左手指甲弥漫性色素沉着；B. X 线微区分析黑甲有钙、铅（8.15%）和硫

Figure 23-20-1　A. The diffuse pigmentation of the fingernails of left hand; B. EDXM of the dark fingernail showed calcium, lead（8.15%）and sulfur

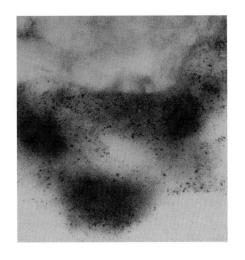

图 23-20-2　角质细胞膜表面有铅电子致密小颗粒
(×14 000)

Figure 23-20-2　Electron dense small geanules distribution along the membrane of keratinocyte(×14 000)

21. 纵行红甲
Longitudinal erythronychia

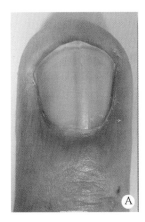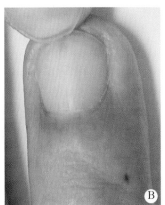

图 23-21-1　A. 外观形态正常,其指甲大致在正中处可见 1.5mm 宽纵行红线,始于甲母质,沿甲纵轴方向向甲游离缘延伸;B. 按压后红线完全消失

Figure 23-21-1　A median longitudinal red band presented in the nail,approximate1.5mm inwidth. It was from nail matrix extending to free margin of nail(A)and it vanished upon a slight pressing(B)

22. 甲变色
Chromonychias

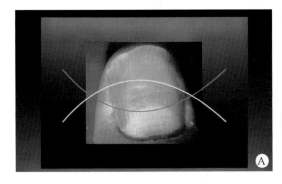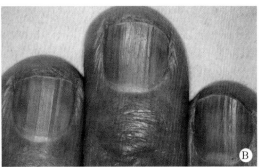

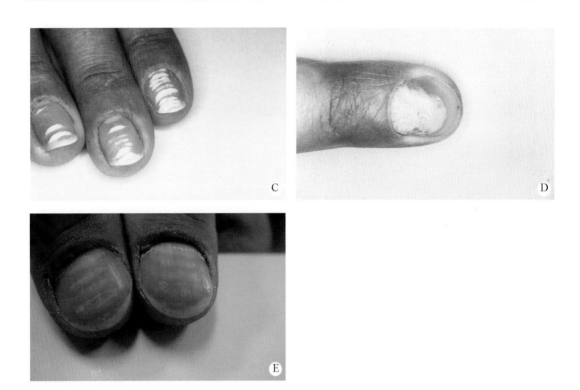

图 23-22-1   A. Zaias 对甲的描述：黄线以下为甲半月区域,红线以上为远端甲皱襞区域；B. 甲银质沉积；C. 点状白甲；D. 假性白甲；E. Mee 线

Figure 23-22-1   A. Zaias statement：the shaps of the lunula（yellow line on the scheme）,the shap of the proximal nail fold （red line on the scheme）；B. Argyria of the nails；C. Leukonychia punctata；D. Pseudoleukonychia；E. Mee's lines

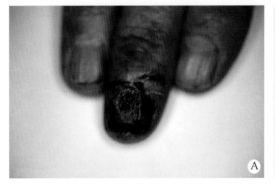

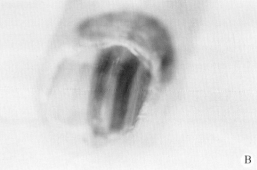

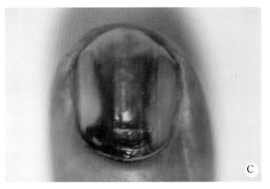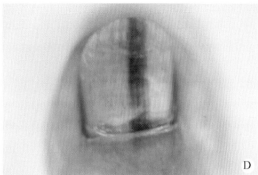

图 23-22-2 A. 恶性黑素瘤引起甲板呈弥漫性黑色；B. 转移性黑素瘤引起的纵形黑甲，Hutchinson's 征阳性；C. 原位黑素瘤引起的纵形黑甲，Hutchinson's 征阴性；D. 先天性黑素细胞痣引起的纵形黑甲

Figure 23-22-2 A. Diffuse black color of the nail plate due to malignant melanoma (MM)；B. Longitudinal melanonychia(LM) due to M. M. Hutchinson's sign positive；C. LM due to MM. Hutchinson's sign negative；D. LM due to congenital melanocytic nevus of the nail

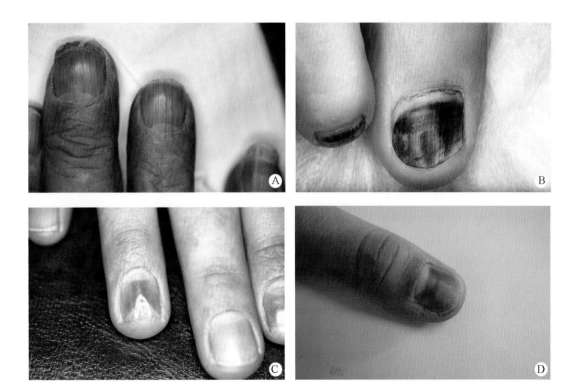

图 23-22-3 A. 蓝甲系缺氧所致的甲蓝色改变；B. 聚维酮碘溶液引起甲板呈弥漫性棕色改变；C. 滥用阿莫罗芬涂膜剂引起甲板呈弥漫性紫褐色改变；D. 绿甲系假单胞菌属感染引起的甲绿色改变

Figure 23-22-3 A. Blue nails due to hypoxia；B.Diffuse brown color of the nail plate due to Betadine solution；C. Diffuse brown-purple color of the nail plate, due to mal-use of Amorolfine lacquer；D. Green nail due to Pseudomonas infection

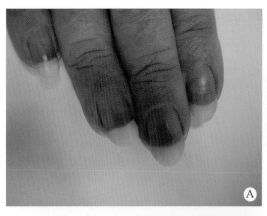
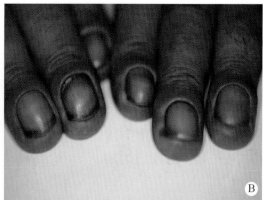
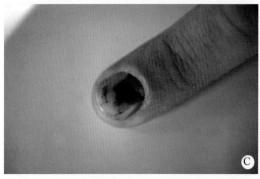

图 23-22-4　A. 橙色甲；B. 黄甲综合征；C. 甲床出血所致黑色甲床

Figure 23-22-4　A. Orange nails；B. Yellow nail syndrome；C. Black nail due to hemorrhage

23. 甲下裂片形出血

Splinter haemorrhages

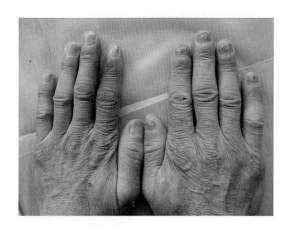

图 23-23-1　右手 5 个指甲远端线状、红褐色裂片形出血，左手指甲正常

Figure 23-23-1　Non-blanchable, reddish-brown, linear haemorrhages involving the distal half of the right five nails, All the left fingernails are normal

24. 颈部皮脂腺增生
Sebaceous hyperplasia of the neck

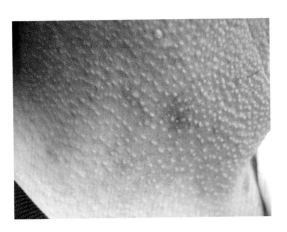

图 23-24-1　颈部有许多直径 2～6mm 黄色小丘疹簇集

Figure 23-24-1　Numerous small yellowish papules 2-6 mm in diameter on the neck

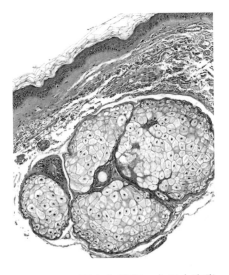

图 23-24-2　真皮上部有一个巨大皮脂腺(HE 染色,×40)

Figure 23-24-2　A large sebaceous gland in the upper dermis(HE stain,×40)

25. 阴囊皮脂腺增生
Sebaceous gland hyperplasia on the scrotum

图 23-25-1　阴囊表面有皮色或淡黄色丘疹

Figure 23-25-1　The fresh-colored or yellowish papules on the scrotum

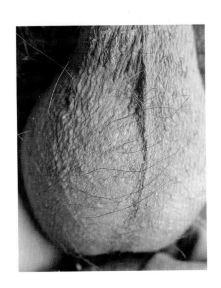

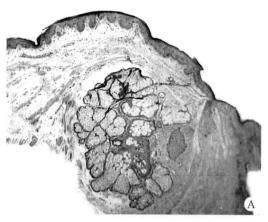
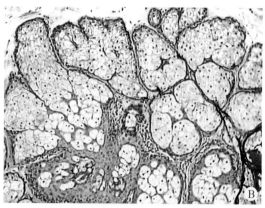

图 23-25-2　真皮内有增生的皮脂腺,分化良好的皮脂腺小叶,中心有扩张的皮脂腺导管(HE 染色,A×40; B×200)

Figure 23-25-2　Marked hyperplasia of sebaceous gland with well differentiated labules and a central dilated sebaceous gland duct in the dermis(HE stain,A×40,B×200)

26. 老年皮脂腺过度增生
Senile sebaceous hyperplasia

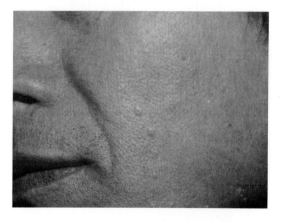
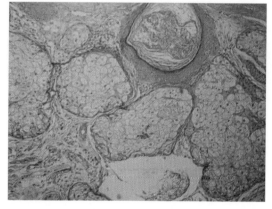

图 23-26-1　左颊有多数黄色小隆起的脐凹状结节
Figure 23-26-1　Several elevated,small,soft,yellow-ish umbilicated nodules on the left cheek

图 23-26-2　真皮有增生的成熟皮脂腺并构成若干小叶
Figure 23-26-2　A geatly enlarged,mature sebaceous gland composed of several lobes in the dermis

27. 烧伤后表皮内皮脂腺增生
Sebaceous hyperplasia within epidermis after scald

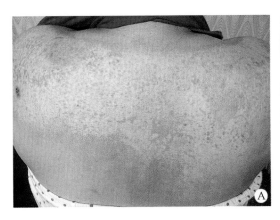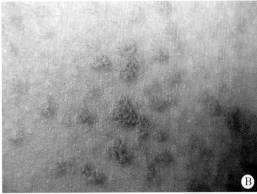

图 23-27-1　A. 上背部大的脱色素斑片内许多直径 2～5mm 红褐色丘疹；B. 背部半圆形丘疹

Figure 23-27-1　A. Many brown papules 2-5 mm in diameter on the large depigmented macula on the upper back；B. Semicircular papules on the back

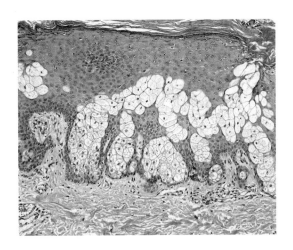

图 23-27-2　表皮中下部许多成熟的皮脂腺，轻度棘层肥厚(HE 染色，×100)

Figure 23-27-2　Many mature sebaceous glands were present in the middle and lower epidermis(HE stain, ×100)

第 24 章
内分泌障碍性皮肤病
Endocrine Skin Diseases

1. 胫前黏液性水肿
Pretibial myxedema

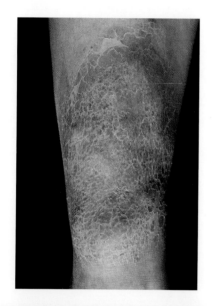

图 24-1-1　胫前大片浸润性棕色斑块,表面角化增厚,毛孔扩大,斑块表面可见直径 3cm 结节

Figure 24-1-1　A large brown infiltrate plaques with hyperkeratosis and a nodular 3 cm in diameter in pretibial region

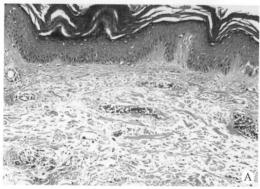
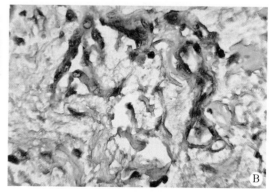

图 24-1-2　A. 表皮角化过度,间有角化不全,颗粒层增厚,真皮胶原纤维间大量黏蛋白沉积(HE 染色,×40); B. 阿申蓝染色阳性(阿辛蓝染色,×100)

Figure 24-1-2　A. Hyperkeratosis and parakeratosis, thickened granular layer, deposition of mucinosis in the dermis between collagen fibrae(HE stain, ×40); B. Positive stain with alcian blue(Alcian blue stain, ×100)

2. 皮肤钙质沉着症
Calcinosis cutis

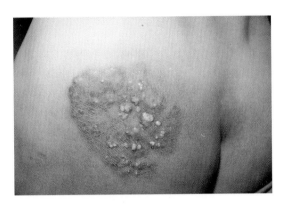

图 24-2-1 左侧臀部外上方 15cm × 15cm 褐色斑块,其上散在绿豆至蚕豆大小黄白色结节,质硬

Figure 24-2-1 A brown plaque 15cm in diameter on the outside of left buttock, associated with white-yellow nodules on it

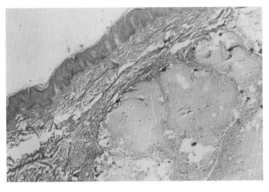

图 24-2-2 表皮轻度萎缩,真皮深层可见均质状、大小不等、团块状钙化物(HE 染色,×40)

Figure 24-2-2 Slight atrophy of the epidermis, variously sized calcific masses in the deep dermis (HE stain, ×40)

3. 阴囊特发性皮肤钙沉着症
Idiopathic calcinosis of the scrotum

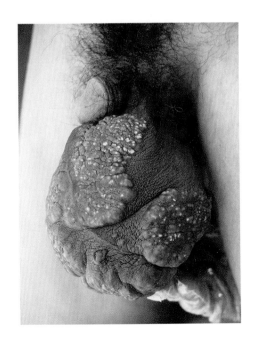

图 24-3-1 阴囊上由多数结节组成的大片斑块损害,斑块境界清楚,边缘隆起

Figure 24-3-1 Numerous firm yellowish subcutaneous nodules beneath the scrotal skin

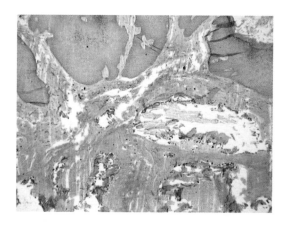

图 24-3-2　表皮呈乳头瘤样增生,真皮层内多处有深蓝色、无定形、团块状物质,胶原广泛增生、纤维化(HE染色,×100)

Figure 24-3-2　Many globular bluish nodules containing an amorphous and homogenous deposits of calcium with epidermal papilomatous hyperplasia in the dermis (HE stain, ×100)

4. 单侧痣样黑棘皮病
Unilateral nevoid acanthosis nigricans

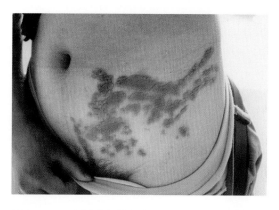

图 24-4-1　左侧腹部黑褐色疣状皮损,呈天鹅绒样外观

Figure 24-4-1　Dark-brown warty lesion, velvet-like appearance on the left abdomen

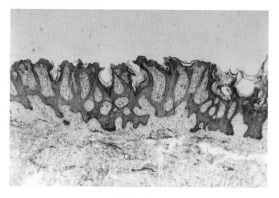

图 24-4-2　表皮角化过度,乳头瘤样增生,乳头间凹陷处棘层肥厚,乳头顶部及两侧表皮变薄(HE染色,×100)

Figure 24-4-2　Hyperkeratosis and papillomatosis, the dermal papillae project upward as fingerlike projections, the valleys between the papillae mild to moderate acanthosis, the thick of stratum malpighii at the tips of the papillae and on the sides of the protruding papillae thinned(HE stain, ×100)

5. 恶性黑棘皮病

Malignant acanthosis nigricans

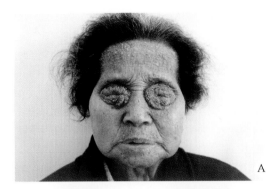

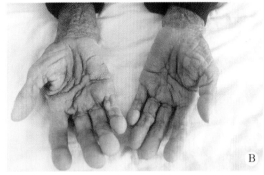

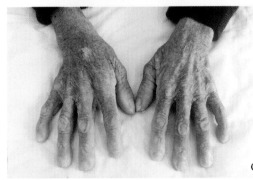

图 24-5-1　A. 面部散在米粒大角化性丘疹，双眼睑结膜增生，呈疣状，睑结膜外翻，眼裂缩小；B、C. 双手皮肤粗糙、增生、肥厚，呈"天鹅绒样"或"牛肚样"，指端呈轻度杵状

Figure 24-5-1　A. Numerous small keratotic papules on the face, warty palpebral conjunctiva, ectropion and eye opening reducing; B, C. Coarse, thickened and hyperplasia skin as velvety on the both hands, with slight digital clubbing

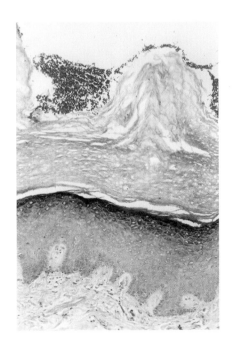

图 24-5-2　表皮角化过度，基底层色素增加，真皮上部血管扩张，少量炎性细胞浸润(HE 染色，×40)

Figure 24-5-2　Hyperkeratosis, basal layer hyperpigmentation, dilated vessels and a few inflammatory infiltrate in the upper dermis (HE stain, ×40)

6. 恶性黑棘皮病合并胃贲门腺癌

Malignant acanthosis nigricans complicated by gastric adenocarcinoma

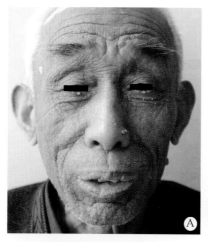
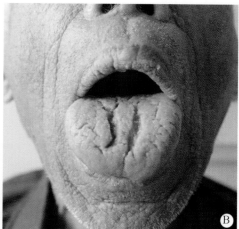
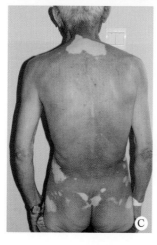
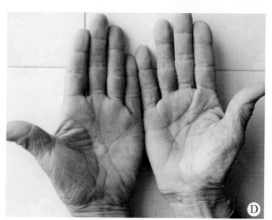

图 24-6-1 A. 面部弥漫性色素沉着和绒毛样增厚；B. 皱襞舌；C. 躯干和头面部许多不规则脱色斑片；D. 掌跖牛胃样皮损

Figure 24-6-1 A. Dirty-looking appearance with diffuse hyperpigmentation and velvety thickening on his face; B. The thickened and furrowed tongue; C. Many irregular depigmented patches on his head and trunk; D. Diffuse velvety thickening and prominent ridges of the palms

7. 高雄激素血症-胰岛素抵抗-黑棘皮病综合征
Hyperandrogenism, insulin resistance and acanthosis nigricans syndrome

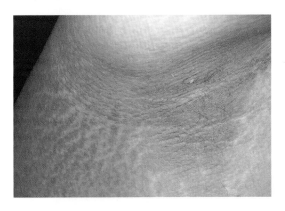

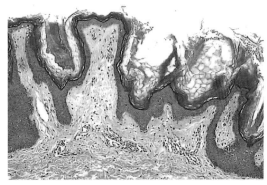

图 24-7-1 腋下皮肤灰棕色或黑色色素沉着,表面干燥、粗糙,如天鹅绒样增厚

Figure 24-7-1 Hyperpigmentation, dryness, coarse, like the papillary hypertrophy on the axillae

图 24-7-2 真皮乳头向上突起呈指状,乳头间凹陷,表皮呈轻度棘层肥厚,并充满角质,乳头顶部及乳头突起侧表皮变薄(HE 染色,×40)

Figure 24-7-2 The dermal papillae project upward as fingerlike projections, the valleys between the papillae mild acanthosis and filled with keratotic material, the stratum malpighii at the tips of the papillae and on the sides of the protruding papillae is thinned (HE stain, ×40)

8. 坏死松解游走性红斑与胰高糖素瘤综合征
Necrolytic migratory erythema (Glucagonoma syndrome)

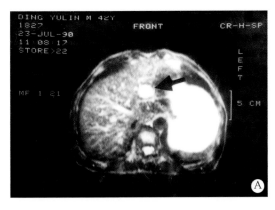

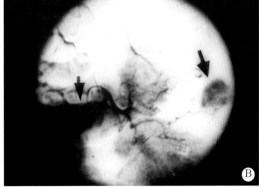

图 24-8-1 A. 胰腺肿瘤(腹部 CT);B. 肝脏肿瘤(腹腔动脉及胰动脉数字减影动脉造影效果)

Figure 24-8-1 A. Tumor in pancreas; B. Tumor in liver

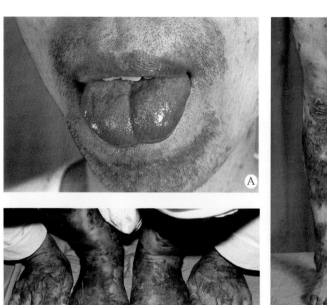
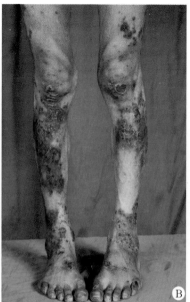

图 24-8-2　A. 口腔黏膜充血,舌呈鲜红色,有浅糜烂及水肿; B. 下肢见对称性红斑、糜烂、渗出及结痂,痂呈薄漆片状,表面有光泽; C. 手足背红斑、粗糙、脱屑、色素沉着,为糙皮病样皮损

Figure 24-8-2　A. Oral mucosa engorgement, vermeil tongue with erosions and edema; B. Symmetric erythema, erosions, effusion and crust with nitid on the lower limbs; C. Erythema, coarseness, desquamation and hyperpigmentation on the dorsa of hands and feet

第 25 章
代谢、营养障碍性皮肤病
Metabolic and Nutritional Skin Diseases

1. 结节性黄瘤病并发主动脉瓣狭窄
Tuberous xanthoma associated with aortic stenosis

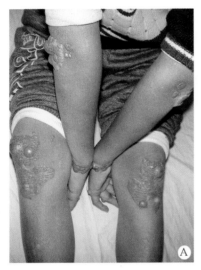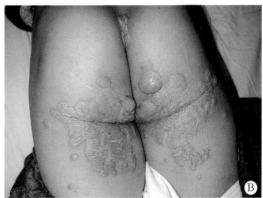

图 25-1-1　指关节、腕关节、肘关节、膝关节伸侧及臀部对称分布黄色或黄红色结节,部分融合成斑块,表面尚光滑

Figure 25-1-1　Symmetric yellow nodules partly confluent on the extension of finger,wrist,elbow,knee joint(A) and stern(B)

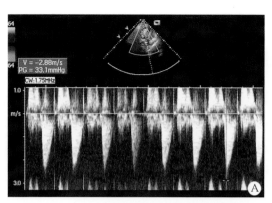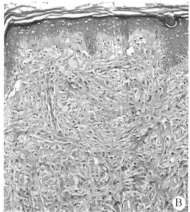

图 25-1-2　A. 通过主动脉瓣的血流速率为 2.88m/s，主动脉瓣跨瓣压差为 4.4kPa（33.1mmHg），提示主动脉瓣狭窄；B. 真皮内见大量泡沫细胞浸润（HE 染色，×200）

Figure 25-1-2　Flow velocity was 2.88m/s through the aortic valve, the pressure gradient of aortic valve was 4.4kPa, in the aortic stenosis by color Doppler ultrasound; B. Considerable foam cells in the dermis (HE stain, ×200)

2. 播散性黄瘤

Xanthoma disseminatum

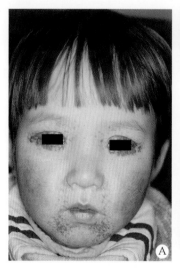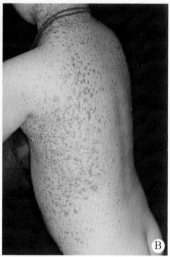

图 25-2-1　A. 面部、颈部可见 1～5mm 大小棕红及浅黄色丘疹；B. 皮损数目多，泛发于面颈、躯干及四肢

Figure 25-2-1　Numerous disseminated orange and yellow brown papules with smooth appearance over the face, neck, trunk and limbs(A,B)

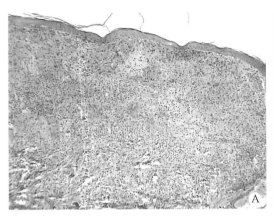

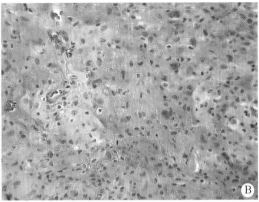

图 25-2-2　A. 表皮大致正常,真皮内可见弥漫性组织细胞浸润,细胞胞质丰富,浅染,部分细胞呈泡沫化
(HE 染色,×40);B. 见少许多核巨细胞,未见典型 Touton 多核巨细胞,局部混有淋巴细胞浸润 (HE 染
色,×100)

Figure 25-2-2　A. Numerous histiocytes and foam cells infiltrate in the dermis(HE stain,×40);B. A few multinucleated giant cells and lymphocytes without Touton giant cell in the dermis (HE stain,×100)

3. 类脂蛋白沉积症
Lipoid proteinosis

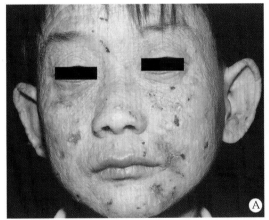

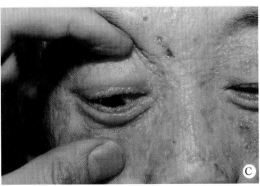

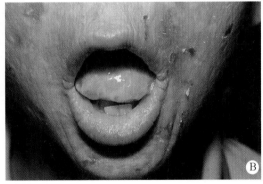

图 25-3-1　A. 面部皮肤弥漫性半透明状蜡样增厚的基础上可见红斑,表皮剥蚀、萎缩和瘢痕;B. 唇、舌黄色浸润,舌大而硬,不能伸出口外;C. 沿上、下睑缘呈串珠状排列着蜡样丘疹

Figure 25-3-1　A. Numerous, skin-colored, waxy papules on the face, with acneiform scarring; B. The yellow white macroglossia with infiltration and hard on palpation, and the patient was unable to protrude it beyond the margins of the lips; C. Papules arranged like beads on a string on the upper and lower eyelid margins

185

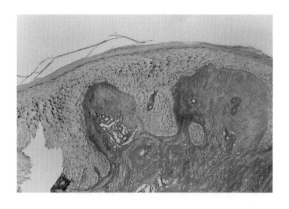

图 25-3-2　真皮乳头层无定形物质 PAS 染色强阳性（×100）

Figure 25-3-2　An amorphous hyaline material in the papillary dermis(×100)

4. 类脂质渐进性坏死
Necrobiosis lipoidica

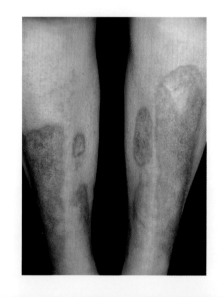

图 25-4-1　双侧胫前大小不等的类圆形暗红色斑块，互不融合，边界清楚，表面光滑呈釉状，中央部分轻微凹陷、萎缩，局部浅静脉曲张和毛细血管扩张

Figure 25-4-1　Various size，oval violaceous plaques with slightly atrophic and telangiectases in the center on the both pretibia

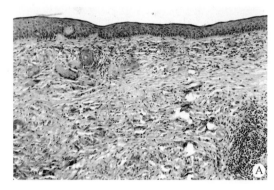

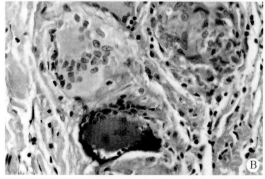

图 25-4-2　表皮萎缩，真皮可见一胶原变性灶，周围有多核巨细胞、上皮样细胞、淋巴细胞和浆细胞浸润，真皮与皮下组织交界处见多个多核巨细胞(HE 染色，A，×100，B，×400)

Figure 25-4-2　The epidermal atrophy，and collagen degeneration，multinucleated giant cells，epithelioid cells，lymphocytes and plasm cells infiltrate in the dermis，multiple multinucleated giant cells locate between the demis and the subcutaneous tissue (HE stain A，×100，B，×400)

5. 幼年性黄色肉芽肿

Juvenile xanthoma（nevo-xanthoendothelioma）

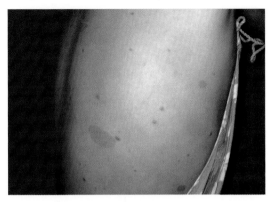

图 25-5-1　散在浅黄色扁平丘疹,并见数处咖啡斑

Figure 25-5-1　Multiple buff flat papules and several café macules

6. 面部苔藓样型幼年黄色肉芽肿

Juvenile xanthogranuloma with lichenoid appearance

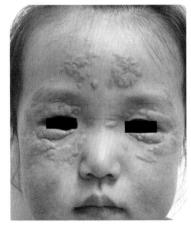

图 25-6-1　面部弥漫性黄褐色斑块,浸润肥厚,间有黄色丘疹

Figure 25-6-1　Diffused red-brown papules with infiltration, as well as some solitary yellow nodules among the papules over her face

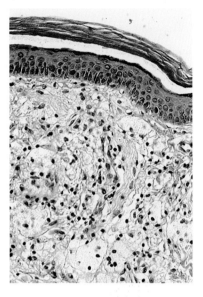

图 25-5-2　真皮浅层及中部大量组织细胞和泡沫细胞浸润,伴有少量淋巴样细胞(HE 染色,×400)

Figure 25-5-2　Numerous histocytes, foam cells and a few lymphoid cells infiltrate in the upper and middle dermis (HE stain, ×400)

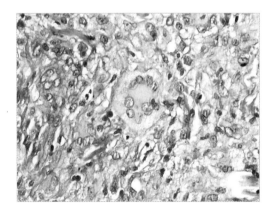

图 25-6-2　典型的 Touton 巨细胞(HE 染色,×400)

Figure 25-6-2　Typical Touton giant cells (HE stain, ×400)

7. 渐进性坏死性黄色肉芽肿
Necrobiotic xanthogranuloma

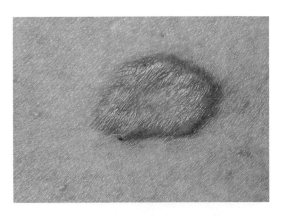

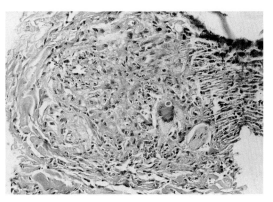

图 25-7-1　圆形斑块呈暗红黄色,中心萎缩,边缘隆起

Figure 25-7-1　Round xanthomatous plaques with central atrophy and elevated edge

图 25-7-2　真皮内渐进性坏死和肉芽肿反应(HE 染色,×200)

Figure 25-7-2　Xanthogranulomatous pictures accompanied with necrobiosis in the dermis(HE stain,× 200)

8. 成人单发黄色肉芽肿
Solitaty adult xanthogranuloma

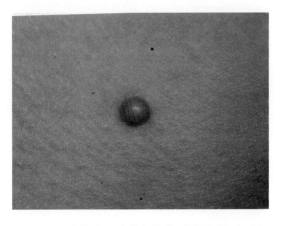

图 25-8-1　颈部有一淡黄色结节,表面光滑,有毛细血管扩张

Figure 25-8-1　A light yellow nodule on the neck

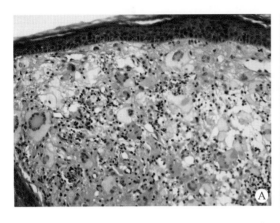

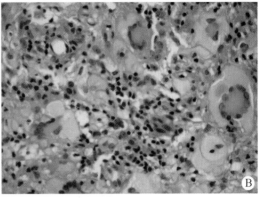

图 25-8-2　A. 表皮萎缩,真皮以泡沫细胞为主的炎症细胞浸润,散在淋巴细胞有 Touton 巨细胞(HE 染色,×100);B. Touton 巨细胞胞核呈花环状排列,胞质呈泡沫状(HE 染色,×150)

Figure 25-8-2　A. Epidermal atrophy and numerous foam cells and lymbhocytes associated with Touton giant cell in the dermis (HE stain,×100);B. The Touton giant cell has nuclei lain in ring surrounded by foamy cytoplasm(HE stain,×150)

9. 先天性红细胞生成性卟啉病
Congenital erythropoietic porphyria

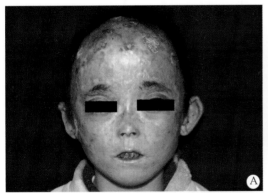

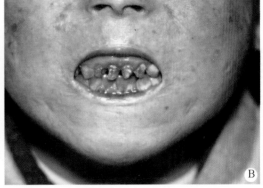

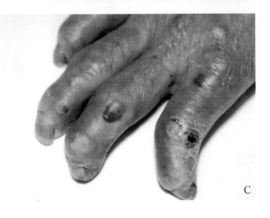

图 25-9-1　A. 面容老态,面部毳毛增多,皮肤色素沉着,散在萎缩性瘢痕,局部有厚痂、血痂;耳郭瘢痕明显,部分残缺,鼻部变小、削尖;B. 口唇变薄,口周有放射状沟纹,自然光下多个门牙、切牙呈棕红色;C. 手指上可见数个黄豆大的血疱,手指变短,指端毁形,多个指间关节僵硬变形

Figure 25-9-1　A、B. Old facial appearance, hypertrichosis, hyperpigmentation, mutilating scar, part loss of auricle, nose diminishing, lip attenuation, actinomorphic lines around mouth, and multiple erythrodontia; C. Deformities of extremity end, several soybean sized blood blister on the fingers

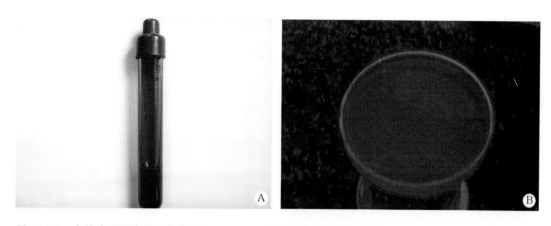

图 25-9-2   自然光下尿液呈红葡萄酒色；B. Wood 灯下尿液呈淡红色荧光

Figure 25-9-2   A. Wine urine in the normal light; B. Urine pink fluorescence when exposed to a Wood's light

10. 皮肤异色病样淀粉样变病

Poikiloderma-like cutaneous amyloidosis

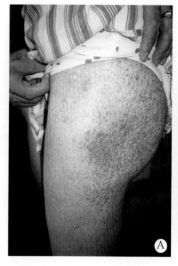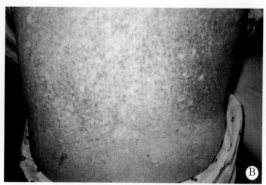

图 25-10-1   A. 左侧背部皮肤呈灰白花斑样改变；B. 并见密集成片米粒大黄褐色扁平丘疹

Figure 25-10-1   A, B. Poikilodermatous skin and lichenoid papules on the left back

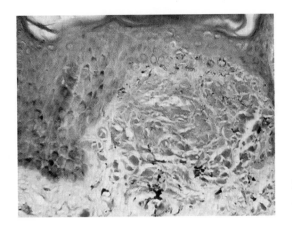

图 25-10-2 真皮乳头内呈现蓝紫色的沉淀物为染色阳性的物质(结晶紫染色,×100)

Figure 25-10-2 Deposits of amyloid in the uppermost dermis (Methyl violet stain,×100)

11. 结节型皮肤淀粉样变性
Nodular amyloidosis

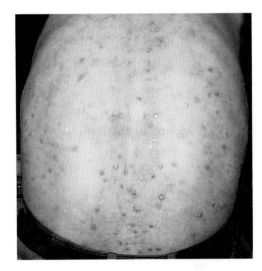

图 25-11-1 背部散在绿豆至黄豆大褐色结节

Figure 25-11-1 Several brown nodules on the back

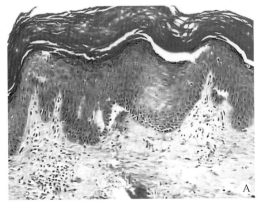
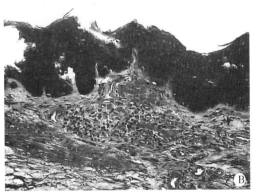

图 25-11-2 A. 角化过度,棘层肥厚,真皮乳头均质红染色淀粉样蛋白沉积(HE 染色,×200);B. 紫红色物质沉积在真皮浅层(结晶紫染色,×200)

Figure 25-11-2 A. There are hyperkeratosis and epidermal hyperplasia. Dermal papillae are rounded eosinophilic amorphous amyloid(HE stain,×200);B. Red masses of amyloid are present in the upper dermis(Violet stain,×200)

12. 黏液水肿性苔藓
Lichen myxedematosus

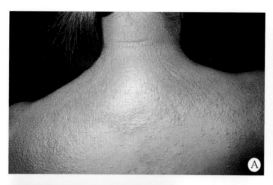

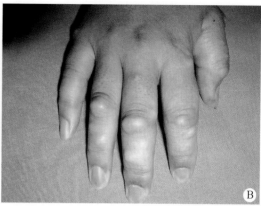

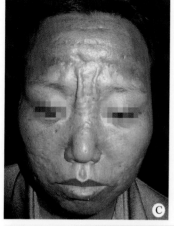

图 25-12-1 A. 淡红色和黄色丘疹分布在项部；B. 肤色结节在指背；C. 浸润斑块在面部

Figure 25-12-1 A. The pale-red or yellowish papules on the nape; B. The flesh-colored nodules on the fingers; C. infiltrate plaques on the face

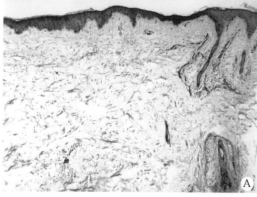

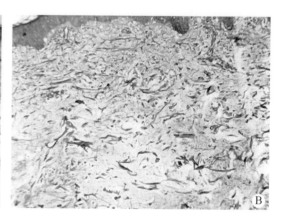

图 25-12-2 A. 真皮内有大小不一不着色的空隙(HE 染色，×40)；B. 在胶原纤维束间有弥漫的黏蛋白沉积(阿新蓝染色，×400)

Figure 25-12-2 A. There are unstained spaces of various sizes in the dermis(HE stain, ×40); B. The diffuse infiltration with mucin among the collagen bundles(Alcin blue stain, ×400)

13. 硬化性黏液水肿性苔藓

Scleromyxedema

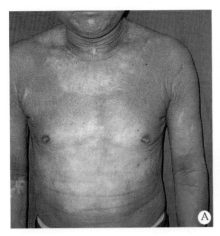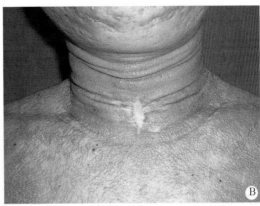

图 25-13-1 A. 躯干、上肢皮肤弥漫肥厚、浸润性斑块；B. 颈部、胸部许多苔藓样丘疹

Figure 25-13-1 A. Thickened skin and infiltrated plaques over the trunk and the upper arm; B. Multiple lichenoid papules on the neck and chest

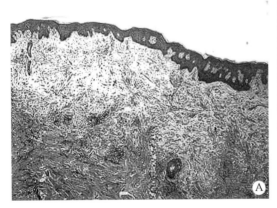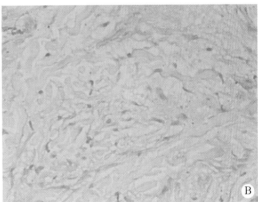

图 25-13-2 A. 真皮上部胶原稀疏、水肿(HE 染色,×100);B. 胶原纤维之间见黏蛋白沉积(阿新蓝染色,×100)

Figure 25-13-2 A. Sparseness and edema of collagen in the upper dermis(HE stain,×100); B. Mucin deposition between the collagen bundles (Alcian blue stain,×100)

14. 毛囊黏蛋白病
Follicular mucinosis

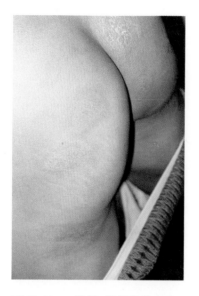

图 25-14-1　臀部、骶部数片红斑，轻度浸润

Figure 25-14-1　Several infiltrate erythemas on the buttock and sacrum

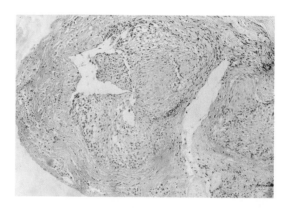

图 25-14-2　阿新蓝染色在毛囊上皮及毛囊周围呈明显阳性反应（阿新蓝染色，×100）

Figure 25-14-2　Deposition of mucin in the outer root sheath（Alcian blue stain，×100）

15. 网状红斑黏蛋白病
Reticular erythematous mucinosis

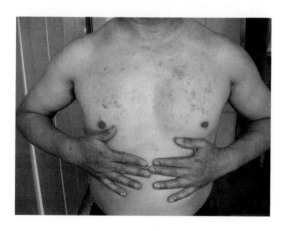

图 25-15-1　前胸、上肢有网状红色斑块及斑片，散在少量丘疹

Figure 25-15-1　Reticular erythematous maculopapular lesion on the upper chest

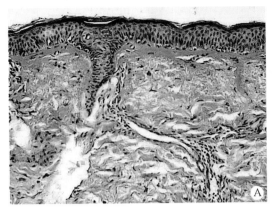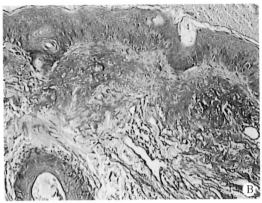

图 25-15-2 A. 真皮轻度水肿,血管及毛囊周围有淋巴细胞浸润(HE 染色,×200);B. 真皮胶原束之间有黏蛋白沉积(阿新蓝染色,×200)

Figure 25-15-2 A. Perivascular and perifollicular lymphocytic infiltration in the upper reticular dermis(HE stain,×200);B. Mucin deposition between collagen bundles (Alcian blue stain,×200)

16. 皮肤局灶性黏蛋白病
Cutaneous focal mucinosis

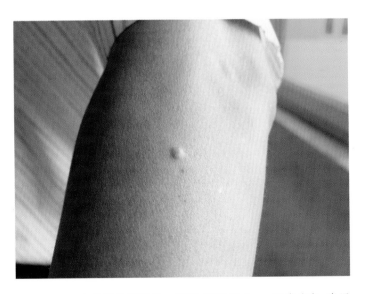

图 25-16-1 左前臂外侧可见一结节,直径约 4mm,正常皮色,半透明,表面光滑,境界清楚

Figure 25-16-1 A well-circumscribed translucent skin-colored nodule 4 mm in diameter with smooth surface on the extensor surface of left arm

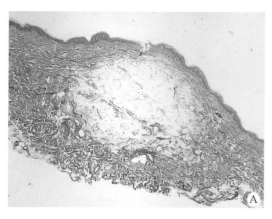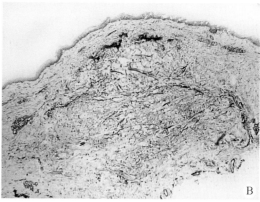

图 25-16-2　A. 真皮中上部充满比较疏松的无定形物质,界限不清,无包膜,周围成纤维细胞增多,胶原增生(HE 染色,×40);B. 真皮中上部可见明显紫色异染区(阿新蓝染色,×100)

Figure 25-16-2　A. Loose formless substance with uncircumscribed in the middle dermis, fibroblast increasedly and collagen hyperplasia (HE stain, ×40); B. Markedly purple metachrometic area in the middle dermis (Alcian blue stain, ×100)

17. 肢端持续性丘疹性黏蛋白沉积症
Acral persistent popular mucinosis

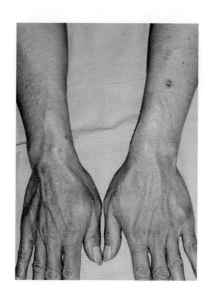

图 25-17-1　双前臂,双手背对称性分布多发大小不一的半透明丘疹

Figure 25-17-1　Numerous waxy papules are symmetrically on both arns and dosors of both hands

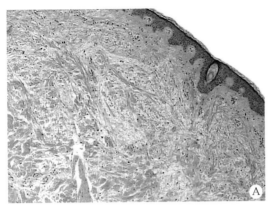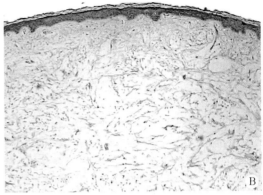

图 25-17-2　A. 真皮浅层、中层胶原纤维间隙增大,胶原纤维减少(HE 染色,×40);B. 真皮中黏蛋白沉积(阿新蓝染色,×40)

Figure 25-17-2　A. The collagen fibers in the reticular dermis are widely separated by deposits of mucin(HE stain,×40);B. The deposits of mucin in the upper and middle dermis(Alcian blue stain,×40)

18. 烟酸缺乏症
Pellagra

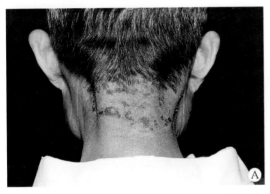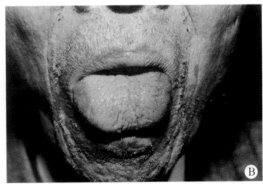

图 25-18-1　A. 颈项部可见边界清楚的水肿性暗紫红斑,皮肤增厚,表面有黑褐色厚痂;B. 口腔黏膜糜烂、浅表溃疡,舌质淡红,表面有沟纹

Figure 25-18-1　A. Erythema with scaling greasily,sharply defined amaranth macules and skin thick on neck;B. Oral mucosa erosion and small ulcer in the mouth

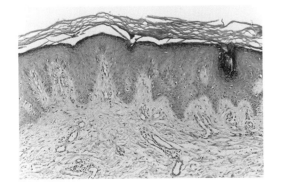

图 25-18-2　表皮角化过度,颗粒层增厚,棘层肥厚,皮突延长。真皮浅层血管周围少量淋巴细胞和组织细胞浸润(HE 染色,×40)

Figure 25-18-2　Hyperkeratosis, thickened granular layer and acanthosis, elongation of the rete ridges, a few lymphocytes and histocytes infiltrate perivascular in the upper dermis(HE stain,×40)

19. 胡萝卜素血症
Carotenemi

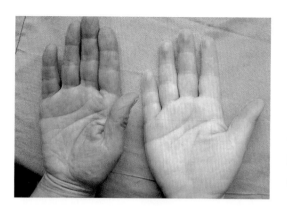

图 25-19-1　双手掌皮肤黄染,呈橘黄色

Figure 25-19-1　Yellowish orange pigmentation of the skin on right palm(left side)

20. 糖原贮积病Ⅰ型
Type Ⅰ glycogenosis

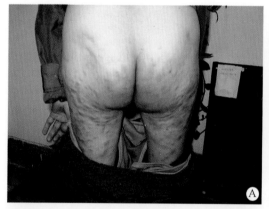

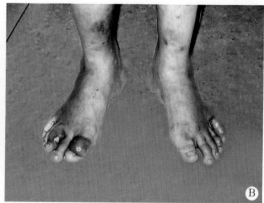

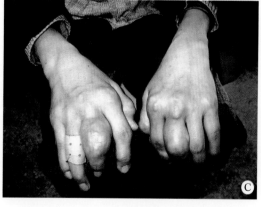

图 25-20-1　A. 臀、股部大小不等结节;B. 足部暗红色结节;C. 手指关节处许多结节

Figure 25-20-1　A. Numerous nodules on the both buttocks and thigh; B. Wine nodules on the feet; C. Many nodules on the knuckle

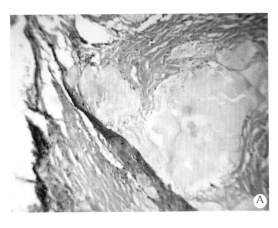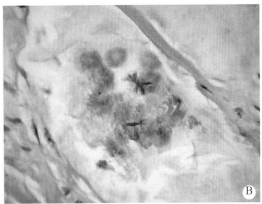

图 25-20-2　A. 真皮内均质状红色团块(HE 染色, ×100)(甲醛液固定); B. 真皮内棕色尿酸盐结晶,呈放射状(HE 染色, ×400)(无水乙醇固定)

Figure 25-20-2　A. Homogeneous red masses in the dermis(HE stain, ×100); B. Brown uric acid crystal with actinomorphic in the dermis(HE stain, ×400)

21. 褐黄病

Ochronosis

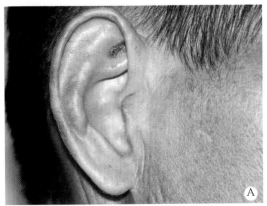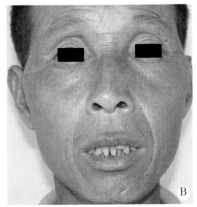

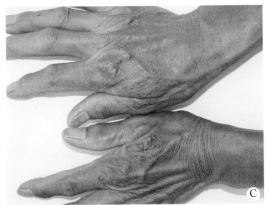

图 25-21-1　A. 耳郭内侧蚕豆大小棕褐色斑块;B. 双颧部、鼻梁和上唇淡绿至深褐色斑疹,边界不清;C. 双手背针头至粟粒大小褐黑色坚实性丘疹

Figure 25-21-1　A. Horse-bean-sized brown plaques on the inner auricle; B. Greenish and brown maculae with obscure boundary on the cheekbones, nasal bridge and the upper lip; C. Firm black brown papules on the dorsal of both hands

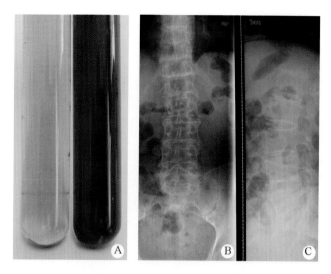

图 25-21-2   A. 新鲜尿液加入 10％NaOH 溶液后颜色迅速变为黑色；B. 腰椎 X 线检查：腰椎骨质疏松；C. 椎间盘钙化，椎间盘突出

Figure 25-21-2   A. The color of fresh urine rapidly became black after addition of 10％ NaOH solution；B. Spine X-ray: Showed osteoporosis of lumbar vertebrae；C. calcification and protrusion of intervertebral disc

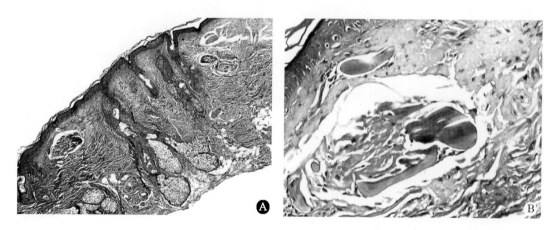

图 25-21-3   A. 表皮轻度萎缩、变薄，真皮内胶原纤维变性，胶原束肿胀，胶原束间棕黄色、均质状团块样物质沉积；B. 甲苯蓝染色示团块状物质呈黑色

Figure 25-21-3   A. Slight epidermal atrophy and thinning, degeneration of collagen fibers, collagen bundle swelling, deposition of yellow-brown boluses between collagen; B. Toluene blue staining showed that the mass material was black

第 26 章
色素障碍性皮肤病
Disturbances of Pigmentation

1. 色素型分界线
Pigmentary demarcation lines

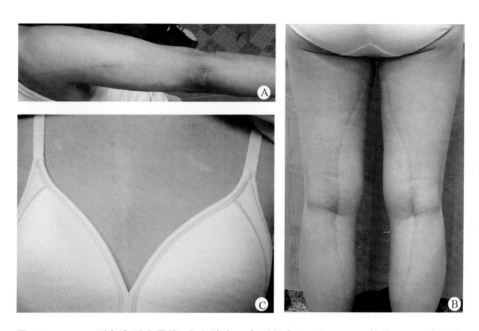

图 26-1-1　A. A 型色素型分界线：左上肢有一条形褐色斑，宽 0.5cm，长约 20cm，表面光滑；B. B 型色素性分界线：从脚后跟延伸到臀皱褶处对称性分布长约 58cm，宽 15～20cm 的色素沉着带，色素区域内侧缘清楚，而外侧缘逐渐变淡至正常肤色；C. C＋E 型色素型分界线：胸部沿前正中线自胸骨切迹至乳头水平见色素减退性条纹，两侧胸部见对称性分布的色素减退性斑片

Figure 26-1-1　A. A pigmentary band, approximately 0.5cm × 20cm distributes over the left upper limb(Type A)；B. Type B pigmentary demarcation lines：58cm × (15-20) cm band-like pigmentation symmetrically distributed over the flexor aspects of the lower limbs. The medial borders of the pigmented areas were sharply demarcated, but the lateral borders merged imperceptibly into normal skin；C. The type C dermacation line was a hyperpigmented line seen over the mild-portion of the chest. Type E displayed two obliquely oriented hypopigmented macule occurring bilaterally on the lateral aspect of the chest

2. 黄褐斑
Melasma

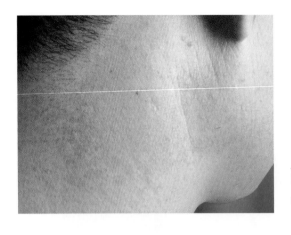

图 26-2-1　颈项部有不规则褐色沉着斑

Figure 26-2-1　A brown irregular hyperpigmented macule on the neck

3. 泛发性雀斑样痣病
Generalized lentiginosis

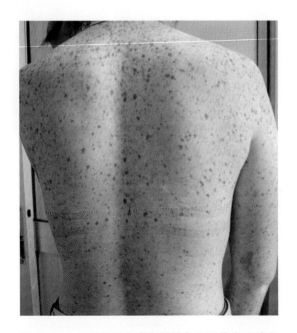

图 26-3-1　躯干有很多雀斑样褐色斑不伴有系统异常

Figure 26-3-1　Multiple lentigines occured on the trunk without systemic abnormalities

4. 多发性黑子综合征
Multiple lentigines syndrome(LEOPARD syndrome)

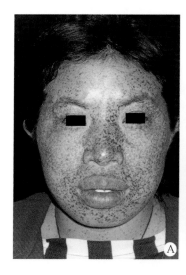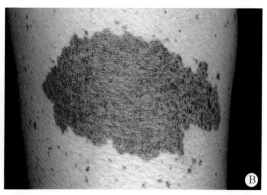

图 26-4-1　A. 面部有很多棕黑色小斑；B. 左下肢有一大片棕色斑，其表面有黑色丘疹
Figure 26-4-1　A. Nurmorous small dark brown macules on the face; B. A large brown plaque on the left limb associatel with dark papules on it

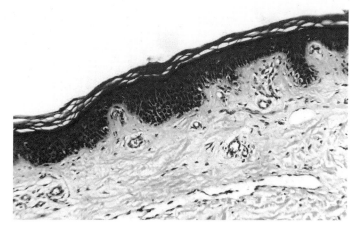

图 26-4-2　表皮轻度角化过度，棘层肥厚，基底层色素增多，真皮有噬色素细胞(HE 染色，×400)
Figure 26-4-2　Light hyperkeratosis, acanthosis and hyperpigmentantion in basal layer of epidermis, melanophage in the dermis (HE stain, ×400)

5. 补骨脂素长波紫外线雀斑样痣

PUVA lentigo

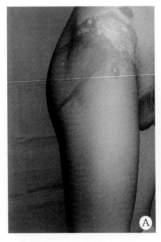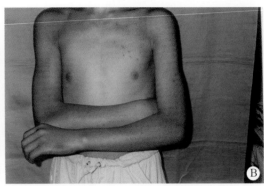

图 26-5-1　A. 表面红肿，四周色素沉着；B. 全身散在褐色至黑色星状斑点

Figure 26-5-1　A. Hyperpigmentation around swelling erythema；B. Generalized brown to black speckle

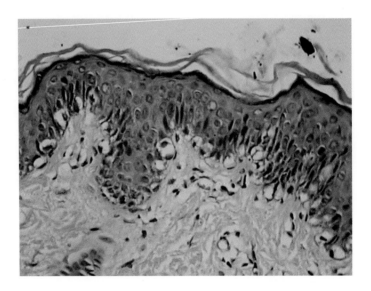

图 26-5-2　基底层透明细胞增加，可见双核透明细胞（HE 染色，× 400）

Figure 26-5-2　The basal clear cells marked increase with some binuclear clear cells（HE stain，× 400）

6. 非典型阴茎雀斑样痣

Atypical penile lentigo

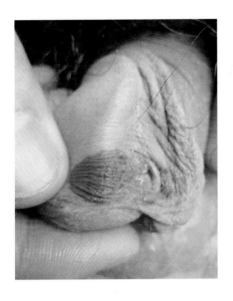

图 26-6-1　龟头处约 1 cm×1 cm 大黑斑

Figure 26-6-1　A black macula in a size of 1 cm×1 cm on the glans penis

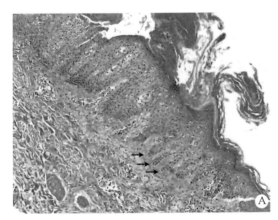

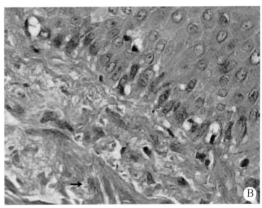

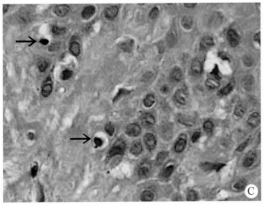

图 26-6-2　A. 表皮突向下伸长呈杵状 (HE 染色，×40)；B. 基底层细胞色素明显增多，黑素细胞数量增加，真皮内可见噬黑素细胞(HE 染色，×200)；C. 部分黑素细胞呈现异型性(HE 染色，×400)

Figure 26-6-2　A. Elongation of the rete ridges（HE stain，×40）；B. Hyperpigmentation of the basal cell layer with increase in the number of melanocytes. The dermis contained some large melanophages（HE stain，×200）；C. A few heterotypic melanocytes occurred in the superficial and middle epidermis（HE stain，×400）

7. 巨大先天性黑素细胞痣
Giant congenital melanocytic nevus

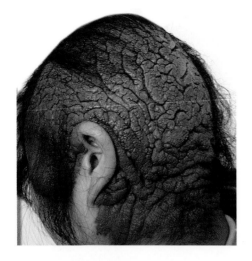

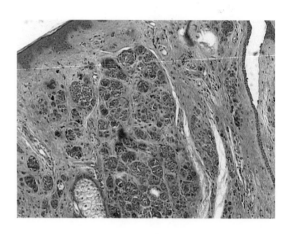

图 26-7-1　左侧头皮凹凸不平,似脑回状,表面色素沉着,有少量黑色短粗毛

Figure 26-7-1　Large pigmented cerebriform masses on the scalp covered with a few black short hairs

图 26-7-2　真皮内大小不等、形态不一的痣细胞巢(HE 染色,×40)

Figure 26-7-2　Variously sized nevus cell nests in the dermis (HE stain,×40)

8. 太田痣
Nevus of Ota

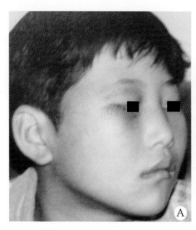
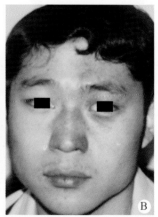

图 26-8-1　A. ⅠA型:上下眼睑有色素斑; B. ⅠB型: 颧部有色素斑

Figure 26-8-1　A. Type ⅠA: Spotted pigmentation limited to the upper and lower eyelids; B. Type ⅠB: Spotted pigmentation limited to the zyomatic region

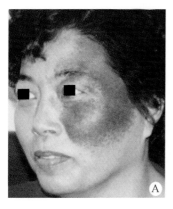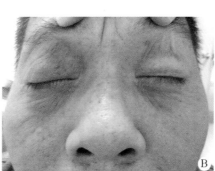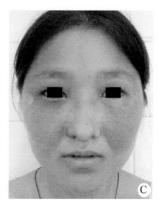

图26-8-2　A. Ⅱ型:眼睑,颧部和鼻有色素斑;B. Ⅲ型:眼睑,颧部,鼻和奥有色素斑;C. Ⅳ型:两侧面部有褐青色沉着斑

Figure 26-8-2　A. Type Ⅱ:Spotted pigmentation limited to the eyelids zyomatic and nose region;B. Type Ⅲ: Spotted pigmentation limited to the eyelids zyomatic,nose region and forehead;C. Type Ⅳ:Bilateral pigmentation involves both sides of the face

9. 太田痣合并鲜红斑痣
Nevus Ota associated with nevus flammeus

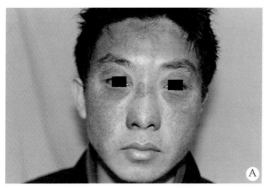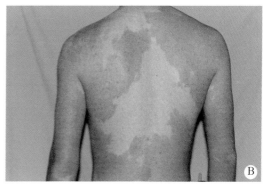

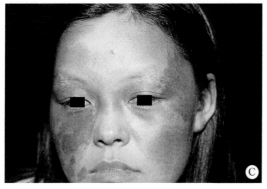

图26-9-1　A. 面部双侧对称黑褐色斑片;B. 双上肢及手部、胸部和肩胛部、背部,腰骶部有大片红斑; C. 面部黑褐色斑片双侧对称,分布范围为额部、眼周

Figure 26-9-1　A. Symmetrical bluish and brownish macules on the face; B. Red patches on the upper limbs, hands, chest, shoulder blade, waist and sacrum; C. Symmetrical brownish macules on the forehead and periorbital

10. 伊藤痣
Naevus of Ito

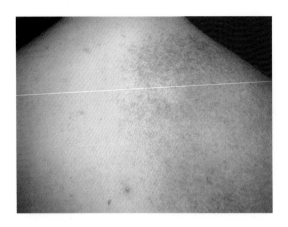

图 26-10-1　右上背及肩部褐青色斑

Figure 26-10-1　Bluish and brownish maculae on the right scapular and deltoid regions

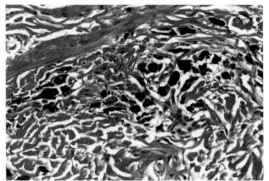

图 26-10-2　真皮中部胶原纤维之间散在圆形、椭圆形或梭形黑素细胞(HE 染色，×100)

Figure 26-10-2　Round, oval or fusiform melanocytes scatter among the collagen bundles in the dermis (HE stain, ×100)

11. 伊藤痣上继发白斑(集晕痣与晕皮炎现象于一体)
Partial depigmentation arised in the Nevus of Ito: the halo nevus and halo dermatitis in the same patient

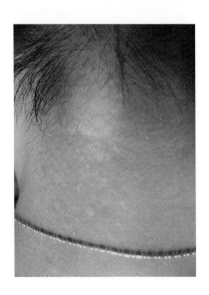

图 26-11-1　左颈部三色带，自体后正中线向外依次呈瓷白色、蓝灰色和最外层的黄蓝色。色素异常区带下方见点状及多角形、碎纸屑样色素减退斑

Figure 26-11-1　From the midline to the left side of the neck, there presented triphasic pigmentary changes as porcelain-white, sky-blue and blue-brownish outermost in general. Multiple depigmented and confetti-like spots or polygonal patches sized 2-5 mm were sparsely distributed the low part of the discoloration zone

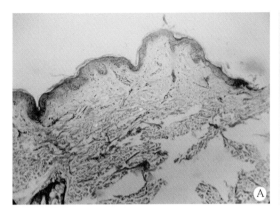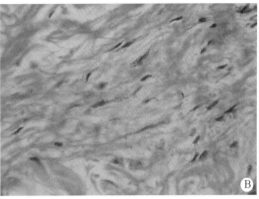

图 26-11-2　A. 真皮浅层和中层血管周围淋巴细胞浸润(HE 染色, ×40); B. 真皮中层胶原纤维之间可以残存的纺锤形黑素细胞, 长轴走向与皮肤表面平行(HE 染色, ×400)

Figure 26-11-2　A. Slight perivascular lymphocytic infiltration in the superficial and mid-dermis (HE stain, × 40); B. Residue spindle shaped melanocytes are sparsely scattered between the collagen bundles in the mid-dermis, whose axis parallel to the skin surface (HE stain, × 400)

12. 面部褐青色痣
Acquired bilateral nevus of Ota-like macules

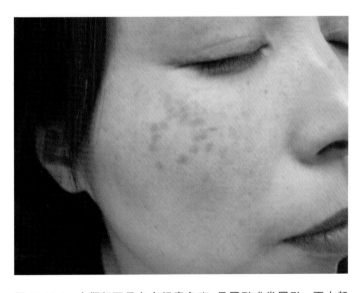

图 26-12-1　右颧部可见多个褐青色斑, 呈圆形或类圆形。面中部三角形烟灰色斑, 颜色不均匀, 鼻背部浅褐色, 眼内侧角处呈黑色或青褐色, 边界不规则

Figure 26-12-1　Somecircular or class circle brown spos presented on the right zygomati

209

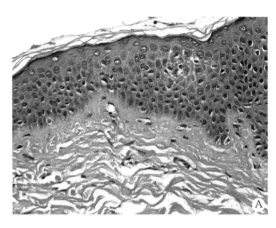 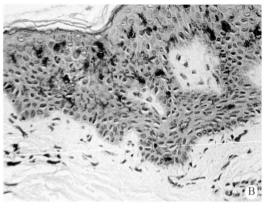

图 26-12-2　角质形成细胞的黑素增加,表皮突未见延长,而有大量的黑素细胞.一些分散的、双极的或不规则的黑素细胞和部分黑素沉着物出现在网状真皮层(A. HE 染色,×200;B. S100 染色,×200)

Figure 26-12-2　A. Increased melanin in the keratinocytes, and excessive numbers of melanocytes. were present in the epidermis, (HE stain, ×200); B. A few scattered, bipolar or irregular melanocytes and some melanin deposits were noted in the reticular dermis(S100 stain, ×200)

13. Becker 痣中并发痤疮

Acne vulgaris superimposed on the Becker's nevus

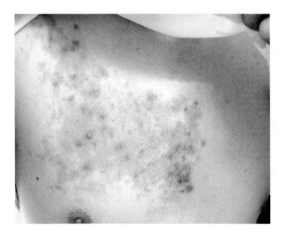

图 26-13-1　右前胸褐色斑片,其中毳毛比周围稍粗。在色素沉着斑中有粉刺、多发性毛囊性炎性丘疹及数个囊肿,但周边皮肤无上述皮损

Figure 26-13-1　Brownish macules presented on the right chest. The hair in the macules was slight thicker than normal. Comedones, inflammatory follicular papules and cysts were strictly confined to the pigmented macules

14. 双侧分布的色素性毛皮痣合并颈部白色纤维丘疹病

Bilateral Becker nevus associated with white fibrous papulosis of the neck

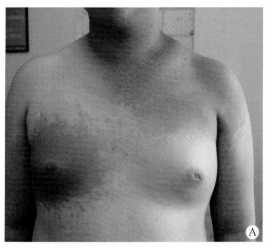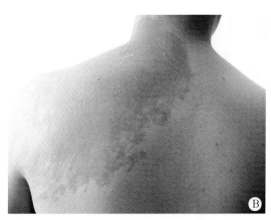

图 26-14-1　A. B 左颈部、肩胛、胸前、上肢片状不规则黄褐色至深褐色色素沉着斑片，皮损中央呈黑褐色，密集分布长约 2 cm 粗黑毛发

Figure 26-14-1　A. B There are light or dark brown patchs and hypertrichotic on the neck, the anterior chest, scapular and the left upperarm, with many pachy hairs about 2 centimeters on it

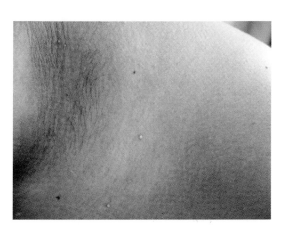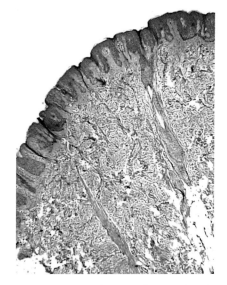

图 26-14-2　颈部左侧皮损可见散在的圆形、黄白色，非毛囊性丘疹

Figure 26-14-2　Discrete, non-follicular and round pale papules on the left patch

图 26-14-3　棘层肥厚，基底层色素增加，真皮中上部胶原明显增生、致密。立毛肌数量增多(HE 染色，×40)

Figure 26-14-3　there were acanthosis and hyperpigmented in the basal cell layer associated with thickened collagen bundles in the dermis and the arrector pili muscles were increased in number and size (HE stain, ×40)

15. Becker 综合征
Becker's syndrome

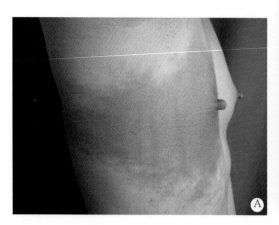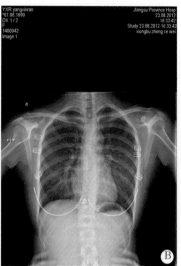

图 26-15-1　A. 右侧胸背有一大片境界清楚褐色斑伴少数 1～2mm 长毳毛,合并乳房发育不良;B.
脊柱侧弯

Figure 26-15-1　A large sharply demarcated hyperpigmentedmacula with a few longer vellus hairs 1-
2mm long on the right chest and back associated with breast dysplasia（A）and scoliosis（B）

16. 神经皮肤黑变病
Neurocutaneous melanosis

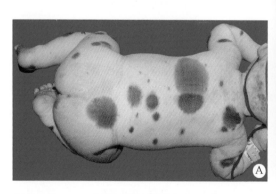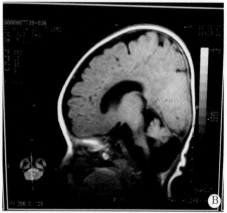

图 26-16-1　A. 背部及四肢可见多个巨大先天性色素痣；B. 头颅 MR 显示:双侧侧脑室扩大,小脑
延髓池扩大,第四脑室扩大,脑积水,符合 Dandy-Walker 畸形

Figure 26-16-1　A. Multiple giant congenital melanotic nevi on the back and extremities；B. Magnetic
resonance imaging showed：enlarged lateral ventricles，cerebellomedullary cistern and epicele，to-
gether with hydrocephalus suggest Dandy-Walker malformation

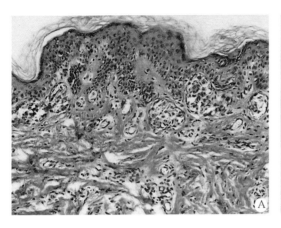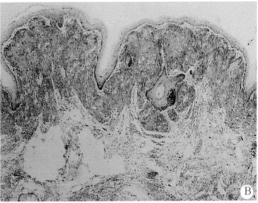

图 26-16-2 A. 表皮基底层及真皮浅层可见痣细胞呈巢状分布,部分痣细胞巢延及真皮深层,围绕附属器分布,可见成熟现象,未见核分裂象,真皮浅层单一核细胞片状浸润,并有嗜黑素细胞;B. 痣细胞显示 HMB45 染色(+)

Figure 26-16-2 A. Nested nevocytes were observed in the basal layer and the superficial dermis; Some infiltrated around appendages in lower dermis, Some nevocytes were mature without karyokinesi; B. Nevocytes were positive for HMB45 antibody

17. 进行性肢端黑变病

Acromelanosis progressive

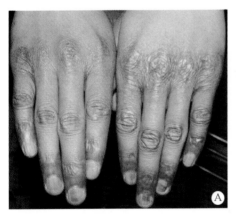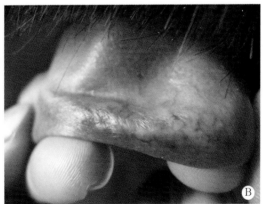

图 26-17-1 双手(A)及耳郭(B)可见弥漫性暗褐色斑疹及斑片,指间关节背侧可见黑褐色色素性条纹,指甲见纵行的黑色色素线,耳郭呈现蛛网状线状褐色斑

Figure 26-17-1 Diffuse dark brown patches on the acral areas of the fingers(A) and both auricles (B); Brown striated pigmentation on the nails and flexor aspects of interphalangeal joints; Spider web like brown maculae on the auricles

213

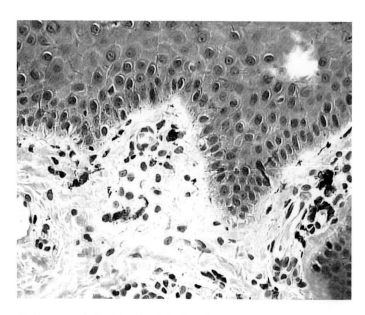

图 26-17-2　表皮基底层黑素细胞增多,透明细胞呈簇状,色素增加,基底细胞无液化变性,真皮浅层见大量噬色素细胞及黑素颗粒,轻度淋巴细胞浸润(HE 染色,×400)

Figure 26-17-2　Increased melanocytes in basal layer; Cluster of pigmented clear cells in basal layer; No liquefaction degeneration in basal cells; In addition to mild lymphocytic infiltration, many melanophages and melanin granules in the dermis(HE stain, ×400)

18. 眶周黑皮病
Periobital melanosis

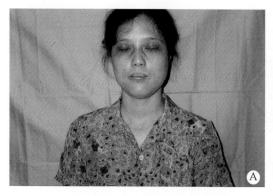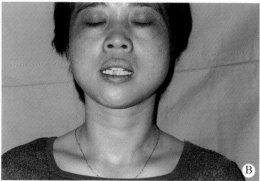

图 26-18-1　A. 轻度眶周色素沉着(姐姐);B. 轻度眶周色素沉着(妹妹)

Figure 26-18-1　A. Mild periorbital hyperpigmentation(sister); B. Mild periorbital hyperpigmentation(younger sister)

19. 北村网状肢端色素沉着症
Reticulate acropigmenttion of Kitamura

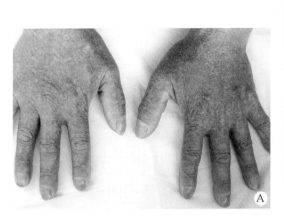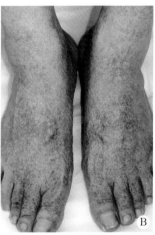

图 26-19-1　轻微内凹的色素斑发生于双手背(A)和双足背(B)毗邻形成网状

Figure 26-19-1　Slightly depressed hyperpigmented macules on the both dorsal hands (A) and feet(B) which form a reticulate pattern

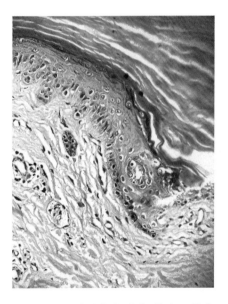

图 26-19-2　表皮角化过度,基底层黑素增多(HE 染色,×200)

Figure 26-19-2　Epidermal hyperker-ato-sis and hyperpigmentation of the basal layer (HE stain,×200)

20. 大疱性先天性皮肤异色症
Congenital poikiloderma with bullae

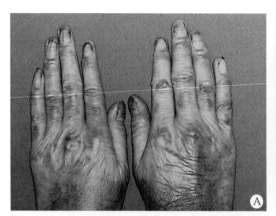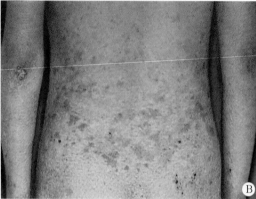

图 26-20-1　A. 手背皮肤萎缩伴甲营养不良；B. 腰背部皮肤异色改变

Figure 26-20-1　A. Skin atroply on the dorsum of hands with dystrophic nail；B. Poikiloderma on the waist and back

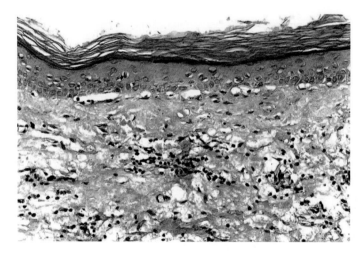

图 26-20-2　表皮萎缩，基底细胞液化变性，毛细血管周围有炎性细胞浸润（HE 染色，×100）

Figure 26-20-2　Epidermal atrophy and hydropic degeneration of basal cells, an inflammatory infiltrate is found around the capillary walls (HE stain, ×100)

21. 皱褶部网状色素沉着症
Dowling-Degos disease

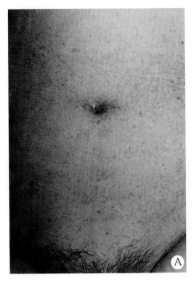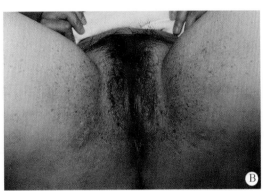

图 26-21-1　A. 腹部褐色斑点；B. 股内侧、外阴部对称性色素沉着斑，融合成网状

Figure 26-21-1　A. Dark brown spots on the abdomen; B. Symmetric confluent reticular pigmented macules on the vulva and inner aspects of thighs

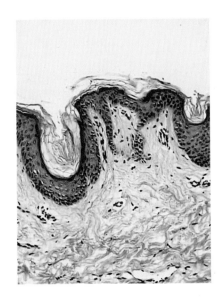

图 26-21-2　表皮角化过度，棘层肥厚，表皮突延长，基底层色素增加，真皮层小血管周围炎性浸润，周围有嗜黑素细胞(HE 染色，×100)

Figure 26-21-2　Marked follicular plugging and rete ridge elongation with hyperpigmentation along basal layer. Perivascular lymphohistiocytic infiltration with melanophages in the papillary dermis(HE stain，×100)

22. 遗传性对称性色素异常症并发掌跖角化病

Dyschromatosis symmetrical hereditaria with palmoplantar keratoderma

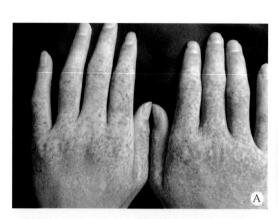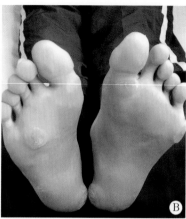

图 26-22-1   A. 双手指背及掌背多发性、对称性色素减退斑,其中散在粟粒至黄豆大黑褐色斑片,混杂呈网状;B. 双足跟、足跖及第 1、5 趾腹有半圆形淡黄色半透明角化性斑块

Figure 26-22-1   A. Multiple and symmetricl hyperpigmented and hypopigmented macules on the extensor surface of fingers and hand back; B. Symmetric hyperkeratosis on the soles and heels

23. 家族性进行性色素沉着

Familial progressive hyperpigmentation

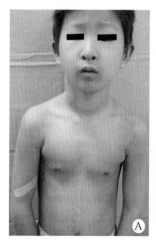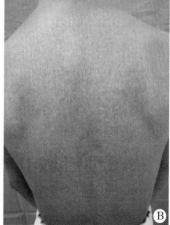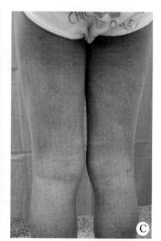

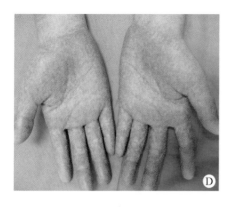

图 26-23-1 几乎累及全身的泛发性色素沉着,胸部和腹部(A),肩部、背部和腰部(B),下肢(C),手掌(D)
Figure 26-23-1 Extensive hyperpigmented spots covered almost of her body,especially on his perioral area,neck,corpus linguae,thoracic region and abdominal part (A),shoulders,back and lumbar parts (B),lower limbs(C),palms (D)

24. 家族进行性色素沉着和色素减退
Familial progressive hypo-and hyperpigmentation

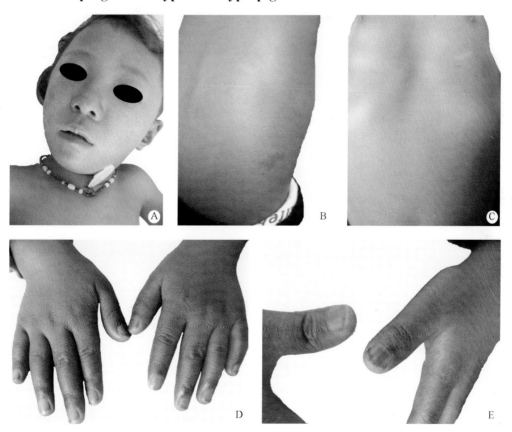

图 26-24-1 A. 脸部网状色素沉着斑;B、C. 胸背部深褐色皮肤上,出现不规则的深色咖啡斑和桉树叶样白斑;D. 指关节上显著的色素沉着;两侧拇指纵行黑甲(多条带状);E. 两侧拇指纵行黑甲(多条带状)

Figure 26-24-1 A. Reticulate network of hyperpigmented macules over the face; B,C. Some irregular heavily café-au-lait spots and Ash-leaf-like white macules were superimposed on the uniformly deep bronze-brown skin. Lesions on the chest(A);Lesions on the back(B); D. Markedly hyperpigmented skin over the knuckles; Longitudinal melanonychia (multiple bands) in her both thumbs; E. Longitudinal melanonychia (multiple bands) in her both thumbs

25. 遗传性泛发性色素异常症
Dyschromatosis universalis hereditaria

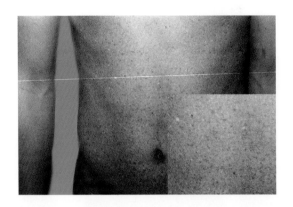

图 26-25-1　腹部有色素沉着斑间以色素减退斑

Figure 26-25-1　Generalized hyperchromic macules mingled with achromic macules on the abdomen

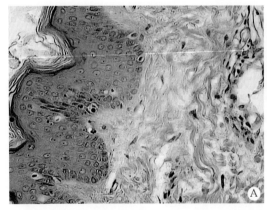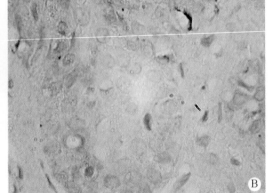

图 26-25-2　A. 色素沉着斑中基底层和棘层下部细胞黑素明显增加(HE 染色,×400);B. 色素减退区黑素细胞胞质内阳性颗粒少见或缺如,个别细胞核染色阳性(HE 染色,×400)

Figure 26-25-2　A. Heavily stained melanin pigments in the basal layer of the epidermis in the hyperchromic macule (HE stain,×400); B. Melanin pigments are reduced or absent with normal numbers of melanocytes in the achromic area(HE stain,×400)

26. 伴巨大黑素小体表现的遗传性对称性色素异常症
Hereditary symmetrical dyschromatosis with melanin macroglobules

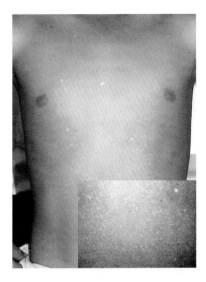

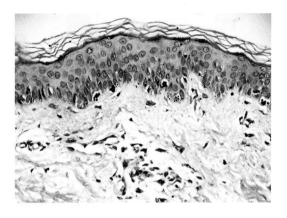

图 26-26-2　基底层色素增多,黑素细胞内普遍可见多个 1～3μm 大小黑素颗粒滞留。全层角质形成细胞内偶见巨大黑素细胞,真皮内少量嗜色素细胞
Figure 26-26-2　Hyperpigmentation was found in basilar layer. 1-3μm melanin macroglobules were detained in the melanocytes or keratinocytes above. Melanophages were noted in the dermis

图 26-26-1　乳房下胸腹部见弥漫性灰色色素,其中夹杂粟米至绿豆大小色素减退斑
Figure 26-26-1　Diffused grayish macules on the abdominal skin were interspersed with hypopigmented macules,which were sized as maize to green bean

27. 线状和旋涡状痣样过度黑素沉着病
Linear and whorled nevoid hypermelanosis

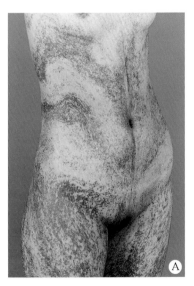

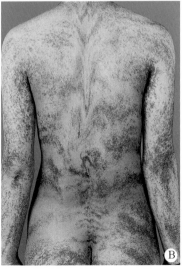

图 26-27-1　躯干及四肢淡褐色或深棕色沿 Blaschko 线分布的条状或旋涡状排列的色素沉着斑
Figure 26-27-1　Linear and whorled hyperpigmentation following the lines of Blaschko on the trunk and limbs

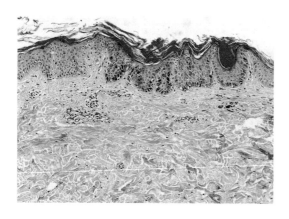

图 26-27-2　表皮角化过度,基底层明显色素增加和黑素细胞增多,真皮上部少量嗜黑素细胞(HE 染色,×100)

Figure 26-27-2　Hyperkeratosis, increased pigmentation and melanocytes in the basal layer, a few melanophage in the upper dermis (HE stain, ×100)

28. 点彩样色素沉着斑
Pointillist melanotic macules

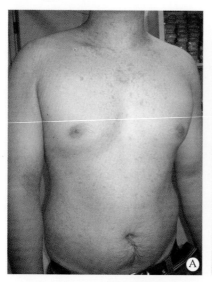
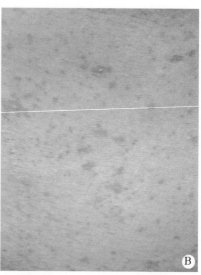

图 26-28-1　躯干、颈及四肢见成百数千个色素斑,播散性分布,以胸部最多见(A)。色素斑针头大小,群集处呈星形或鸡爪形斑,就像一黑色人体点彩画(B)

Figure 26-28-1　The macules were evenly dark colored in such an impressive way of distinct, stellate or claw-like borders(A). The spots were uniformly pin sized, oval or round, whereas the bizarre macules varied ranges from 0. 1 cm to several centimeters in diameter(B)

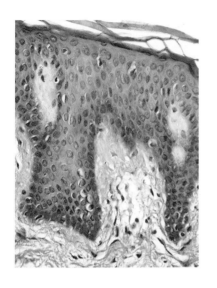

图 26-28-2　基底层黑素显著增加，形成眼线征。真皮乳头见少数局灶性嗜色素细胞，其余正常（HE 染色，×400）

Figure 26-28-2　Remarkable basilar hyperpigmentation (pigmented eye linear sign) without melanocytic hyperplasia. The dermis was almost normal except foci melanophages in the papillary dermis (HE stain, ×400)

29. 获得性真皮黑素细胞增生症
Acquired dermal melanocytosis

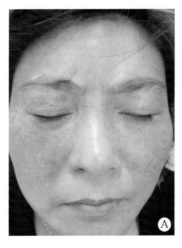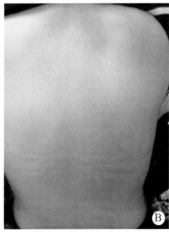

图 26-29-1　泛发性多发性灰蓝色斑在面部（A）和背部（B）

Figure 26-29-1　Generalized multiple blue-gray maculae on the face (A) and back (B)

223

30. 意外粉粒沉着病
Accidental tattoos

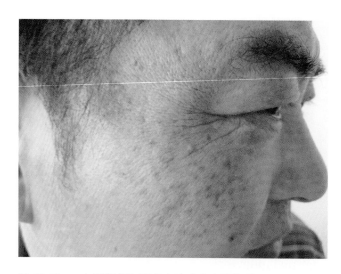

图 26-30-1　右侧颊部和颞部有淡蓝色和黑色斑

Figure 26-30-1　Light blue and dark maculae on the right cheek and temple

31. 波纹状融合性网状乳头瘤
Rippling lesions of confluent and reticulated papillomatosis

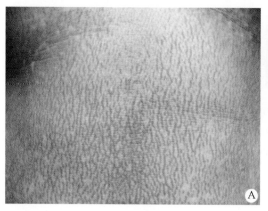 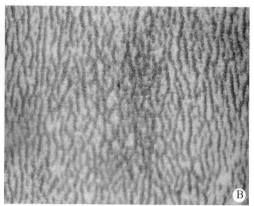

图 26-31-1　腰腹部见黑褐色波纹状皮损（A）；皮损主要为角化性丘疹融合成波纹状条纹垂直分布（B）

Figure 26-31-1　The lesions mainly involved the waist and the abdemon(A)；A closer inspection of the lesions reveals successive,mutiple and keratotic papules,which were vertically rippled(B)

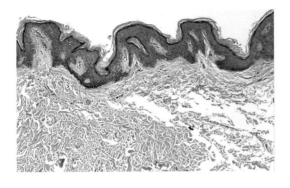

图 26-31-2 表皮网篮状角化过度及轻度乳头瘤样增生,真皮浅层血管周围单一核细胞浸润
Figure 26-31-2 In the epidermis, there was notable basketwaved hyperkeratosis and mild papillomatosis. Mononuclear cells infiltrated superficial small vessels in the dermis

32. 先天性巨大色素痣并发白癜风
Giant congenital pigmented nevus complicated with vitiligo

图 26-32-1 胸腹部原黑斑皮损上有色素脱失斑
Figure 26-32-1 Depigmented patches surrounded by black patches on the chest and abodoman

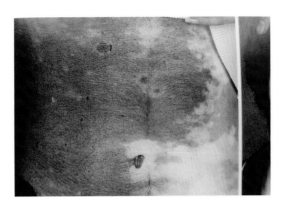

33. 三色白癜风
Trichrome vitiligo

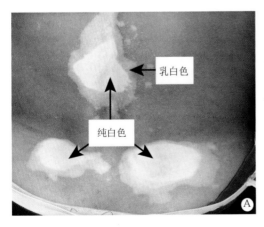

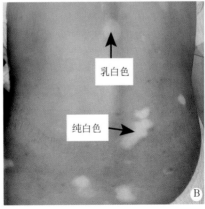

图 26-33-1 A. 皮损中央呈纯白色,其周围绕以淡于正常肤色、宽窄不一的浅白色"中间带"; B. 背部散在分布小片皮损,上部为点或小片浅白色皮损,中部皮损呈纯白色,右下方一处皮损上部为纯白色、下部呈浅白色
Figure 26-33-1 A. White macule or patch in the center, surrounded by intermediate milky white zone, normal appearing skin color at the periphery; B. White lesions with partially milky white color occurred on the bases of normal skin

34. 节段型五色白癜风
Pentachrome vitiligo in a segmental pattern

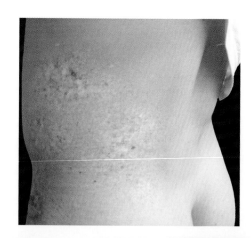

图 26-34-1 左腹部和腰部色素脱失和色素沉着性斑
Figure 26-34-1 Multiple depigmented and hyperpigmented macules on the lumbar areas

35. 炎症性白癜风
Inflammatory vitiligo

图 26-35-1 脱色斑边缘略隆起, 呈红色
Figure 26-35-1 The depigmented macule with a raised edematous red border

36. 儿童无色素性痣
Nevus depigmentosus in children

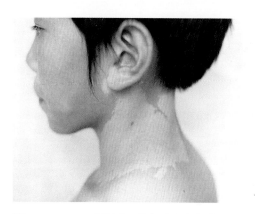

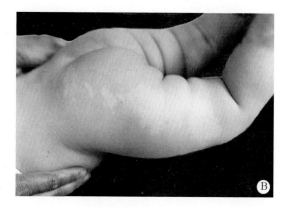

图 26-36-1 A. 左耳垂至颈部淡白色色素减退斑点; B. 左臀部至大腿色素减退斑
Figure 26-36-1 A. Isolated pattern of nevus depigmentosus shows serrated border; B. Segmental pattern of nevus depigmentosus shows serrated border

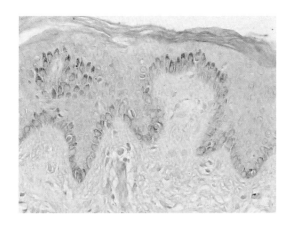

图 26-36-2　基底层黑素细胞无明显减少（HMB45 抗体染色，×100）

Figure 26-36-2　No obvious change is seen in the numbers of melanocytes in the basal layer（HMB45 antibody stain,×100）

37. 星状自发性假瘢

Stellate spontaneous pseudoscars

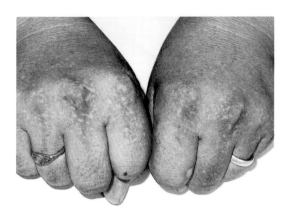

图 26-37-1　双手背有星状或线状色素减退斑

Figure 26-37-1　The white,scarlike,stellate and linear lesions on both dorsa of hands

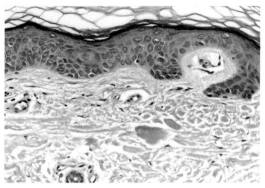

图 26-37-2　表皮角化过度,部分表皮下部色素增加,真皮浅层少量炎细胞浸润和弹性纤维变性（HE 染色，×150）

Figure 26-37-2　Epidermal hyperkeratosis and hyperpigmentation in the basal layer,a few of cell infiltration and degeneration of elastic fiber in the upper dermis（HE stain,×150）

第 27 章
先天性、遗传性皮病 Genodermatoses

1. 色素失禁合并不完全唇裂
Incontinentia pigmenti with unilateral complete cleft lip

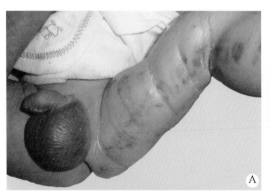
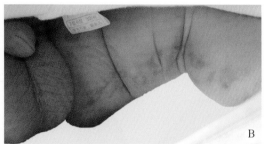
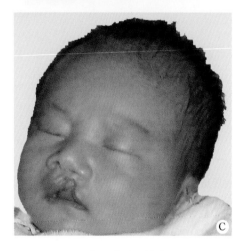

图 27-1-1　A. 左下肢后侧从臀区到足踝线状红斑；B. 45d 时线状色素沉着性斑点和条纹，没有浸润；C. 单侧不完全性唇裂（术前）

Figure 27-1-1　A. A linear erythematous eruption with superimposed vesicles on the left mid-posterior leg from the infragluteal region to the boy's ankle; B. At the age of 45 days, linear weakly pigmented spots and streaks without infiltration were noticed; C. Preoperative image where the left unilateral complete cleft lip can be observed

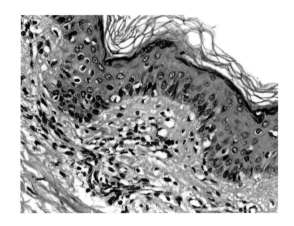

图 27-1-2 色素性皮损的病理：表皮角化不良细胞，基底层色素颗粒增多。真皮层大量嗜黑素细胞，基底膜正常（HE 染色，×200）

Figure 27-1-2 Histological features of the pigmented lesion. The epidermis was remarkable because of its dyskeratotic cells and increased melanin in the basal cell layer. Large numbers of melanin-laden macrophages were present in the dermis. The basement membrane was normal（HE stain，×200）

2. 色素失禁伴乳房发育不良

Incontinentia pigmenti associated with an undeveloped breast

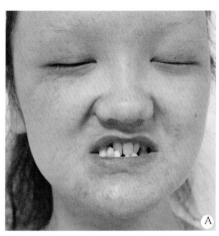
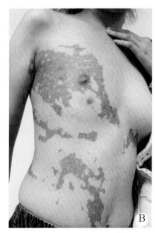
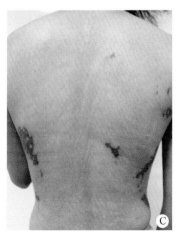
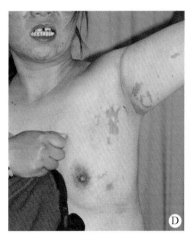

图 27-2-1 A. 高额、窄鼻、眶周和口周色素沉着，圆锥形尖牙，眉毛的中外侧稀疏；B. 右侧腋下、胸肋部网状和线状色素沉着斑，右侧乳房发育不全，两个乳头；C. 背部 V 形色素沉着线；D. 女孩的妈妈上门牙间隙较大，左肩部和胸部黑褐色斑

Figure 27-2-1 A. The girl with a high forehead, a narrow nose, periorbital and perioral hyperpigmentation, and some short, conical and pointed teeth. Her eyebrows were absent laterally and sparse medially; B. Many hyperpigmented maculae appeared either in a reticulated or linear arrangement on her right axillary fold, sternocostal area. Undeveloped right breast with two hypoplastic nipple-areola complexes; C. Some V-shaped hyperpigmented linear lesions on her back; D. The girl's mother with median diastema between the maxillary central incisors and some brown-black patches and mottles on her left shoulder and sternocostal area

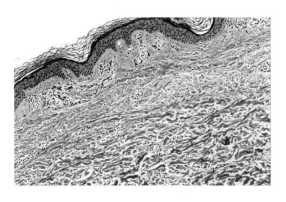

图 27-2-2　色素沉着皮肤的病理检查:轻度的角化过度,基底层色素颗粒增多,皮肤附属器(汗腺、毛发、皮脂腺)缺如,真皮浅层血管周围散在双极或不规则的嗜黑素细胞(HE 染色,×200)

Figure 27-2-2　Histopathologic features of a hyperpigmented skin. Slight hyperkeratesis, increased melanin in the basal layer, and excessive melanocytes. No skin appendages including sweat glands, hair follicles and sebaceous glands were observed. (HE stain, ×200)

3. 家族性慢性良性天疱疮
Familial chronic benign pemphigus

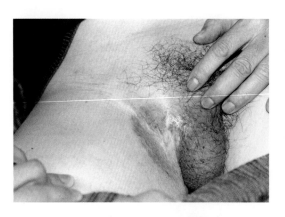

图 27-3-1　右侧腹股沟红斑、浸渍、糜烂

Figure 27-3-1　Erythemas, macerates and erosions on the right groin

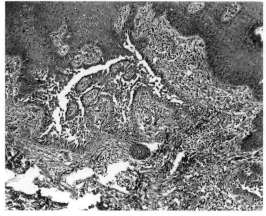

图 27-3-2　表皮基底层上方有一个腔隙,真皮乳头突向腔内呈绒毛状,腔内有棘层松解细胞,真皮浅层有炎性细胞浸润(HE 染色,×100)

Figure 27-3-2　Suprabasal lacunae with elongated papillae protrude upward in the the bulla forming villi and acantholysis cell in the bulla cavity, inflammatory infiltrate in the upper dermis (HE stain, ×100)

4. 单纯型大疱性表皮松解症：Weber-Cockayne 亚型
Epidermolysis bullosa simplex：Weber-Cockayne

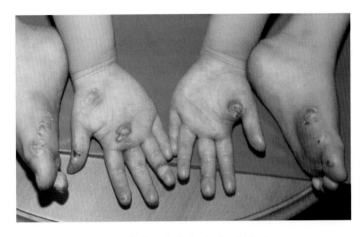

图 27-4-1　手掌、足部有黄豆大水疱、血疱，疱壁厚

Figure 27-4-1　Soybean sized blisters with thick wall on the palms and soles

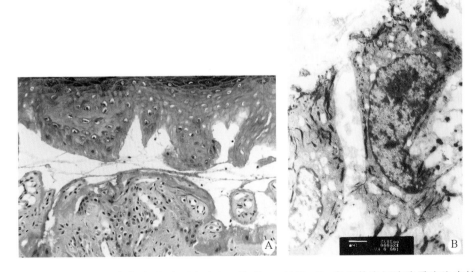

图 27-4-2　A. 表皮细胞水肿，表皮下水疱(HE 染色，×100)；B. 表皮基底细胞胞质空泡变性(透射电镜×6000)

Figure 27-4-2　A. Subepidermis blisters, associated with edema of epidermis cell (HE stain，×100)；B. Vacuolization in the basal cells (TEM，×6000)

5. 常染色体隐性遗传的 Hallopeau-Siemens 型营养不良型大疱性表皮松解症

Hallopeau-Siemens type of recessive dystrophic epidermolysis bullosa

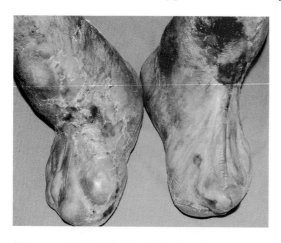

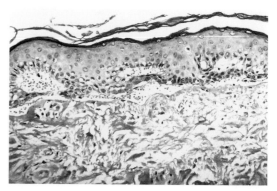

图 27-5-1　双足十趾融合形成袜套样并趾

Figure 27-5-1　Fusion of 10 toes into mittenlike deformities and complete loss of finger nails with scarring

图 27-5-2　表皮下水疱形成（↑）（HE 染色，×20）

Figure 27-5-2　A subepidermal blister(↑)(HE stain, ×20)

6. 胫前大疱性表皮松解症

Pretibial epidermolysis bullosa

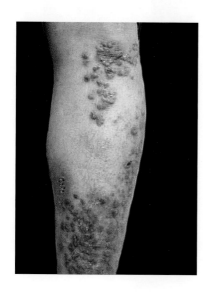

图 27-6-1　胫前有较多紫红色结节及斑块,部分区域有绿豆大的水疱,疱壁紧张

Figure 27-6-1　Multiple violaceous nodules and plaques, some mung bean-sized blisters on the pretibial

232

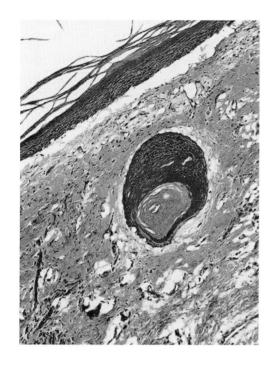

图 27-6-2　表皮角化过度，表皮真皮交界处可见裂隙形成，真皮浅层毛细血管扩张及轻度结缔组织增生，管周有少量淋巴细胞浸润，真皮中上部可见数个囊肿样结构，囊壁为复层鳞状上皮（HE 染色，×100）

Figure 27-6-2　Hyperkeratosis associated with the cavity forming between the epidermis and dermis, the dilated capillaries and slight hyperplasia of connective tissue in superficial dermis, a few lymphocytes infiltrate in perivascular, and several cystoid structures, which walls consisting of squamous epithelium（HE stain，×100）

7. 痒疹样显性遗传营养不良型大疱性表皮松解症
Prurigo-like inherited epidermolysis bullosa

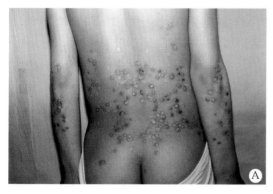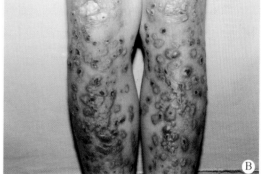

图 27-7-1　A. 腰背部有散在的圆形、椭圆形隆起呈暗棕红色的痒疹样结节、斑块；B. 膝部形成条索状瘢痕和肥厚斑块

Figure 27-7-1　A. Round or oval, brownish red nodules and plaques on the waist and back；B. Funicular scars and thick plaques on the knees

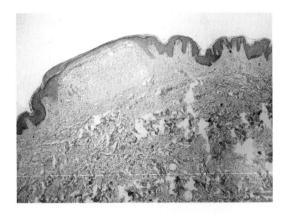

图 27-7-2　表皮变薄、变平,基底细胞液化变性,有典型的粟丘疹结构(HE 染色,×40)

Figure 27-7-2　Epidermis atrophy, liquefication degeneration of the basal layer with typical milia structure (HE stain, ×40)

8. Siemens 大疱性鱼鳞病
Ichthyosis bullosa of Siemens

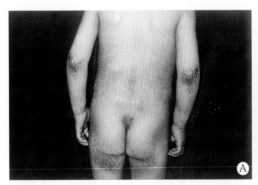
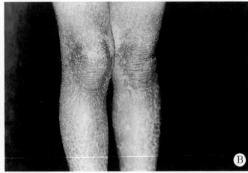

图 27-8-1　A. 全身皮肤明显角化过度,右侧腰围片状脱皮区; B. 下肢明显角化过度,左膝关节内侧片状脱皮区

Figure 27-8-1　A. Marked hyperkeratosis on the whole skin, mauserung peeling of the skin on the right waist; B. Marked hyperkeratosis on the both lower limbs, mauserung peeling of the skin on the flexures of left knee

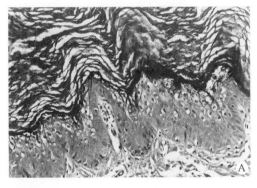
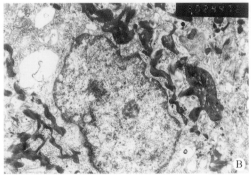

图 27-8-2　A. 角化过度和颗粒层细胞水肿(HE 染色,×200); B. 透射电镜下颗粒层细胞内高密度团块聚集(×5000)

Figure 27-8-2　A. Hyperkeratosis and swollen granular cells (HE stain, ×200); B. High electron-density conglomeration in the granular layer (TEM, ×5000)

9. 表皮松解性角化过度（大疱性先天性鱼鳞病样红皮病）

Epidermolytic hyperkeratosis（Bullous congenital ichthyosiform erythroderma）

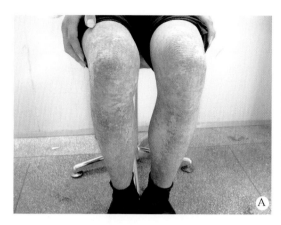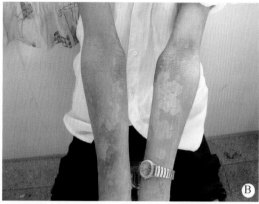

图 27-9-1　A. 双下肢见灰色或深褐色斑块，表面干燥，覆盖肥厚性鳞屑，部分呈疣状，膝关节伸侧形成沟状角化过度；B. 双上肢灰褐色干燥鳞屑斑，肘关节处形成沟状角化过度

Figure 27-9-1　A. Grey or brown, dryness plaques with thickened scales, partly verrucous scaling on the lower limbs, furrowed hyperkeratosis on the extensor of knees; B. Grayish brown macules with dryness scales on the upper limbs, furrowed hyperkeratosis on the elbow joint

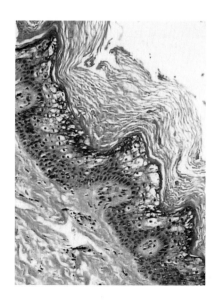

图 27-9-2　角质层呈板层状排列，颗粒层增厚，棘层上部与颗粒层胞质皱缩，核周空泡化，病变处细胞边界不清，可见大小不等腔隙，呈表皮松解性角化过度改变（HE 染色，×100）

Figure 27-9-2　Horny layer arrangement in lamellar, thickened granular layer containing irregularly shaped keratohyaline granules, and perinuclear haloes, epidermal cells detach in the granular cell layer (HE stain, × 100)

10. 表皮松解性角化过度鱼鳞病伴侏儒
Epidermolytic hyperkeratosis ichthyosis complicated by dwarf

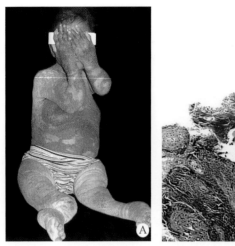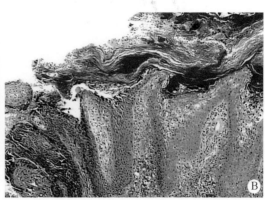

图 27-10-1　A. 全身弥漫性覆盖灰棕色痂皮、鳞屑,边缘高起；B. 表皮角化过度伴角化不全,棘层肥厚,颗粒层中可见裂隙,裂隙内有较多角化不良细胞(HE 染色,×200)

Figure 27-10-1　A. Generalized pale-brownish macules covered crusts and scales with elevated edges on whole body；B. Marked hyperkeratosis and parakeratosis,a fissure filled with some dys-keratotic cell is observed in granular layer of epidermis(HE stain,×200)

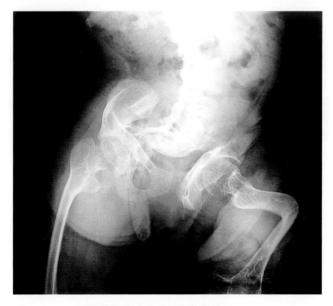

图 27-10-2　双侧股骨发育细小,伴弯曲畸形

Figure 27-10-2　The both fine thighbone with bend deformity

11. 火棉胶婴儿
Collodion baby

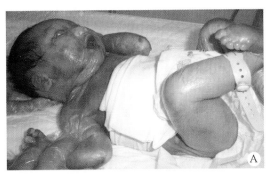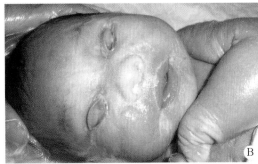

图 27-11-1　A. 新生婴儿全身皮肤包裹在羊皮纸样的膜内,活动受限；B. 眼睑外翻

Figure 27-11-1　A. An infant was born in a constricting parchment-like membrane with that limits motion；B. Ectropion

12. 先天性角化不良
Dyskeratosis congenita

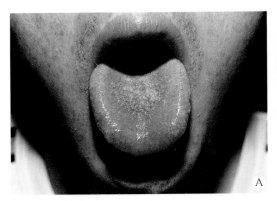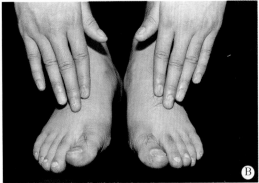

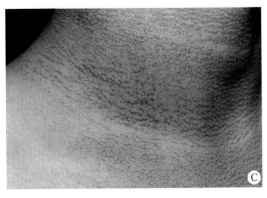

图 27-12-1　A. 舌正中处有一白色增厚斑；B. 指（趾）甲萎缩、纵嵴、部分脱落；C. 颈部条纹或细网状褐色色素沉着斑

Figure 27-12-1　A. Shed leukoplakia on the central of tongue；B. Finger nail and toenail atrophy and vertical stria,partly breaking off；C. Widespread reticulated and hyperpigmented brown patches on the neck

13. 残留性多指症
Rudimentary polydactyly

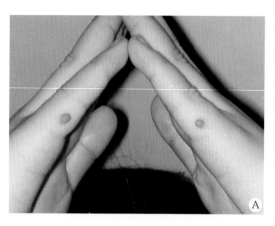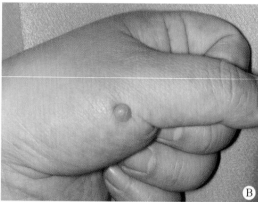

图 27-13-1　A. 双手小指尺侧各见一淡红色结节；B. 左手拇指根部桡侧淡红色半球形结节

Figure 27-13-1　A. Reddish nodules on the ulnar side of the fifth fingers on both hands；B. A reddish hemispherical nodule on the radial aspect of the left thumb

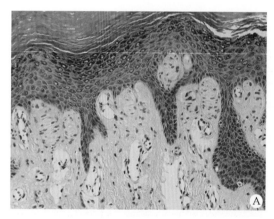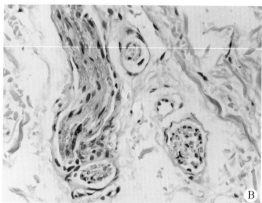

图 27-13-2　A. 真皮乳头层见大量触觉小体及扩张的毛细血管；B. 真皮浅层见较多神经纤维及增生的内皮细胞和毛细血管，真皮网状层见较多神经纤维束，周围见完整的神经束膜

Figure 27-13-2　A. Many Meissner corpuscles and telangiectasias in the dermal papillae；B. Many nerve fibers, proliferating endothelial cells and capillaries in the upper dermis, increased number of nerve fascicles with intact membrane in the reticular dermis

14. 骨膜增生厚皮症
Pachydermoperiostosis

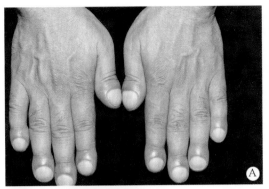
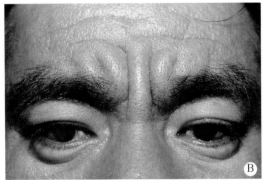

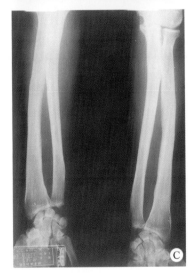

图 27-14-1 A. 十指末端呈杵状膨大；B. 头面部皮肤增厚,形成皱褶；C. 骨皮质增厚

Figure 27-14-1 A. Clubbing of the digits；B. Thickening and furrowing of the skin of the face and scalp；C. The periosteal proliferation ofthe bones of both ulna, radius, tibia and fibula

15. 先天性皮肤缺损
Congenital localized absence of skin

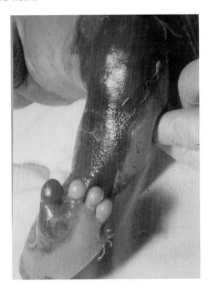

图 27-15-1 生后双小腿和足背有大片糜烂面

Figure 27-15-1 Large eroded areas on both lower legs and dorsa of feet at birth

16. 婴儿肢端纤维瘤病
Infantile digital fibromatosis

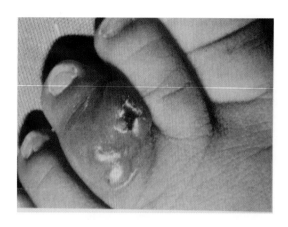

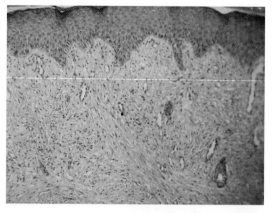

图 27-16-1　左足第 3 趾背有粉红色光滑坚硬结节
Figure 27-16-1　A smooth, hard, pink, monteder nodule on the left third toe

图 27-16-2　真皮上层有大量成纤维细胞增生（HE 染色，×60）
Figure 27-16-2　A large proliferation of spindle-shaped fibroblasts in the upper dermis（HE stain, ×60）

17. 掌跖多发性皮肤纤维瘤
Dermatofibroma

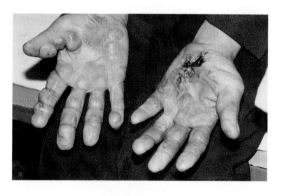

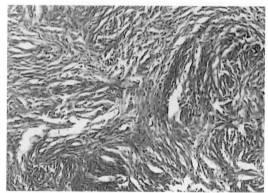

图 27-17-1　几十个呈扁球形、椭圆形、质地坚实的皮色结节
Figure 27-17-1　Numerous round, oval, firm, skin-colored nodules on both palms

图 27-17-2　真皮内纤维组织增生，结节内有纵横交错排列的胶原纤维（HE 染色，×100）
Figure 27-17-2　Fibrous nodules containing collagen fibers irregular arrangement in interwinding in the dermis（HE stain, ×100）

18. 着色性干皮病继发恶性肿瘤
Carcinomas in patients with xeroderma pigmentosa

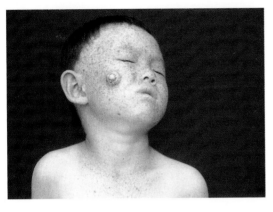

图 27-18-1 面部有点状色素沉着,右侧面部有一肿物,表面呈火山口样

Figure 27-18-1 Mottled pigmentation on the face, a tumor with shallow ulcer on the right face

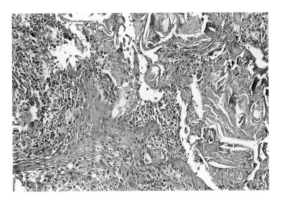

图 27-18-2 继发的鳞状细胞癌,肿瘤与表皮相连,向下深入真皮,境界不清,主要由鳞状细胞组成,细胞异形明显,可见角珠(HE 染色,×100)

Figure 27-18-2 Invasive carcinoma of the epidermis, uncircumscribed tumor consisting of atypical squamous cells and horn pearls in the dermis (HE stain, ×100)

19. 棘状秃发性毛发角化症
Keratosis follicularis spinulosa decalvans

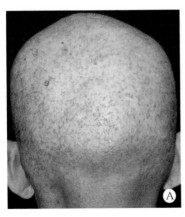

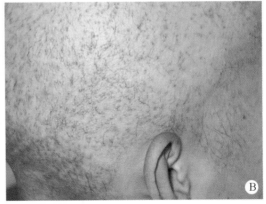

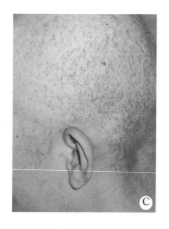

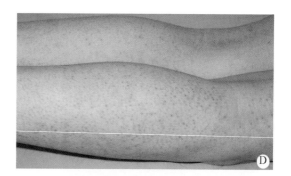

图 27-19-1　A,B,C. 累及整个头皮的瘢痕性脱发,散在许多毛囊性过度角化性丘疹;D. 下肢屈侧毛发角化症

Figures 27-19-1　A,B,C. Extensive cicatricial alopecia involving the entire scalp with follicular hyperkeratotic papules; D. Keratosis pilaris on the flexor surfaces of the lower extremities

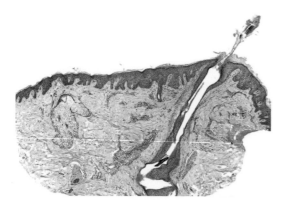

图 27-19-2　毛囊过度角化,毛囊周围轻度纤维化,伴密集慢性炎细胞浸润(HE 染色,×40)

Figure 27-19-2　Follicular hyperkeratosis,mild perifollicular fibrosis with moderately dense chronic inflammatory cell infiltrate(HE stain,×40)

20. 幼年透明蛋白纤维瘤病
Juvenile hyaline fibromatosis

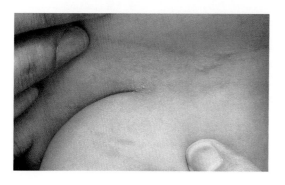

图 27-20-1　右腹股沟枣核大梭形皮下结节

Figure 27-20-1　Fusiform subcutaneous nodules on the right groin

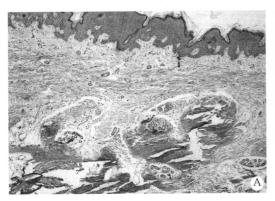
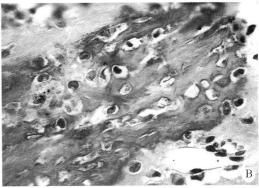

图 27-20-2 A. 肿瘤组织位于真皮内,与周围结缔组织分界清楚,由瘤细胞和基质构成(HE 染色,×40);
B. 肿瘤基质 PAS 染色阳性(PAS 染色,×100)

Figure 27-20-2 A. Tumor cells embedded in the eosinophilic hyaline ground substance with chondroid appearance in the dermis(HE stain,×40); B. PAS positive in tumor stroma (PAS stain,×100)

21. 小斑片三色皮肤征
Cutis tricolor parvimaculata

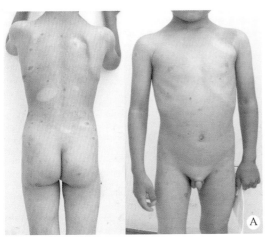
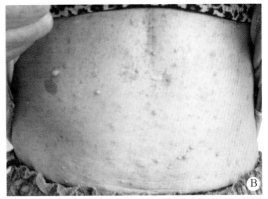

图 27-21-1 A. 出生后,全身散在大小不一的色素沉着斑,在色素沉着斑周围、附近见类似形态的色素减退斑。形成色素沉着斑、色素减退斑及正常皮肤的小斑片三色皮肤;B. 患者母亲腹部神经纤维瘤皮损,腹部见较多牛奶咖啡斑和圆形增生物,其质地较软

Figure 27-21-1 A. Numerous hyperpigmented macules dissseminated on his skin at birth,with small hypopigmented macules serveing as a halo or neighboring. Small patches of hyperpigmentation,hypopigmentation and normally pigmented skin are indictive the diagnosis of cutis tricolor parvimaculata. B. Abdomenal lesions of neurofibromatosis presented in the patient's abdomen. Multiple cafe-au-lait-spots and soft neurofibromas were shown on the abdomen

243

22. 丘疹性弹力纤维离解
Papular elastorrhexis

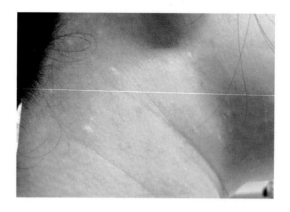

图 27-22-1　下颌及项、枕部白色斑疹及丘疹,呈圆形及多角形

Figure 27-22-1　White indurated macules and papules on the neck and mandibular region. Some are polygonal in shape

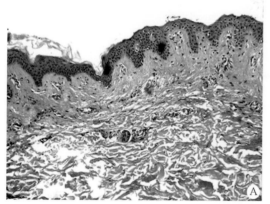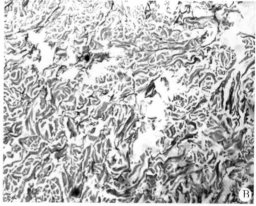

图 27-22-2　A. 棘层轻度增厚,真皮内血管周围淋巴细胞浸润明显,真皮乳头层胶原纤维轻度增生(HE 染色,×100);B. 真皮内弹性纤维明显断裂、减少(Acid orcein 染色,×200)

Figure 27-22-2　A. Pathologically, mild acanthosis, and a perivascular lymphocytic infiltration in the dermis. Collagen fibers increased slightly in the papillary dermis(HE stain,×100); B. Fragmentation and reduction of elastic fiber in the dermis. (Acid orcein stain,×200)

第 28 章
黏膜及黏膜皮肤交界处疾病
Disorders of the Mucous Membranes

1. 梅尔克松-罗森塔尔综合征
Melkersson-Rosenthal syndrome

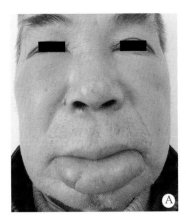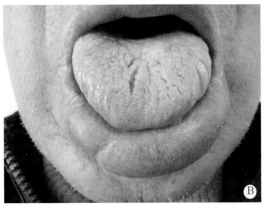

图 28-1-1　A. 左鼻唇沟变浅,口角轻度向右侧偏斜,鼓腮左侧漏气;B. 下唇弥漫性红肿,伸舌稍向右侧偏斜,舌体肥大,舌面有明显沟纹

Figure 28-1-1　A. Left nasolabia shallow fold, slightly rightward commissure; B. Diffuse swelling of the lower lip, tongue slightly skewed to the right, enlarged fissured tongue

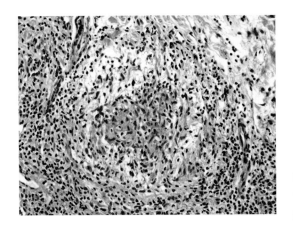

图 28-1-2　真皮深层上皮细胞肉芽肿改变,周围有淋巴细胞浸润(HE 染色,×200)

Figure 28-1-2　Epithelioid granulomas surrounded by lymphocytic infiltration in the deep dermis(HE stain, × 200)

2. 浆细胞性唇炎
Plasma cell cheilitis

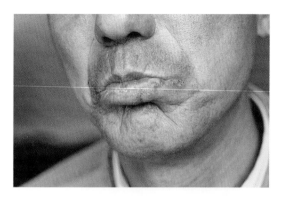

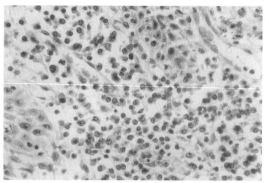

图 28-2-1　下唇有一红色斑块,上覆盖鳞屑和痂

Figure 28-2-1　A dark-red plaque covered with scales and crusts on lower lip

图 28-2-2　真皮内有多数浆细胞和少数淋巴细胞浸润(HE 染色,×500)

Figure 28-2-2　Diffuse infiltration of plasma cells and a few lymphocytes in the dermis(HE stain,×500)

3. 阴茎硬化性淋巴管炎
Sclerosing lymphangiitis

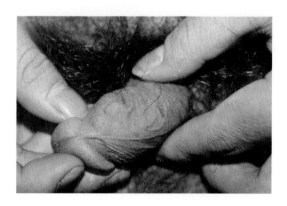

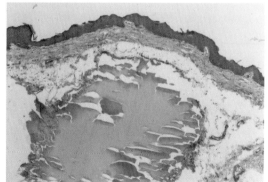

图 28-3-1　包皮内板背侧见皮色半透明条索状物

Figure 28-3-1　A cordlike structure encircling the coronal sulcus of the penis

图 28-3-2　真皮内可见扩张的淋巴管腔,内含均质红染的淋巴液(HE 染色,×40)

Figure 28-3-2　A dilated lymph vessel containing homogeneous lymph liquid in the dermis (HE stain,× 40)

第 29 章
皮肤肿瘤 Tumors of the Skin

一、表皮肿瘤 Epidermal Tumors

1. 棘层松解性角化不良表皮痣
Acantholytic dyskeratotic epidermal nevus

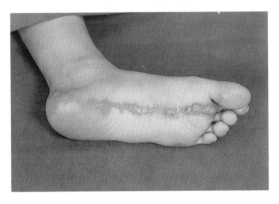

图 29-1-1　左足底第 2 趾端至足跟疣状隆起的丘疹及斑块

Figure 29-1-1　Verruca-like papulars and plaques from the second toe to heel on the left vola pedis

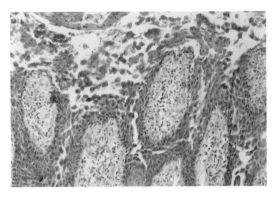

图 29-1-2　基底层上方棘层松解,可见大量角化不良细胞(HE 染色,×200)

Figure 29-1-2　Suprabasal clefts with acantholytic and multiple dyskeratotic cells(HE stain,×200)

2. 棘层松解角化不良性表皮痣并发色素性毛表皮痣

Acantholytic dyskeratotic epidermal naevus complicated by pigmented hairy epidermal naevus

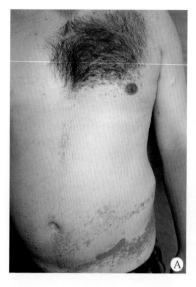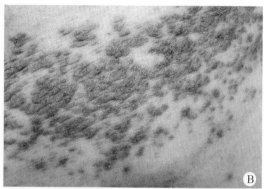

图 29-2-1　A. 左胸片状多毛区,中心部位皮肤纹理较粗,斑片区密集分布的淡红色丘疹,融合成片,左腹部呈带状分布的棕红色疣状丘疹,大部分融合; B. 左侧腹部黄红色毛囊性疣状丘疹,部分融合呈带状分布

Figure 29-2-1　A. A sheet hair with conflenting, damask papules on the left chest, and densely, brown red, verrucous papules partly confluenting arranged in line on the left abdomen; B. Brownish follicle, verrucous papules partly confluenting arranged in line on the left abdomen

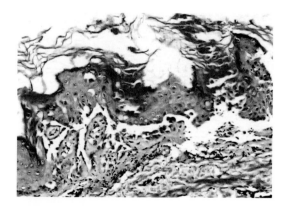

图 29-2-2　表皮呈乳头瘤样增生,有角化过度,基底层上棘层松解和裂隙形成,可见圆体、谷粒(HE 染色, × 100)

Figure 29-2-2　Papillomatosis, hyperkeratosis and focal areas of suprabasal cleft with acantholysis and corps ronds and grains(HE stain, × 100)

3. 泛发性表皮痣
Epidermal nevus

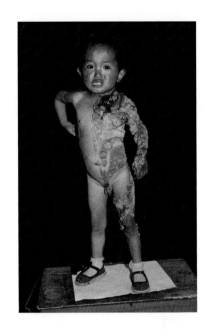

图 29-3-1　左侧颈部、肩、躯干部,左上肢灰褐色角化性疣状增生性皮损,融合成斑块,线状、带状排列,损害偏侧性不超过中线

Figure 29-3-1　Verrucous and hyperkeratotic plaques arranged in linear on the left neck, shoulder, trunk and upper limb

4. 黑头粉刺痣
Comedo naevus

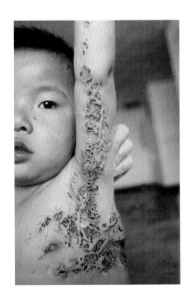

图 29-4-1　左侧胸壁有多数带状分布的黑头粉刺

Figure 29-4-1　Neumerous "black-heads" distributed in band on the left chest

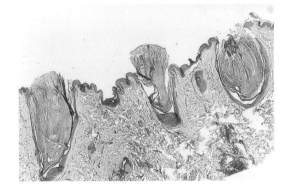

图 29-4-2　在扩张的毛囊口有 3 个角质栓(HE 染色,×200)

Figure 29-4-2　Three keratotic plugs dilate follicular orifice(HE stain,×20)

5. 表皮痣综合征
Epidermal nevus syndrome

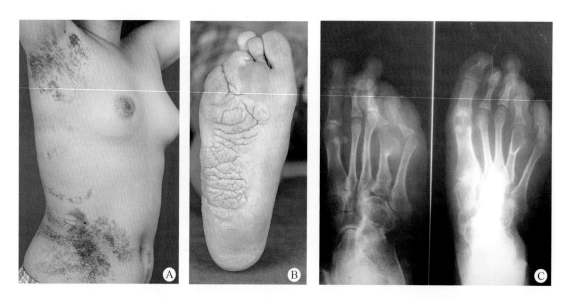

图 29-5-1　A. 右侧腋下、胸部、乳晕及腹部疣状斑块；B. 右足跖皮肤肥厚, 皱褶成沟回状, 第 3 趾呈巨趾, 第 4、5 趾变短；C. 右足多发性骨软骨瘤, 第 3 趾巨趾畸形

Figure 29-5-1　A. Verrucous plaques on the right axilla, chest, periareola and abdomen; B. The soles thickened, the third toe macrodactyly, shortened of the fourth and fifth toe; C. Multiple osteochondroma on the right foot, the third toe macrodactyly

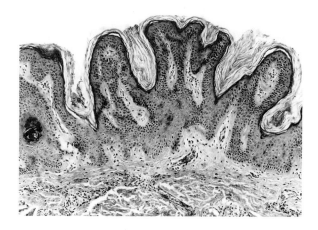

图 29-5-2　表皮角化过度, 棘层肥厚, 基底层色素增加, 真皮浅层血管周围淋巴细胞浸润(HE 染色, ×100)

Figure 29-5-2　Hyperkeratosis, acanthosis, hyperpigmentation of basal layer, and perivascular lymphyocytes infiltrate in the upper dermis (HE stain, ×100)

6. 多发性小丘疹脂溢性角化病
Multiple small papular seborrheic keratosis

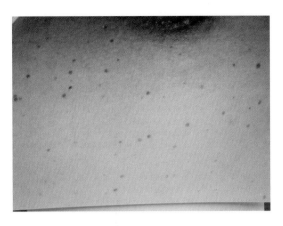

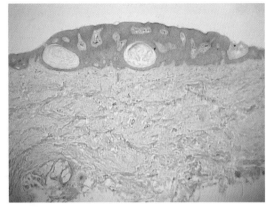

图 29-6-1　胸部和腹部有多数褐色小丘疹

Figure 29-6-1　Numerous small brown papules on the chest and obdomen

图 29-6-2　表皮内有中度棘层肥厚和角质囊肿(HE 染色,×100)

Figure 29-6-2　Moderate acanthosis and horncysts in the epidermis (HE stain,×100)

7. 放线型分布的脂溢性角化病
Seborrheic keratosis distributed along skin cleavage lines

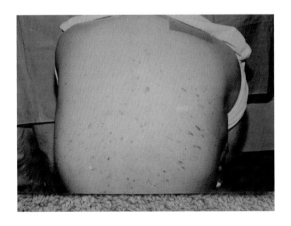

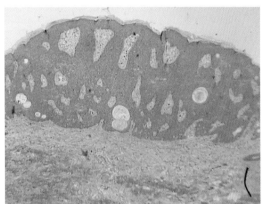

图 29-7-1　背部有棕色纺锤形轻度隆起的丘疹沿皮肤割线分布

Figure 29-7-1　Brownish spindle,slightly raised papules tended to follow skin cleavage lines on lower back

图 29-7-2　表皮内有角化过度,棘层肥厚,角囊肿和基底细胞增殖(HE 染色,×100)

Figure 29-7-2　Hyperkeratosis, acanthosis, horn cysts,and proliferation of basal cells in the epidermis (HE stain,×100)

8. 雨滴状脂溢性角化症
Raindrop-like seborrheic keratoses

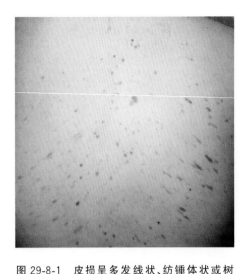

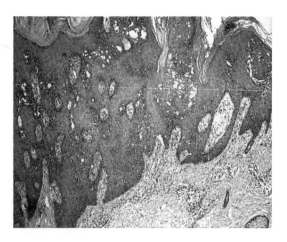

图 29-8-1　皮损呈多发线状、纺锤体状或树叶状,沿皮肤纹理线状或放射状分布

Figure 29-8-1　Multiple linear, spindle-or leaf-shaped eruptions distributed linearly or radially along the direction of skin cleavage lines

图 29-8-2　表皮角化过度,棘层增厚和角囊肿,真皮内有慢性炎症反应。鳞状上皮和基底层细胞增生,棘层细胞增厚(HE 染色, × 100)

Figure 29-8-2　Hyperkeratosis and acanthosis and horn cysts in the epidermis and chronic inflammatory reaction in dermis. The stratum Malpighi showed moderate acanthosis caused by proliferation of squamous and basal cells(HE stain, × 100)

9. 脂溢性角化病和卵状糠秕马拉色菌
Seborrheic keratosis and pityrosporum ovale

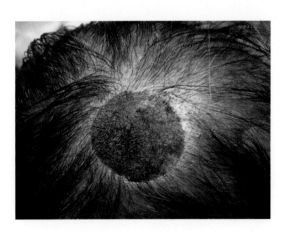

图 29-9-1　头部有一个大黑色角化斑块

Figure 29-9-1　A large black keratotic plaque on the head

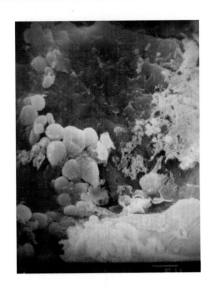

图 29-9-2　扫描电子显微镜发现皮损角质层表面有许多圆形和卵圆形孢子

Figure 29-9-2　Lots of round and oval spores found on the horny layer observed by Scanning electronic microscopy

10. 大细胞棘皮瘤

Large cell acanthoma

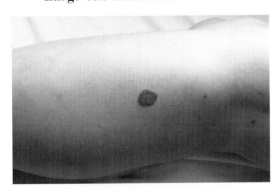

图 29-10-1　小腿外侧轻度隆起的淡褐色斑块

Figure 29-10-1　Light brown plaque on the lateral side of calf

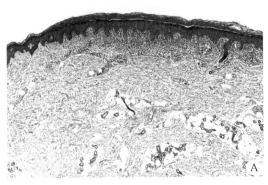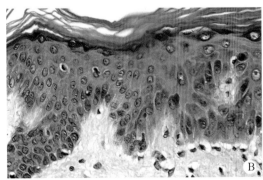

图 29-10-2　A. 表皮增生,棘层肥厚,并伴有明显炎性细胞浸润(HE 染色,×100);B. 棘层肥厚,细胞体积明显增大(HE 染色,×400)

Figure 29-10-2　A. Epidermal hyperplasia, acanthosis and inflammatory cell infiltrate (HE stain, ×100); B. Enlarged keratinocytes and acanthosis (HE stain, ×400)

11. 巨大皮角
Giant cutaneous horn

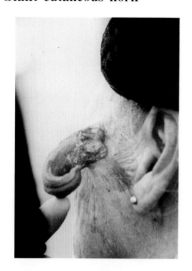

图 29-11-1　皮角呈牛角状,基底暗紫色,表面粗糙
Figure 29-11-1　Ox horn like dark purple lesions with coarse surface

12. 发疹性毳毛囊肿
Eruptive vellus hair cyst

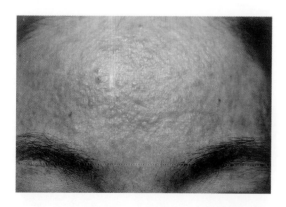

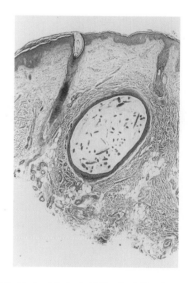

图 29-12-1　额部散在许多毛囊性丘疹,呈灰蓝色,少数丘疹顶端可见脐凹
Figure 29-12-1　Numerous blue hair follicle papules on the forehead, a few papules having umbilicated surface

图 29-12-2　真皮中部囊肿形成,囊壁为鳞状上皮,囊壁较薄,囊内含有许多毳毛的横断面或斜切面(HE 染色,×40)
Figure 29-12-2　Cysts in the upper middermis lined by squamous epithelium, containing numerous transversely or obliquely cut vellus hairs (HE stain, ×40)

13. Pinkus 纤维上皮瘤

Fibroepithelioma of Pinkus

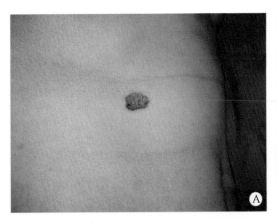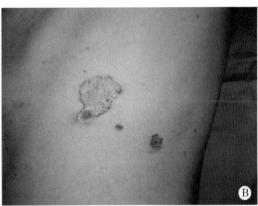

图 29-13-1　两侧腰部见 4 个褐色、淡红色斑,分别为 0.3cm×0.3cm、1cm×1cm、1cm×2cm 和 3cm×4cm 大,较大皮损边缘褐黑色、稍隆起,可见扩张的毛囊口,中央淡红色、轻度萎缩,表面无糜烂、渗出,无浸润

Figure 29-13-1　Four brown or erythrous maculae or patches with a brown-colored, elevated borderline in different size on two sides of the waist. Some dilated follicular orifices are seen in the fringe. The central part of the patches is erythrous and slight atrophy, without erosion and infiltration

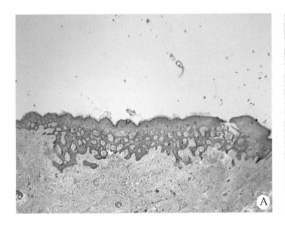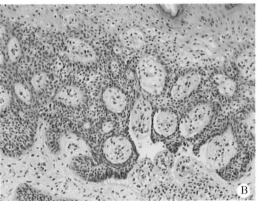

图 29-13-2　A. 轻度角化过度,棘层轻度肥厚(HE 染色,×40);B. 棘层下方大量基底样细胞增生,增生的肿瘤细胞条索伸入真皮毗邻吻合形成网络状,基底细胞胞核大而深染,胞质少,呈嗜碱性,基底层黑素颗粒增多,基底膜完整。真皮中部血管扩张,有以淋巴细胞为主的大量炎症细胞浸润(HE 染色,×200)

Figure 29-13-2　A. Mild hyperkeratosis and acanthosis in the epidermis. (HE stain, ×40); B. Reticulated strands of basaloid cells extending into the dermis. The macronuclei of basal cells are deeply basophilic. There are more melanin granules in basal layers and the basement membrane is integrated. Hemangiectasia and numerous lymphocytes infiltration in the mid-dermis. (HE stain, ×200)

14. Pinkus 纤维上皮瘤合并基底细胞癌
Fibroepithelioma of Pinkus associated with basal cell carcinoma

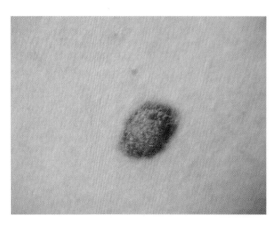

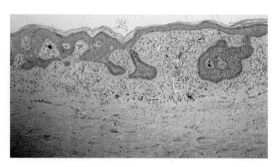

图 29-14-1　Pinkus 纤维上皮瘤患者二年后（图 29-13）腹部和胸部有两个浸润性红斑

Figure 29-14-1　Two years later two infiltrated erythematous patches on the abdomen and chest

图 29-14-2　表皮基底部有向真皮不规则增生的肿瘤细胞组成的团块（HE 染色，×100）

Figure 29-14-2　The tumor showed buds and irregular proliferations of tumor attached to the undersurface of the epidermis(HE stain, ×100)

15. 多发性角化棘皮瘤
Multiple keratoacanthoma

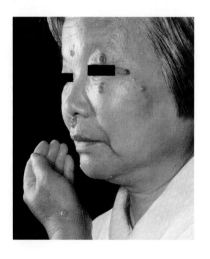

图 29-15-1　13 个坚实半球形 0.5～1.0cm 直径大结节，中心呈火山口状，分布在面部和手腕

Figure 29-15-1　Thirteen firm, dome-shaped nodules 0.5-1.0cm in diameter with a homfilled crater in its center on the face and wrist

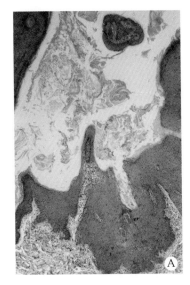
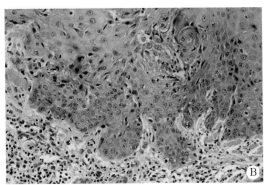

图 29-15-2　A. 一个大而不规则的火山口,中充满角化物质(HE 染色,×40);B. 火山口底部增生的表皮细胞中有核异形和不典型核分裂(HE 染色,×100)

Figure 29-15-1　A. A large, irregularly shaped crater filled with keratin(HE stain, ×40); B. The epidermal proliferatins at the base of creter show nuclear atypia and atypical mitoses(HE stain, ×100)

16. 鲍温病
Bowen's disease

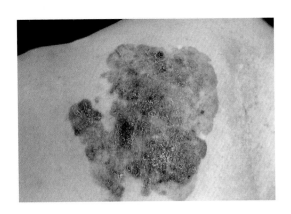

图 29-16-1　左侧肩胛区可见一暗红色斑块,边界清,呈不规则形,基底潮红,上覆少许黄痂和鳞屑

Figure 29-16-1　A sharply defined irregular erythematous with slightly scaly and crust on the left scapular area

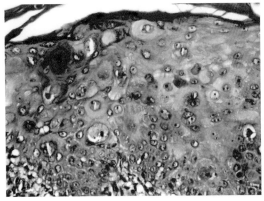

图 29-16-2　表皮角化过度伴角化不全,棘层肥厚,整个表皮排列完全紊乱,许多细胞呈高度不典型性,核的大小、形态和染色深浅不一(HE 染色,×400)

Figure 29-16-2　Hyperkeratosis, parakeratosis and acanthosis, the epidermal cells lie in complete disorder and many of them are atypical showing large and hyperchromatic nuclei (HE stain, ×400)

17. 多发性鲍温病
Multiple Bowen's disease

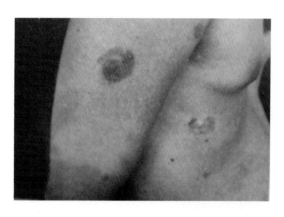

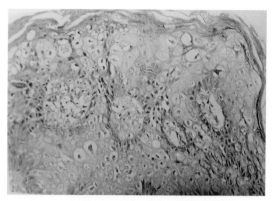

图 29-17-1　上臂、胸、腹散在棕褐色丘疹、斑块,表面浅糜烂、结痂

Figure 29-17-1　Brownish papules and plaques with superficial erosions and crusts on the the upper arm, chest and abdomen

图 29-17-2　表皮细胞大小不一,排列紊乱,见空泡细胞及少数异形核分裂象(HE 染色,×400)

Figure 29-17-2　The cells of the stratum malpighii lie in complete disorder, some of them on vacuolization and atypical mitotic figures (HE stain, ×400)

18. 生殖器 Paget 病
Genital Paget's disease

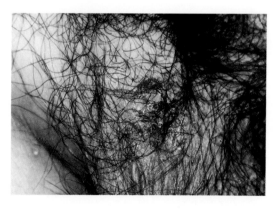

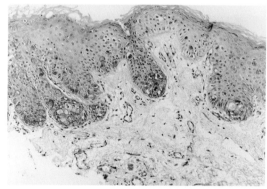

图 29-18-1　阴囊、阴茎、会阴部浸润性红斑或斑块,边界较清楚,其中央有糜烂和浅溃疡

Figure 29-18-1　Infiltrated well-circumscribed erythemas and plaques with central erosion and superficial ulcers on the scrotum, penis and perineum

图 29-18-2　表皮内散在或群集的细胞,其胞体是棘细胞的 1~2 倍大,无细胞棘突,胞质丰富而淡染,呈空泡状,核呈圆形或椭圆形,染色较深,有的细胞核被挤到一边,呈新月状,胞质 PAS 染色阳性(PAS 染色,×200)

Figure 29-18-2　Scattered PAS-positive Paget's cells in the epidermis (PAS stain, ×200)

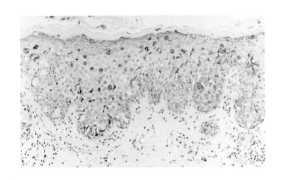

图 29-18-3　免疫组化染色见表皮内散在或群集的上皮膜抗原(EMA)阳性细胞(APC 法,×200)

Figure 29-18-3　Epithelial membrane antigen（EMA）positive cells scatter or group in the epidermis（APC stain,×200）

19. 疣状表皮发育不良继发基底鳞状细胞癌和多发性纤维毛囊瘤

Epidermodysplasia verruciformis associated with basal squamous cell carcinoma and multiple fibrofolliculoma

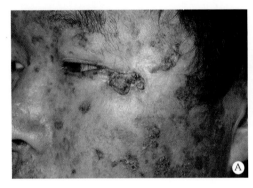
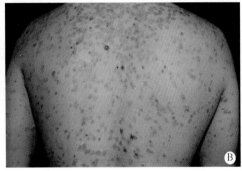

图 29-19-1　A. 左眼下方有一蚕豆大的灰色角化性斑块,中央破溃,边缘隆起；B. 背部见许多绿豆至黄豆大褐色斑片,轻度角化

Figure 29-19-1　A. The size of horsebean grey keratosis plaque with central erosion and margin ridgy；B. The size of mung bean to soybean brown macula with lightly keratosis

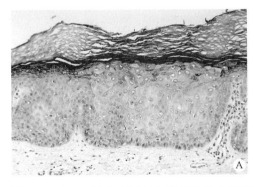
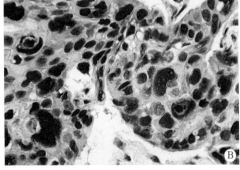

图 29-19-2　A. 表皮角化过度,棘层肥厚,可见较多空泡细胞(HE 染色,×100)；B. 真皮散在基底细胞和鳞状细胞团块,部分细胞核大,呈卵圆形或长形,胞质较少(HE 染色,×400)

Figure 29-19-2　A. Hyperkeratosis,acanthosis and numerous vacuolated cells in the epidermis（HE stain,×100）；B. Irregular nests of basal cells and squamous cells invading the dermis in varying degrees and interspaces between the cell nests（HE stain,×400）

20. 浅表性基底细胞上皮瘤
Superficial basal cell epithelioma

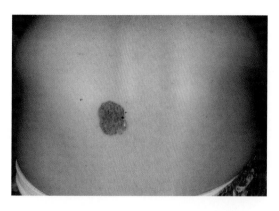

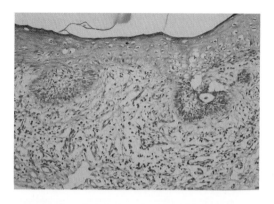

图 29-20-1　背部有紫红色斑,边缘有黑褐色丘疹

Figure 29-20-1　A purplish red patch surrounded by dark bown papules on the back

图 29-20-2　肿瘤团块与表皮相连,团块由基底样细胞构成,团块周围细胞呈栅栏栏状排列(HE 染色, ×200)

Figure 29-20-2　The buds of tumor cells attached to the undersurface of the epidermis. The peripheral cells of tumor show palisade arrangenment (HE stain,×200)

21. 毛囊漏斗形基底细胞癌
Infundibulocystic basal cell carcinoma

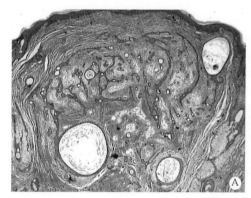

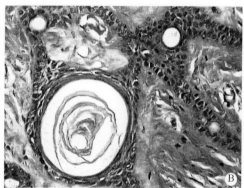

图 29-21-1　A. 真皮内肿瘤境界清除,上皮样细胞条索状增殖相互交织成网状,伴多个毛囊漏斗上皮样结构的囊肿(HE 染色,×40);B. 肿瘤团块中央细胞为胞质丰富淡染的鳞状细胞,而外周细胞为呈栅栏状排列的核深染基底样细胞,囊肿内含角蛋白或毳毛,类似毛囊漏斗部结构,无毛球和毛乳头结构,黏蛋白丰富(HE 染色,×200)

Figure 29-21-1　A. A well-circumscribed,intradermal tumor is composed of many anastomosing cords and strands of epithelial cells with a reticulated pattern,. There are multiple infundibular cystic structures scattered throughout the neoplasm. (HE stain,×40); B. Squamoid cells are present in the central of the tumor with oval pale nuclei,while peripheral cell layer is composed of basaloid cells with hyperchromatic,elongated nuclei in a palisade arrangement,the cyts containing corneocytes or wholly hair are lined by follicular infundibular epithelium,follicular bulbs and papillae are absent with abundant mucin(HE stain,×200)

22. 慢性放射性皮炎继发鳞状细胞癌
Chronic radiodermatitis secondary squamous cell carcinoma

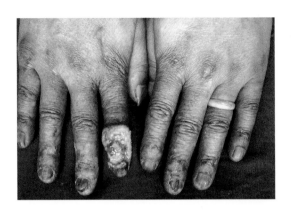

图 29-22-1 双手指背干燥、角化、脱屑、色素沉着，轻度萎缩。多个指甲明显增厚，呈暗褐黄色。右手示指第 1、2 指节伸侧见一溃疡，溃疡周围似肉芽肿样肿胀

Figure 29-22-1 Dryness, keratosis, peeling, hyperpigmentation and slight atrophy, several marked thickened brownish yellow nails, a ulcer on the extensor of the first and second knuckle of index finger

23. 皮肤透明细胞鳞状细胞癌
Cutaneous clear cell squamous cell carcinoma

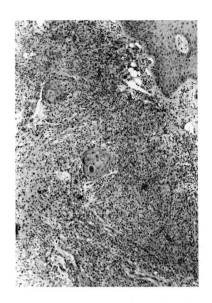

图 29-22-2 表皮不规则增生，未见明显异形性。真皮全层可见多个肿瘤细胞团块，部分团块中央可见角珠，肿瘤细胞呈明显非典型性，可见核分裂象及不对称分裂象（HE 染色，×100）

Figure 29-22-2 Irregular hyperplasia epidermis, many tumor cell masses with marked atypical cells, mitotic figures and atypical mitotic in the whole dermis (HE stain, ×100)

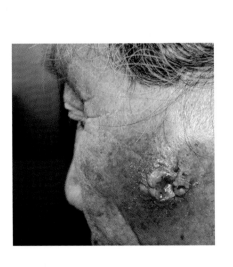

图 29-23-1 左颊部有一个 2cm×2cm 的结节、溃疡
Figure 29-23-1 A 2cm×2cm nodular and ulcer on the left vizard。

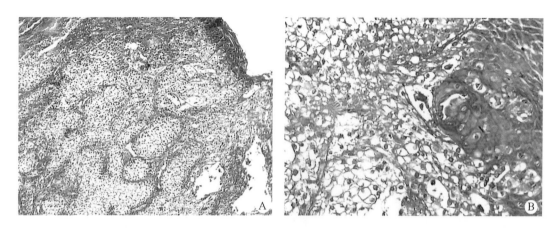

图 29-23-2　癌细胞呈巢状,细胞为多角形,胞质透明,核明显异型(HE 染色,A,×100;B,×400)

Figure 29-23-2　The tumor masses consist of normal squamous cells and of atypical squamous cells which with clear cytoplasm and atypical nuclei (HE stain,A,×100;B,×400)

24. 双侧斑块型粟丘疹

Bilateral milia en plaque

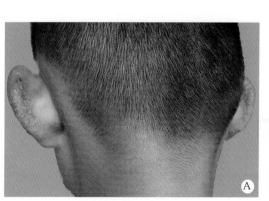
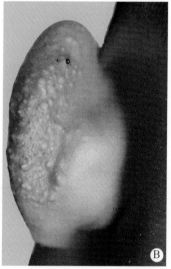

图 29-24-1　A. 双侧耳后可见密集黄白色,轻微红斑上散在少许开放性粉刺;B. 左耳的近观图,红色斑块上许多粟丘疹和黑头粉刺

Figure 29-24-1　A. White yellow cystic lesions scattered within slightly erythematous plaques symmetrically localized on the posterior aspects of both his ears;B. Close view of the left ear. Multiple milia and a few open comedones overlaid the erythematous plaques

25. 外耳道内斑块型粟丘疹

Milia en plaque in bilateral auricular canals

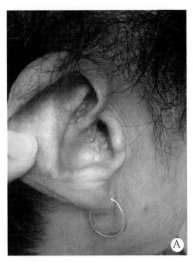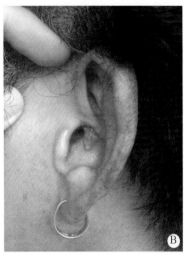

图 29-25-1　双侧外耳道内,基底部红斑上簇集性肤色-灰色丘疹,直径 3～5mm

Figure 29-25-1　Grouped skin-coloured to gray papules,3 to 5 mm in diameter on erythematous background,symmetrically located at the end points of the bilateral auricular canals

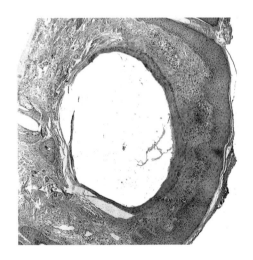

图 29-25-2　见复层鳞状上皮包裹的表皮下囊肿,周围有中度的淋巴细胞浸润(HE 染色,×100)

Figure 29-25-2　A well-formed cyst just beneath the epidermis was enveloped by the stratified squamous epithelium and surrounded by a moderate lymphocytic infiltration (HE stain,×100)

26. 多发性发疹性粟丘疹
Multiple eruptive milia

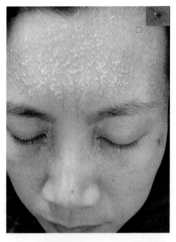

图 29-26-1　面部密集分布的白色丘疹,尤其在额部和双侧鼻唇沟处

Figure 29-26-1　Multiple monomorphic white papules distributed on her face,especially on her forehead and bilateral infraorbital regions

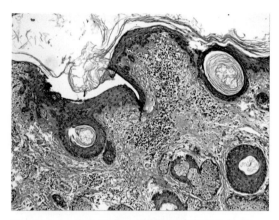

图 29-26-2　表皮下囊肿,囊壁为复层鳞状上皮(HE 染色,×100)

Figure 29-26-2　Some well-formed cysts just beneath the epidermis enveloped by a stratified squamous epithelium (HE stain,×100)

27. 四黑头扩张孔
Dilated pore with four comedos

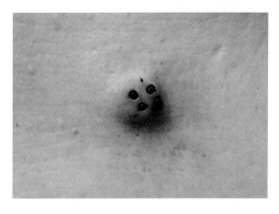

图 29-27-1　躯干上部有一个有 4 个开放性黑头粉刺的丘疹

Figure 29-27-1　A solitary popular with four open comedos on the trunk

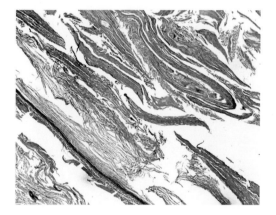

图 29-27-2　扩张孔中充满大量角质(HE 染色,×100)

Figure 29-27-2　A dilated pore was filled with cornified debris(HE stain,×100)

28. 倒置性毛囊角化病
Inverted follicular keratosis

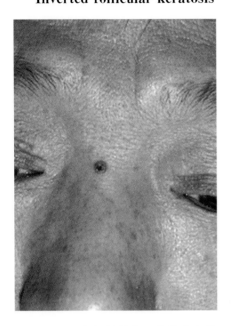

图 29-28-1　鼻梁根部有一米粒大角化性丘疹,呈灰褐色,界限清楚,中央破溃,表面结黑色痂

Figure 29-28-1　A millet-sized, well-circumscribed dust-colour papule with central erosions and black crust on the base of nose bridge

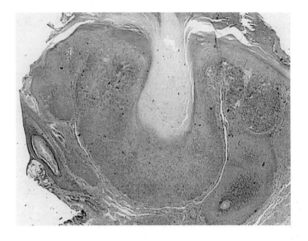

图 29-28-2　可见角质栓的陷窝,壁部由鳞状上皮覆盖,周边部为基底样细胞,中央为外毛根鞘细胞,形成鳞状漩涡,增生组织周围有毛囊结构(HE 染色,×20)

Figure 29-28-2　Keratin-filled invaginations covered with squamous epidermis, around basaloid cells, formation of squamous eddies and follicular structures(HE stain, ×20)

二、皮肤附属器肿瘤 Tumors of the Epidermal Appendages

30. 皮脂腺痣
Facial nevus sebaceous

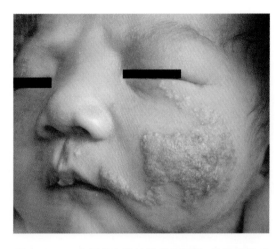

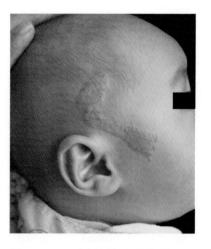

图 29-30-1　左面部多发性棕黄色斑块，呈蟹足样或"W"形

Figure 29-30-1　Multiple, brown-orange plaques on the left side of the baby's face presented as a creeping crab or the letter "W" shape

图 29-30-2　右侧颞部和颧部镰刀形黄红色斑块

Figure 29-30-2　A sickle-shaped yellowish-red plaque was located on the right temple and the pars zygomatica

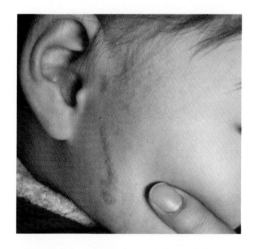

图 29-30-3　右侧耳前区钩形黄红色斑块

Figure 29-30-3　The plaque arranged in a linear pattern on the right preauricular region, presented as a hook-shape

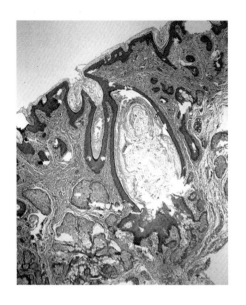

图 29-30-4 病理上,表皮轻度角化过度,伴有角质栓。真皮浅层可见基底样团块和条索,真皮中部许多成熟的皮脂腺(HE 染色,×100)
Figure 29-30-4 Histologically, there was slightly hyperkeratinization of the epidermis as well as multiple keratinous plugs. A few basaloid clumps and chords in the superficial layer of dermis and numerous mature sebaceous glands in the mid-dermis were observed. (HE stain, ×100)

31. 皮脂腺痣合并大汗腺囊腺瘤

Nevus sebaceus with apocrine cyst adenoma

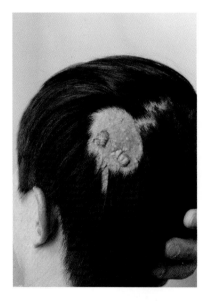

图 29-31-1 头部淡黄色斑块,其上有糜烂面
Figure 29-31-1 A flaxen plaque with erosions on scalp

267

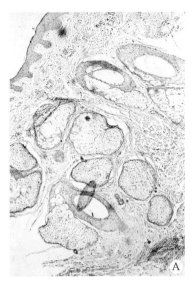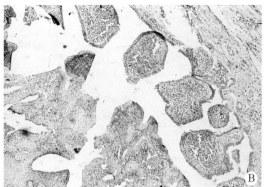

图 29-31-2　A. 与毛囊相连的皮脂腺小叶大量增生(HE 染色,×100);B. 表皮呈乳头瘤样增生,真皮内囊腔壁由两层构成,内层显示顶浆分泌(HE 染色,×100)

Figure 29-31-2　A. Numerous mature sebaceous glands in the upper dermis (HE stain,×100);B. Papillomatosis in the epidermis, a cystic invagination lined by two rows of cells, decapitation secretion of the nearest luminal cells (HE stain,×100)

32. 乳晕皮脂腺增生

Sebaceous hyperplasia around nipple

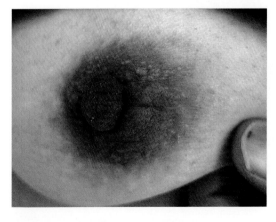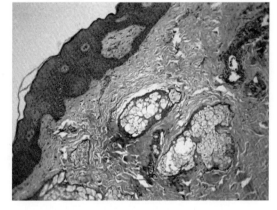

图 29-32-1　右乳晕散在多个肤色结节

Figure 29-32-1　Numerous skin color nodules around the right nipple

图 29-32-2　真皮浅层可见增生的皮脂腺小叶(HE 染色,×100)

Figure 29-32-2　Several enlarged sebaceous lobules in the upper dermis(HE stain,×100)

33. 线状皮脂腺痣综合征
Linear nevus sebaceous syndrome

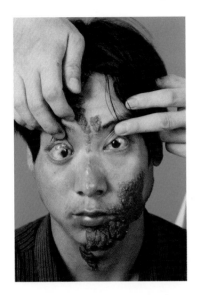

图 29-33-1　左眼球呈上转位,上方球结膜充血,增生的组织沿上方球结膜向角膜浸润,左侧面部不规则分叶状棕黑色肿物,表面粗糙,凹凸不平

Figure 29-33-1　Lesions of nevus sebaceous located in the midline of the scalp and on both sides of the face, pterygium of bilateral conjunctivae with high myopic retina

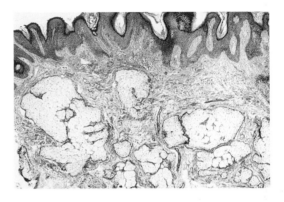

图 29-33-2　表皮呈乳头瘤样增生,角化过度,皮脂腺过度增生呈结节状(HE 染色,×100)

Figure 29-33-2　A large numbers of sebaceous glands and papillomatous hyperplasia of the epidermis with hyperkeratosis(HE stain,×100)

34. 大汗腺囊瘤
Apocrine hidrocystoma around nipple

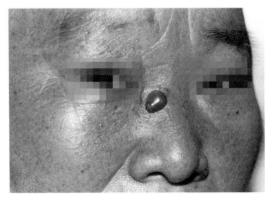

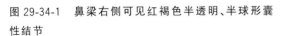

图 29-34-1　鼻梁右侧可见红褐色半透明、半球形囊性结节

Figure 29-34-1　A rufous translucent nodule of cystic consistency on the right of bridge of nose

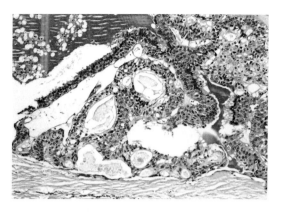

图 29-34-2　瘤体为大汗腺分泌部分的增生性腺瘤，位于真皮内，有较大的囊腔，衬以两层囊壁细胞，内层分泌细胞呈高柱状，顶端有顶浆分泌（HE 染色，×100）

Figure 29-34-2　The dermis contains several large cystic spaces into which papillary projections often extend, the inner surface of the wall and the papillary projections lined by a row of secretory cells of variable height showing "decapitation" secretion indicative of apocrine secretion (HE stain, ×100)

35. 恶性小汗腺汗孔瘤
Malignant eccrine poroma

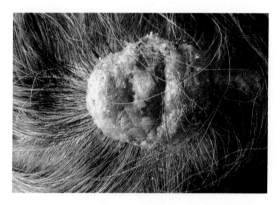

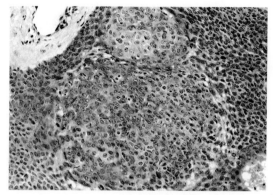

图 29-35-1　头皮见一核桃大肿块，边界清楚，色暗红，表面破溃，基底潮湿，表面凹凸不平

Figure 29-35-1　A well-circumscribed, walnut sized, brownish red nodule with erosions and wet base on the scalp

图 29-35-2　周围基底样细胞体积较小，呈立方形，排列紧密，中央不典型嗜伊红鳞状细胞体积较大，核深染，有明显异形性（HE 染色，×200）

Figure 29-35-2　Tumor locate in the epidermis, composed most of basel like cells and some atypically eosinophilic squamous cells scattered as masses (HE stain, ×200)

36. 带状疱疹样分布的多发性小汗腺螺旋腺瘤
Multiple eccrine spiradenomas in a linear or zosteriform distribution

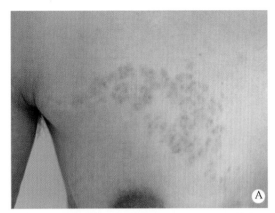

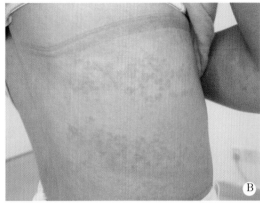

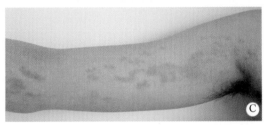

图 29-36-1 右侧胸前(A)、腰腹部(B)、上肢屈侧(C)条带状紫红色斑疹,沿肋间神经或肢体纵轴分布

Figure 29-36-1 Zosteriform distribution of purple maculae on the right chest(A),aspect side of upper limb(B), waist and abdomen (C) along the intercostal nerve or long axis of limb

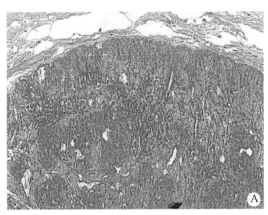

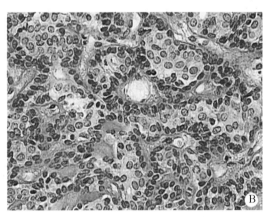

图 29-36-2 A. 真皮深部一个大的和多个小的境界清楚的瘤细胞团块,周围有纤维包膜(HE 染色,×100);B. 瘤组织由两种细胞组成,一种细胞核大、淡染,位于细胞团块中央,另一种细胞核小、深染,排列在瘤细胞索周边,部分瘤细胞排列成玫瑰花样,并可见少数小管腔(HE 染色,×100)

Figure 29-36-2 A. A large and many small, well-circumscribed, dermal nodule comprised of tumors surrounded by fibrous membrane(HE stain, ×100); B. Tumors were composed of cells with large, lightly stained nuclei located in the center of the tumor, and some cells with small, darkly stained nuclei around the Tumor. Some tumor cells are arranged in rose pattern with a few small lumens(HE stain, ×100)

37. 汗管瘤合并粟丘疹
Syringoma associated with milium-like lesions

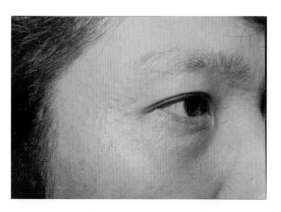

图 29-37-1　颞部有孤立的丘疹,部分丘疹合并粟丘疹

Figure 29-37-1　Solitary papules and papules associated with milium-like lesions on the temple

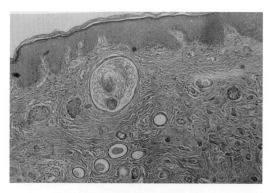

图 29-37-2　真皮有角质囊肿,其下方有多数含有胶样物质的囊管和上皮细胞 (HE 染色,×100)

Figure 29-37-2　A keratin-filled cyst in the papillary dermis. Below are numerous cystic ducts containing colloidal material and epithelial strands (HE stain,×100)

38. 发疹型汗管瘤
Eruptive syringoma

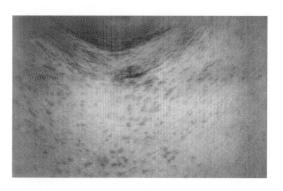

图 29-38-1　颈下至前胸泛发黄色、黄褐色实质性丘疹,隆起于皮面

Figure 29-38-1　Numerous yellow and snuffcolored papules on the neck to prothorax

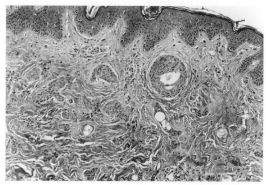

图 29-38-2　真皮浅层散在上皮细胞条索和细胞巢,部分细胞巢中见形成囊腔的腺管样结构(HE 染色,×200)

Figure 29-38-2　Epithelial cords and cell islands in the upper dermis,part of cells are lands containing ductal structures(HE stain,×200)

39. 粟丘疹样表现的外阴汗管瘤

Milia-like syringoma

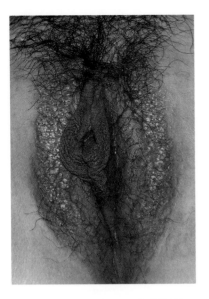

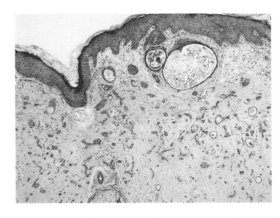

图 29-39-1　双侧大阴唇密集粟粒至绿豆大肤色丘疹,部分丘疹顶端可见淡白色小丘疹,不融合

Figure 29-39-1　The dense skin-colored papules size of millet to mung bean on the both of labia majora

图 29-39-2　表皮角化过度,棘层轻度肥厚,真皮浅层可见角质囊肿,真皮全层散在大小不一的囊腔,腔内有嗜酸性无定形物,可见许多实性细胞条索(HE染色,×40)

Figure 29-39-2　Hyperkeratosis,keratin cysts in superficial dermis,cystic ductal lumina filled with acidophil and many cells cords (HE stain,×40)

40. 泛发性发疹性透明细胞汗管瘤

Generalized eruptire clear-cell syringoma

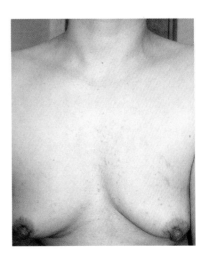

图 29-40-1　颈、躯干淡褐色或肤色 1～2mm 大的小丘疹

Figure 29-40-1　Multiple,small,skin-colored or slightly yellowish, soft papules 1mm or 2mm in size on the neck and trunk

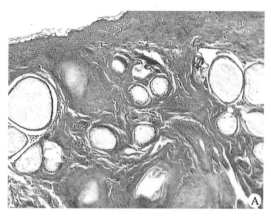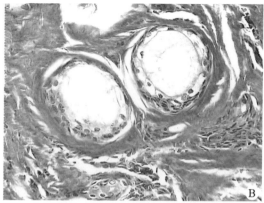

图 29-40-2　A. 真皮有数个小导管,细胞岛形状不规则,大小不一(HE 染色,×100);B. 细胞岛多由透明细胞组成(HE 染色,×400)

Figure 29-40-2　A. The dermis contains several small ducts, cell islands that are irregular in shape and of varing size(HE stain,×100);B. these islands composed of clear cells(HE stain,×400)

41. 乳头状汗管囊腺瘤
Syringocystadenoma papilliferum

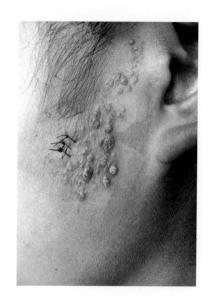

图 29-41-1　左耳前密集粟粒至黄豆大淡红色丘疹,部分中心有脐凹

Figure 29-41-1　Many pink papules on the left preauricular,some of them had an umbilicated center

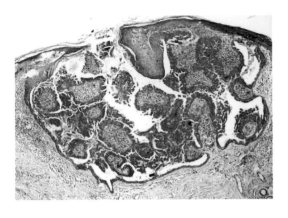

图 29-41-2　表皮呈囊状凹陷,囊腔内有很多绒毛状突起(HE 染色,×40)

Figure 29-41-2　Cystic invaginations in the epidermis, numerous papillary projections extend into the lumen of the cystic invagination(HE stain,×40)

42. 鼻翼部毛囊瘤
Trichofolliculoma

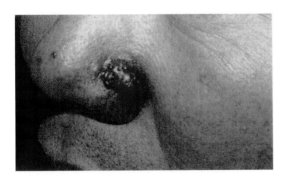

图 29-42-1　左鼻翼部淡红色肿块,中央凹陷见毳毛

Figure 29-42-1　Slightly reddish nodules on the left nasolabial folds with vellous hairs in a central pore

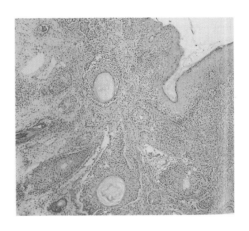

图 29-42-2　真皮内可见多个角化囊肿,囊内可见双折光的毛干(HE 染色,×50)

Figure 29-42-2　Numerous keratinous cysts in the dermal,hair shaft with double refraction in the cysts (HE stain,×50)

43. 微囊肿性附属器癌
Microcystic adnexal carcinoma

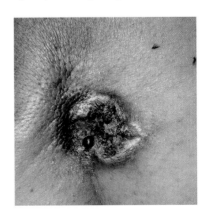

图 29-43-1　胸部右侧浸润性硬斑块,表面结黑褐色痂,皮损与胸壁固定

Figure 29-43-1　An indurated and unmovable plaque with a black crust on its surface on the right chest

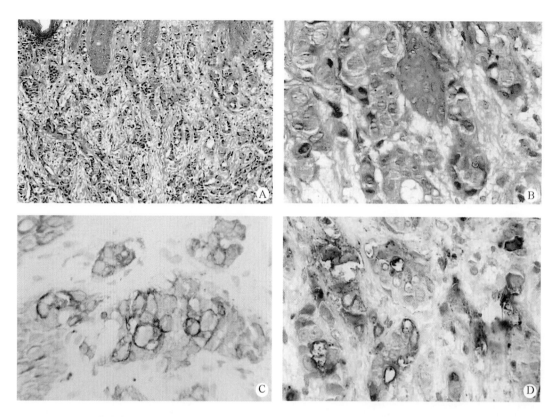

图 29-43-2　A. 表皮角化过度,真皮内肿瘤细胞排列成索状、腺样、小梁状(HE 染色,×100);B. 肿瘤组织周围成基底样细胞排列,中央有鳞状上皮分化(HE 染色,×400);C. 肿瘤细胞 AE1/AE3 阳性(En Vision法,×400);D. 部分肿瘤细胞 CEA 阳性(En Vision 法,×400)

Figure 29-43-2　A. Hyperkeratosis,tumor cells arrangement in funicular,cord and adnoid structures (HE stain,×100); B. Sparse solid islands of squamous cells surrounded by basaloid cells (HE stain,×400); C. Tumor cells AE1/AE3 positive (En Vision method,×400); D. Part tumor cells CEA positive (En Vision method,×400)

44. 孤立性毛发上皮瘤
Solitary trichoepithelioma

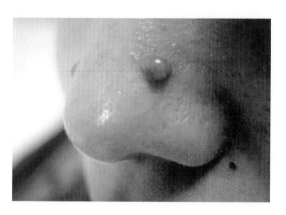

图 29-44-1　左侧鼻翼有一绿豆大半球形丘疹,呈淡褐色

Figure 29-44-1　A mung bean-sized, half ball, light brown papule on the left nosewing

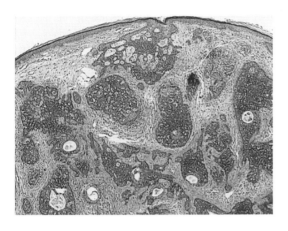

图 29-44-2　真皮内可见较多基底样细胞团及相互交织的细胞索,部分细胞团块内可见角囊肿,周边细胞排列呈栅栏状(HE 染色,×40)

Figure 29-44-2　Numerous basaloid cell masses and cell cords containing horn cysts arranged in network in the dermis(HE stain, ×40)

45. 多发性毛发上皮瘤
Multiple trichoepitheliomas

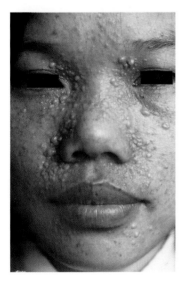

图 29-45-1　面部许多大小不一的结节,呈半球形,肤色,半透明,以面中部居多

Figure 29-45-1　Multiple, varying sized, rounded, shiny, slightly translucent, flesh-colored nodules on the face, especially on the central face

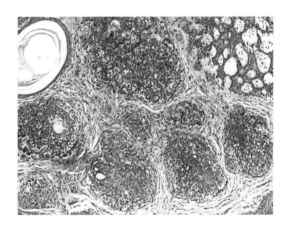

图 29-45-2　真皮由许多基底样细胞构成的细胞团块,可见角囊肿及幼稚毛囊(HE 染色,×100)

Figure 29-45-2　Numerous masses of basaloid cells in the dermis, and keratinous cysts and infantile follicle (HE stain, ×100)

277

46. 水疱型钙化上皮瘤
Calcifying epithelioma with a bulla appearance

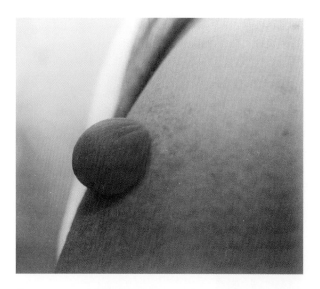

图 29-46-1　左上臂中段伸侧见一约 2.0cm×2.5cm 半透明厚壁水疱,疱壁褶皱

Figure 29-46-1　A wrinkled, purplish, thick-walled, translucent, bulla 2. 0 cm × 2. 5cm in diameter on the left upper arm

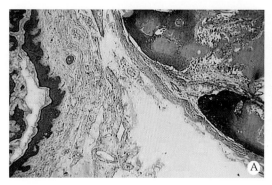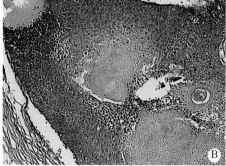

图 29-46-2　A. 表皮与肿瘤细胞岛之间真皮水肿明显,淋巴管数目增多,高度扩张成大小不等薄壁管腔,腔内充满淋巴液(×100); B. 细胞岛由外至内可见典型的嗜碱性细胞、过度细胞和影细胞,影细胞小叶中央见小钙化区(×400)

Figure 29-46-2　A. The marked edema between epidermis and tumor, marked dilated thin-walled lymph vessels filled with lymph fluid(×100); B. The cell islands consisting of basophilic cells, transitional cells, and "shadow" cells with small calcifying areas(×400)

47. 结缔组织增生性毛发上皮瘤
Desmoplastic trichoepithelioma

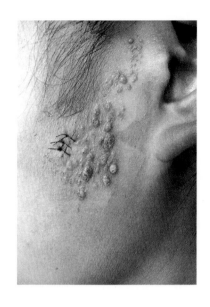

图 29-47-1　头顶部一淡红色环形斑块,边缘轻度隆起,中央有一约黄豆大淡红色丘疹,表面光滑,无毛发,周围轻度萎缩

Figure 29-47-1　Damask, annular plaque with raised border and a damask papules in the center on the scalp

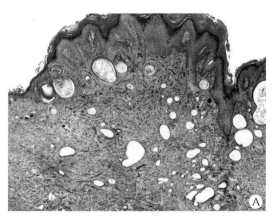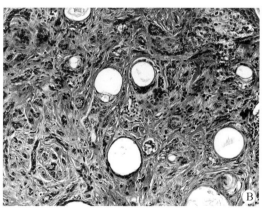

图 29-47-2　A. 表皮轻度增生,真皮浅层许多大小不一的角质囊肿和嗜碱性细胞条索,周围胶原纤维增生(HE 染色, ×40);B. 真皮内多数小角质囊肿,部分角质囊肿的表皮细胞向毛囊分化,形成逗号样结构,形似汗管瘤,细胞呈束状分布,由 1～3 层嗜碱性基底样细胞组成,胶原明显增生,并形成裂隙(HE stain, ×100)

Figure 29-47-2　A. Horn cysts with various size and a strand of basaloid tumor cells in the upper dermis, and considerable amounts of collagen fibers (HE stain, ×40); B. Numerous small horn cytsts in the dermis, narrow strands of basaloid cells and epidermoid cyts infiltrated a fibrotic stroma (HE stain, ×100)

48. 小汗腺血管样错构瘤
Eccrine angiomatous hamartoma

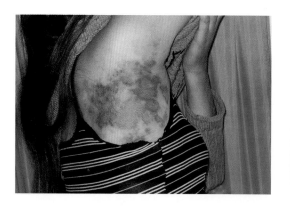

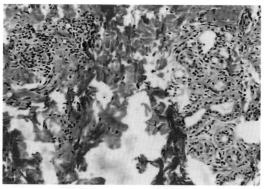

图 29-48-1　淡褐红色多环状斑片,边缘稍隆起,皮损内可见多个毛囊性丘疹

Figure 29-48-1　Bluish multi-annular macules with elevated edges, numerous follicular papules in lesions

图 29-48-2　真皮深层有多数扩张的血管,在扩张的血管附近有多数囊性扩张的汗管(HE 染色,×400)

Figure 29-48-2　Dilated blood vessels in the lower dermis, nearby numerous dilated ducts of eccrine glands (HE stain, ×400)

49. 透明细胞汗腺瘤
Clear cell hidradenoma

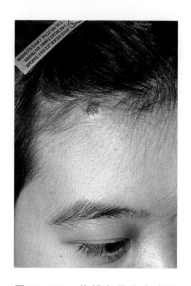

图 29-49-1　前额有甲盖大淡红色结节,界限清楚,表面破溃结痂

Figure 29-49-1　A well-circumscribed, rosiness nodule with crust on the forehead

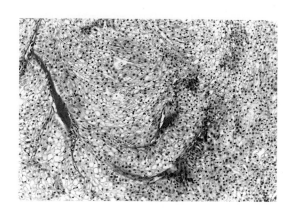

图 29-49-2　肿瘤由透明细胞和多角形细胞组成,两种细胞间有明显过渡,并可见腺腔样裂隙(HE 染色,×100)

Figure 29-49-2　The tumor consisted of polyhedral cells and clear cell, with transitional cells between these two varieties and cystic and lumina spaces (HE stain, ×100)

50. 乳头状汗管囊腺瘤
Syringocytadenoma papilliferum

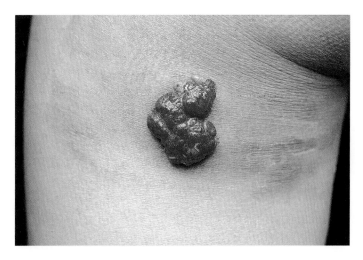

图 29-50-1　在大腿的后部有一个孤立的红色肿物

Figure 29-50-1　A solitary red tumor on the flex aspect of the left leg

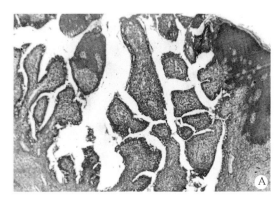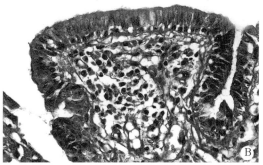

图 29-50-2　A. 多数绒毛突向内褶的腔隙(HE 染色, ×100);B. 腔隙是由 2 层细胞组成的腺上皮(HE 染色, ×400)

Figure 29-50-2　A. Numerous papillary projections into the lumina of the invaginations(HE stain, ×100);
B. The invaginations are lined by glandular epithelium consisted two rows of cells(HE stain, ×400)

51. 乳头状汗管囊腺瘤并发基底细胞上皮瘤
Syringocystadenoma papilliferum complicated by basal cell epithelioma

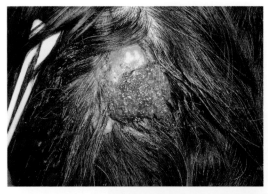

图 29-51-1　头顶有一个红色肿瘤

Figure 29-51-1　A solitary red tumor on the scalp

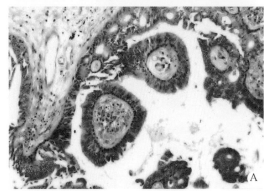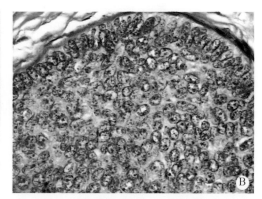

图 29-51-2　A. 腔隙是由 2 层细胞组成的腺上皮(HE 染色，×100)；B. 肿瘤团块细胞的周边细胞核呈栅栏状排列(HE 染色，×400)

Figure 29-51-2　A. The invaginations are lined by glandular epithelium consisted two rows of cells(HE stain，×100)；B. The peripheral cell layer in the masses shows palisade arrangement of nuclei(HE stain，×400)

三、结缔组织肿瘤 Tumors of Fibrous Tissue

52. 上皮样组织细胞瘤
Epithelioid cell histiocytoma

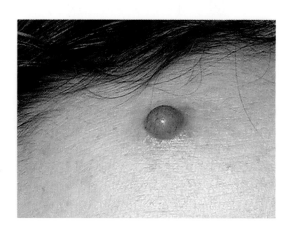

图 29-52-1　额部一半球形紫红色结节，边界清晰

Figure 29-52-1　A well circumscibed protuberant violaceous nodule on the forehead

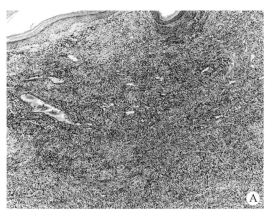
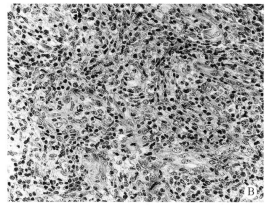

图 29-52-2 A. 肿瘤组织内伴有明显增生扩张的血管,部分区域可见胶原纤维轻度增生(HE 染色,×100);B. 肿瘤主要由上皮样细胞组成,并伴有较多的浆细胞浸润,可见核分裂象(HE 染色,×400)

Figure 29-52-2 A. Marked hyperplasia and dilated vessels in the tumor tissue and slightly collagen fibers hyperplasia (HE stain,×100);B. The tumor is mainly composed of epithelioid cells,and prominent plasma cells with nuclei mitoses (HE stain,×400)

53. 发疹性组织细胞瘤
Eruptive histiocytomas

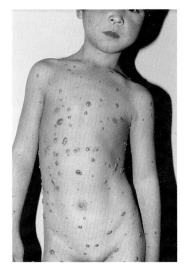

图 29-53-1 躯干有多数肤色到红色丘疹

Figure 29-53-1 Numorous flesh-colored to red papules on the trunk

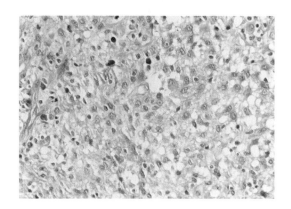

图 29-53-2 真皮内有各型组织细胞构成的浸润(HE 染色,×400)

Figure 29-53-2 An infiltrate composed of various types of histiocytes in the dermis(HE stain,×400)

54. 多中心网状组织细胞增生症
Multicentric reticulohistiocytosis

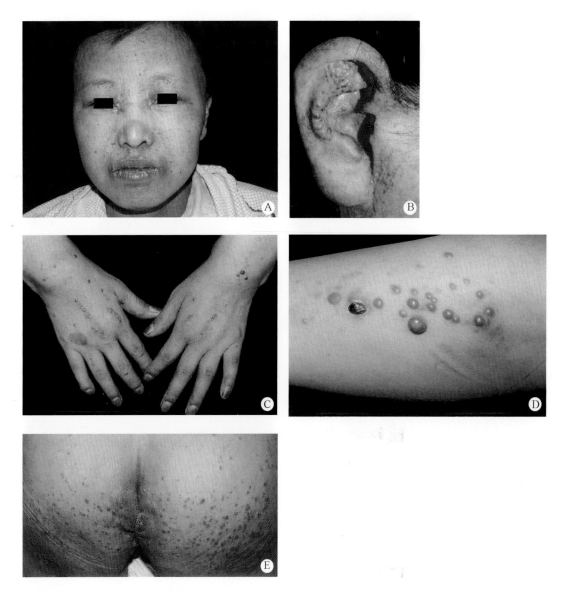

图 29-54-1　丘疹和结节见于面部(A)、耳郭(B)、双手背(C)、肘部(D)、臀部(E)有红色斑块

Figure 29-54-1　There are papules and nodules on the face(A), ears(B)dorsum of hands(C) and elbows(D), erythematous plaques on the battocks(E)

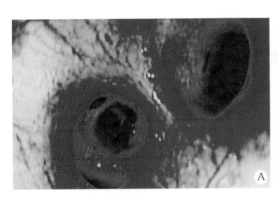
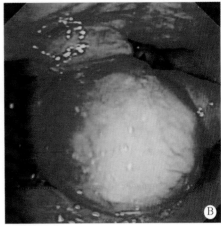

图 29-54-2　A. 支气管内多数结节；B. 咽喉左劈裂处有 1.5 cm×2.0 cm 大赘生物

Figure 29-54-2　A. Neumerous nodules in the bronchus; B. A mass 1.5 cm×2.0 cm in size on the left aryepiglottic fold

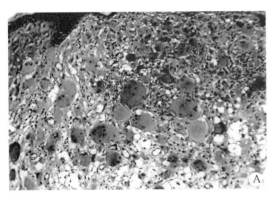
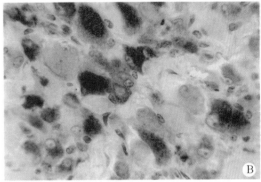

图 29-54-3　A. 真皮内密集组织细胞和多核巨细胞,胞质嗜酸性,呈"毛玻璃样"(HE 染色, ×200); B. 胞质呈棕黄色,CD68 阳性(SP 染色, ×200)

Figure 29-54-3　Histiocytes and multinucleated giant cells with eosinophilic "ground-glass" cytoplasm in the dermis(HE stain, ×200); B. brown-yellow cytoplasm,CD68 postive (SP stain, ×200)

55. 以多发残毁性关节炎为显著表现的多中心网状组织细胞增生症

Multicentric reticulohistiocytosis with arthritis multilans

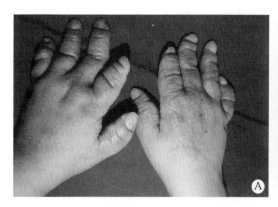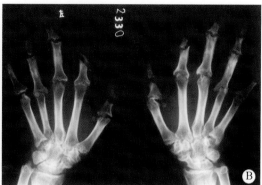

图 29-55-1　双手指短缩畸形；B. 双手诸掌指骨近端骨质破坏、缺损

Figure 29-55-1　A. Deformity of the joints of the both hands；B. Erosions in all proximal interphalangeal joints of both hands

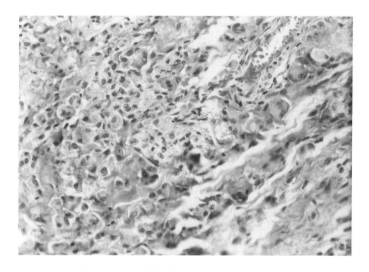

图 29-55-2　真皮内有大而奇形怪状的多核组织细胞,嗜伊红呈"毛玻璃"样外观(HE 染色,×400)

Figure 29-55-2　Large and multinucleated giant cells with eosinophilic granular "ground-glass" cytoplasm are embedded in the stroma of dermis (HE stain,×400)

56. 勒-雪病
Letterer-Siwe disease

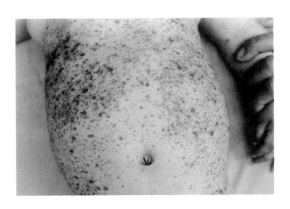

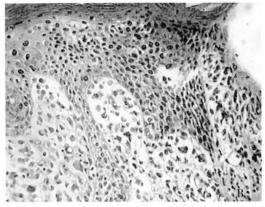

图 29-56-1 胸腹部泛发紫癜和暗红色丘疹,表面有痂或鳞屑

Figure 29-56-1 The petechiae and brownish papules covered with crusts or scales on the chest and the abodoman

图 29-56-2 真皮浅层见单一核细胞浸润,部分细胞移入表皮(HE 染色,×200)

Figure 29-56-2 There is a superficial dermal infiltrate of mononuclear cells, some of them has invaded the epidermis (HE stain,×200)

57. 发疹性朗格汉斯细胞组织细胞增生症
Exanthematous Langerhans cell histiocytosis

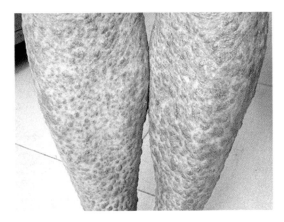

图 29-57-1 下肢密集粟粒至黄豆大的丘疹、结节,大部分呈肤色或淡红色,部分融合,表面无破损

Figure 29-57-1 The foxtail millet to soybean size exanthematous papules and nodules on both low limbs

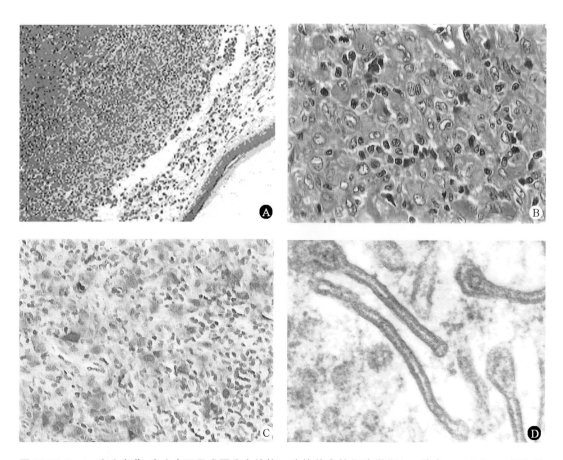

图 29-57-2　A. 表皮变薄,真皮内可见成团分布的较一致的单个核细胞浸润(HE 染色,×100);B. 细胞核形态规则,核大小不一,或多核,核缘弯曲,核畸形或较大的核沟,异染色质增多,边缘细胞器丰富,其间有少量淋巴细胞、中性粒细胞(HE 染色,×400);C. S-100 蛋白呈阳性表达,胞质、胞核黄染(ABC 法染色,×200);D. 电镜下见细胞内有大量的 Birbeck 颗粒,呈棒状,外包单位膜,其内有平行排列的横纹(↑)(×10 000)

Figure 29-57-2　A. Thinned epidermis, masses of mononuclear infiltrate in the dermis, the cells with varying size, pleomorphic, vesicular nuclear(HE, ×100); B. A few lymphocytes, and neutrophils infiltrate(HE, ×400); C. The large histocytic cells infiltrated in the dermis are positive for S-100 (ABC stain, ×200); D. Birbeck granules in the cells under the electron microscopy(×10 000)

58. 播散型 Paget 病样网状细胞增生病
Disseminated pagetoid reticelosis

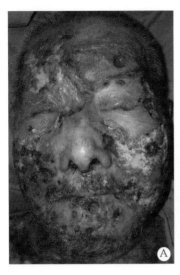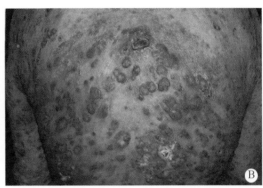

图 29-58-1　A. 面部多数暗红斑块伴鳞屑和结痂；B. 背部多数褐色斑块伴溃疡

Figure 29-58-1　A. Neumerous dark red plaques with scales and crusts on the face;

B. Neumerus brown plaques associated with ulcers on the back

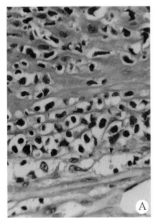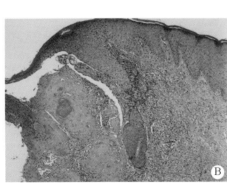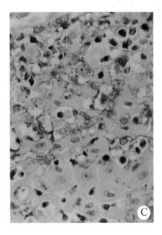

图 29-58-2　A. 表皮内有异型淋巴样细胞浸润,如 Paget 样细胞(HE 染色,×400)；B. 真皮浅层和中层有大量淋巴样细胞浸润,细胞有异型性(HE 染色,×40)；C. CD45 RO 阳性(ABC 法,×400)

Figure 29-58-2　A. Infitrarion of atypical lymphocytes like pagetoid cell in the epidermis (HE stain, × 400);

B. Infiltration of neumerous atypical lymphocytes in the upper and middle dermis (HE stain, × 40); C. CD45 RO is positive (ABC method, × 400)

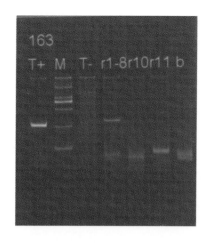

图 29-58-3   T 细胞受体基因重排 TCR-γ 阳性
Figure 29-58-3   T-cell receptor γ is positive

59. 上皮样肉瘤
Epithelioid sarcoma

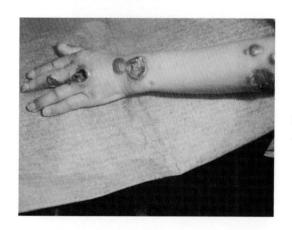

图 29-59-1   上肢暗红色结节，部分结节表面有溃疡
Figure 29-59-1   Brownish nodules associated partly with ulcers on the upper limbs

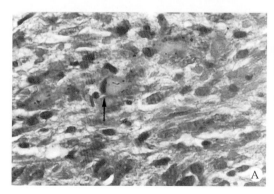

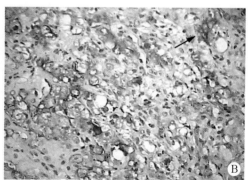

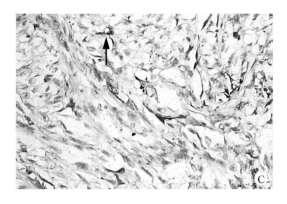

图 29-59-2　A. 不典型上皮样细胞胞质嗜伊红,核有异形性(↑)(HE 染色,×400);B. 肿瘤细胞胞质 CK 表达阳性(↑)(LSAB 法染色,×400);C. 肿瘤细胞胞质 EMA 表达阳性(↑)(LSAB 染色,×400)

Figure 29-59-2　A. Nodular atypical epitheloid cells with eosinophillic cytoplasm and atypical nuclear (↑) (HE stain, ×400); B. Positive staining for cytokeratin (CK) in the tumor cells (LSAB method, ×400); C. Positive staining for epithelial membrane antigen (EMA) in the tumor cells(LSAB,×400)

60. 结节性(假肉瘤性)筋膜炎
Nodular (pseudosarcomatous) fasciitis

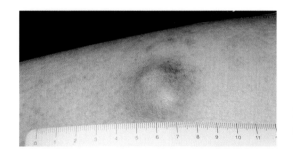

图 29-60-1　左小腿有一个皮下无疼痛和破溃的结节

Figure 29-60-1　A subcutaneous nodule without pain and ulcer on the left leg

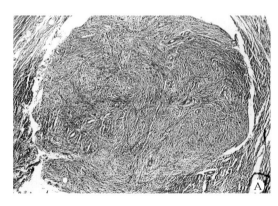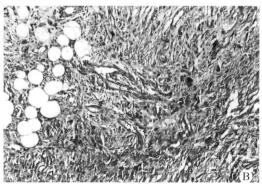

图 29-60-2　A. 真皮及皮下组织有大量梭形细胞增生(HE 染色,×50);B. 有些梭形细胞核外形不规则深染(HE 染色,×250)

Figure 29-60-2　A. Lots of fusiform cells in the dermis and hypodermis(HE stain, ×50); B. Some of fusiform cells has hyperchromatic and irregularly shaped nuclei(HE stain ×250)

61. 先天性隆突性皮肤纤维肉瘤
Congenital dermatofibrosarcoma protuberans

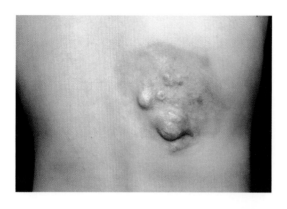

图 29-61-1　背部有一棕褐色萎缩斑,其上有 6 个淡红色光滑结节

Figure 29-61-1　A large brown atrophy patch raised six light red firm smooth nodules on the back

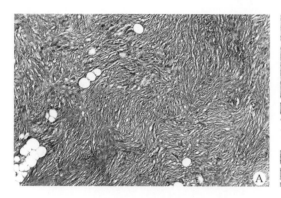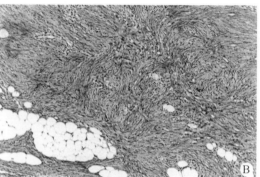

图 29-61-2　A. 致密、单一梭形细胞束呈旋风状排列(HE 染色,×100);B. 瘤细胞胞质 CD34 染色呈阳性(SP 法染色,×100)

Figure 29-61-2　A. Dense, monomorphous, spindle cells arranged in a storiform pattern (HE stain, ×100); B. CD34 positive in cytoplasma of tumor cell (SP stain, ×100)

62. 萎缩斑块样隆突性皮肤纤维肉瘤
Atrophic and plaque-like dermato-fibrosarcoma protuberans

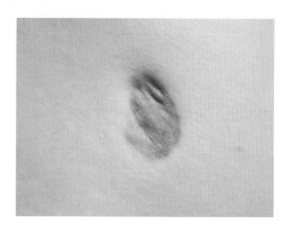

图 29-62-1　右侧腰背部约 3cm×2.5cm 不规则暗红色斑,表面萎缩

Figure 29-62-1　A 3cm×2.5cm irregular dark erythema with atrophic surface on the right lower back

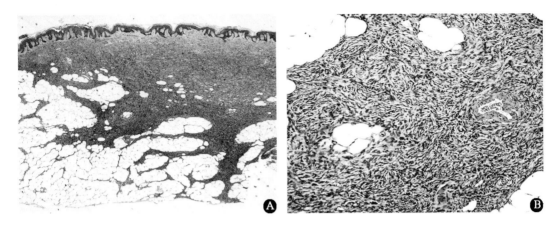

图 29-62-2　真皮及皮下形态和大小均匀一致的梭形细胞,深入和分割皮下脂肪,部分区域梭形细胞呈车辐状排列,少许细胞核大浓染(HE 染色:A,×40;B,×200)

Figures 29-62-2　Monotonous spindle cells in the dermis and subcutaneous tissue,penetrating into the subcutaneous fat; Some cells arranged in cartwheel pattern; A few cells with larger and darker nuclei（HE stain: A,×40;B,×200）

63. 获得性指(趾)部纤维角化瘤
Acquired digital fibrokeratoma

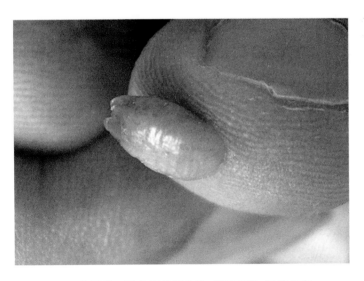

图 29-63-1　右足第 2 趾尖指状增生物,表面光滑,呈淡红色

Figure 29-63-1　A damask,digital neoplasm on the second toe tip of the right foot

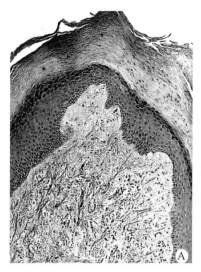
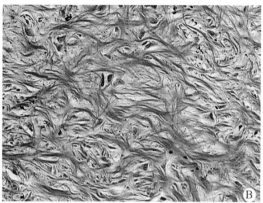

图 29-63-2   A. 表皮角化过度，棘层肥厚，表皮突增宽（HE 染色，×40）；B. 真皮见大量胶原纤维及成纤维细胞增生（HE 染色，×100）

Figure 29-63-2   A. The epidermis shows marked hyperkeratosis and acanthosis with thickened, branching rete ridges（HE stain, ×40）；B. Considerable amount of collagen fibers and fibroblasts in the dermis（HE stain, ×100）

四、脉管组织肿瘤 Tumors of Vascular Tissue

64. 色素血管性斑痣性错构瘤病

Phakomatosis pigmentovascularis

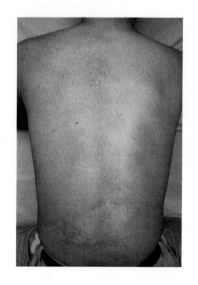

图 29-64-1   背部大片浅灰蓝、暗蓝色斑片，边缘逐渐移行为正常肤色，面积约 40cm×25cm，符合蒙古斑表现，左侧后腰部网状红色斑片，边缘不整，不高出皮面，约 16cm×10cm，符合鲜红斑痣表现

Figure 29-64-1   A grey blue spot about 40cm×25cm on the back, a nevus flammeus about 16cm×10cm on the left waist

65. 匐行性血管瘤
Angioma serpiginosum

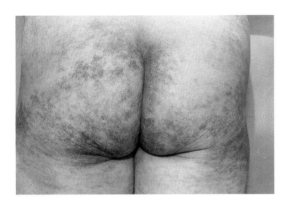

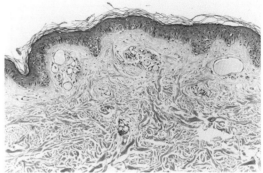

图 29-65-1　臀部可见不规则网状暗红色斑,其上有许多针尖大小紫红色斑点,压之不褪色

Figure 29-65-1　Netlike pattern deeply red maculare and numerous violaceous spots on the buttock

图 29-65-2　真皮乳头和网状层的浅层有扩张和增生的毛细血管(HE 染色,×100)

Figure 29-65-2　Dilated capillaries in the papillae and reticular dermis (HE stain,×100)

66. 反应性血管内皮细胞瘤病
Reactive angioendotheliomatosis

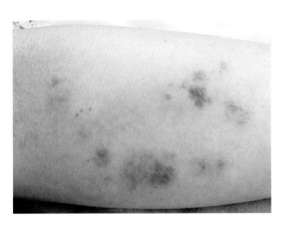

图 29-66-1　左前臂近肘窝处见 6～8 处红斑、丘疹及斑块,较大者达直径 4cm。皮损中可见针尖大小紫癜

Figure 29-66-1　There were 6-8 patches of erythemas,papules or plaques on the antecubital area, the biggest diameter of which was 4cm. There were variable pin-sized purpuras inside

67. 微静脉性血管瘤
Microvenular hemangioma

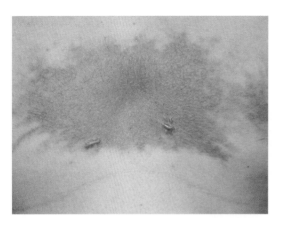

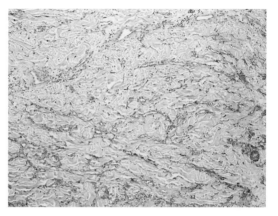

图 29-67-1　胸部有一 7cm×18cm 红斑,边缘不规则

Figure 29-67-1　A 7cm×18cm erythema with irregular border on the chest

图 29-67-2　纤细的胶原间质内裂隙状血管腔(HE 染色,×400)

Figure 29-67-2　Slit-like vascular channels in slightly collagenous stroma. (HE stain,×400)

68. 梭形细胞血管瘤
Spindle cell hemangioma

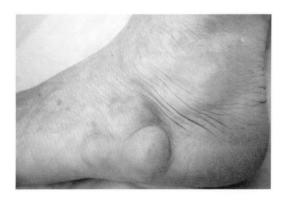

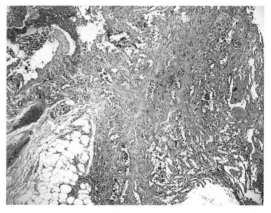

图 29-68-1　左足外侧缘、外踝及左跖部多个肤色或淡红色结节

Figure 29-68-1　Several skin color or reddish nodules on the fibular margin, external malleolus and sole of the left foot

图 29-68-2　真皮中下部见梭形细胞和海绵状血管腔隙构成的团块,海绵状血管腔隙有不规则扩张的薄壁血管窦或裂隙,内衬扁平内皮细胞(HE 染色,×400)

Figure 29-68-2　The tumor composed of spindle tumor cells and cavernous blood vessels with irregular dilated thin-walled sinusoids lined with flattened endothelial cells in the middle and lower dermis(HE stain,×400)

69. 上皮样血管瘤
Epithelioid hemangioma

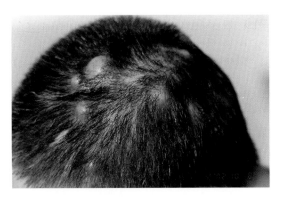

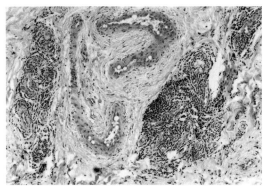

图 29-69-1　头皮左侧可见大小不等的多个结节,暗红色,表面光滑,头发脱落

Figure 29-69-1　Multiple brownish red nodules with smooth surface on the left scalp

图 29-69-2　真皮内可见小叶结构,血管壁及肌层黏液变性,炎性细胞浸润(HE 染色,×200)

Figure 29-69-2　Exuberant proliferation of vessels lined by cuboidal to endothelioid cells and inflammatory infiltration (HE stain,×200)

70. 疣状血管瘤
Verrucous haemangioma

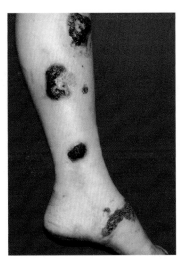

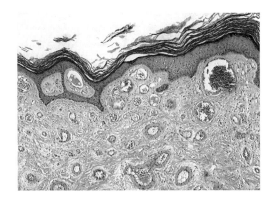

图 29-70-1　沿左小腿内侧分布的暗红色结节和斑块,表面粗糙呈疣状外观

Figure 29-70-1　A group of several well-circumscribed, hyperkeratotic, dark-red, plaques arranged linearly along the inside aspect of left lower extremity

图 29-70-2　表皮角化过度,真皮内增生的血管成团或散在分布,部分血管高度扩张,管腔内充满红细胞(HE 染色,×100)

Figure 29-70-2　Hyperkeratosis of the epidermis and multiple dilated vessels filled with blood in the superficial dermis (HE stain,×100)

71. 丛状血管瘤
Tufted angioma

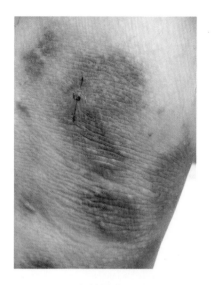

图 29-71-1　左侧腘窝处见暗红色斑块，中央凹陷，边缘隆起呈环状

Figure 29-71-1　Red-brown plaques with thick indurated border and a central depression similar to a doughnut

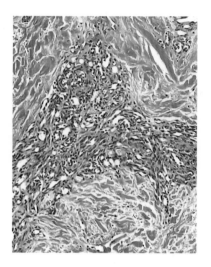

图 29-71-2　真皮内见界限清楚的毛细血管样聚集体(HE 染色，×100)

Figure 29-71-2　Well-circumscribed capillary lobules in the dermis (HE stain，×100)

72. 浅表性血管黏液瘤
Superficial angiomyxoma

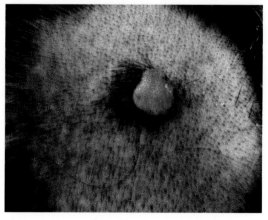

图 29-72-1　头皮一黄豆大(0.5cm×0.5cm)肉红色结节

Figure 29-72-1　A red nodule measuring 0.5cm × 0.5cm on the scalp

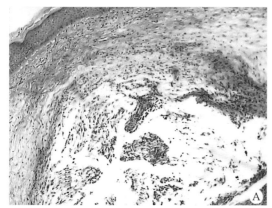

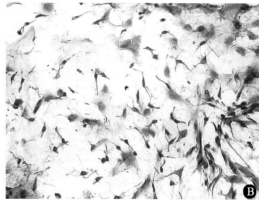

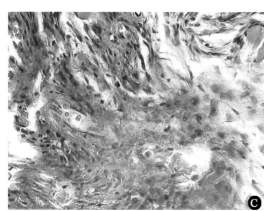

图 29-72-2 A. 肿瘤位于真皮内,界清,有胶原纤维束包绕(HE 染色,×40);B. 整个肿瘤内充满黏液样基质,其间散在星形及纺锤形细胞(HE 染色,×200);肿瘤内和边缘纤维束内有丰富的薄壁小血管(HE 染色,×400)

Figure 29-72-2 A. The tumor located in the dermis, and defined by thick collagen bundles (HE stain, ×40); B. Myxoid stroma fulled the whole tumor, star-and spindle-shaped stromal cells are scattered throughout the tumor (HE stain, ×200); C. Small, thin-wall blood vessels scatter in the tumor and the fibers bundles (HE stain, ×400)

73. 靶样含铁血黄素沉积性血管瘤
Targetoid hemosiderotic hemangioma

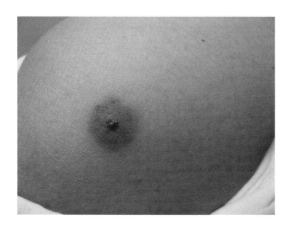

图 29-73-1 左肩胛骨的上方见 1.7cm 靶形皮损,靶中心为 3mm 大小的紫色丘疹,周围见到紫色环,最外为一橘黄色外环

Figure 29-73-1 A 1.7 cm sized, targetoid violaceous papule with an annular violaceous and outmost yellowish ring was noted on the upper part of the left shoulder

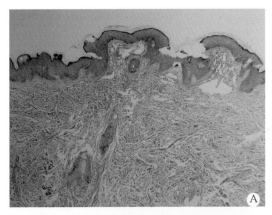
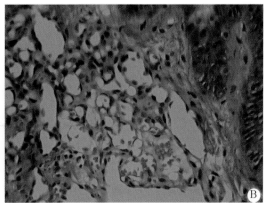
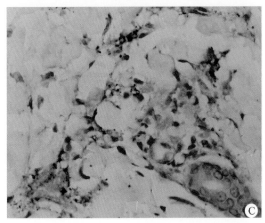

图 29-73-2　A. 真皮浅层见不规则扩张的薄壁管腔呈楔形沿水平面延伸,管腔内含红细胞,部分高度扩张的管腔内充满了均一性、嗜伊红淋巴液。真皮中层的血管走向与浅层血管分布平面成直角或锐角,并被胶原纤维束自然分割,形成狭长的裂隙。血管周围淋巴细胞浸润(HE 染色,×100);B. 真皮浅层红细胞外渗。管腔内皮细胞肿胀,似鞋钉样突向管腔(HE 染色,×400);C. 真皮的胶原束之间含铁血黄素沉积,呈特征性蓝色染色(普鲁士蓝染色,×400)

Figure 29-73-2　A. Histologic evaluation revealed dilated and proliferated capillaries in the superficial dermis. some highly dilated lumens are congested with eosinophilic, homogenous materials. blood vessels or lymphatic vessels run along the directions that parallel the surface of skin. Slit like vessels are located in the middermis and dissected between collagen bundles(HE stain, ×100); B. Vessels are lined with plump, hobnail-like endothelial cells protruding into the lumen. Extravasated erythrocytes is obvious(HE stain, ×400); C. Prussian blue stain for iron high lights abundant hemosiderin deposition between collagen bundles. (Prussian blue stain, ×400)

74. 弥漫性躯体血管角化瘤

Angiokeratoma corporis diffusum

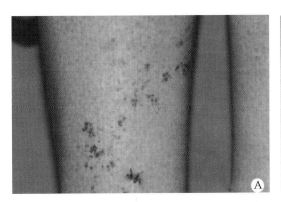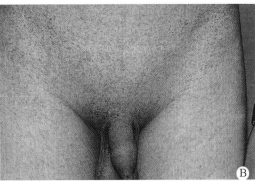

图 29-74-1　A. 左大腿有多数簇集的红色小丘疹；B. 下腹部多数小红色丘疹

Figure 29-74-1　A. Neumerous clusters of ting red papules on the left leg；B. Neumerous ting red papules on the lower abdomen

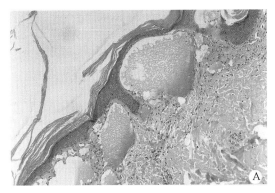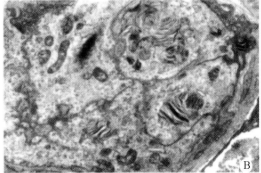

图 29-74-2　A. 真皮乳头层血管扩张，其上方表皮角化过度(HE 染色，×100)；B. 肾小球上皮细胞及系膜细胞肿胀胞质中溶酶体内可见层板状结构小体

Figure 29-74-2　A. Note ectasia blood vessels in the papillary dermis with overlying hyperkeratosis(HE stain, ×100)；B. The concentric in lamellage lysosome of epithelium of renal glomerali

75. 单侧阴囊血管角皮瘤
Unilateral angiokeratoma on the scrotum

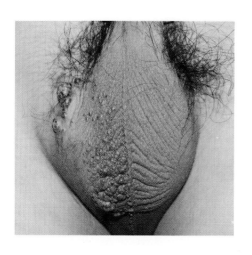

图 29-75-1　右侧阴囊群集紫红色丘疹

Figure 29-75-1　Clusters of mauve papules on the right scrotum

76. 女阴血管角皮瘤
Angiokeratoma on the vulva

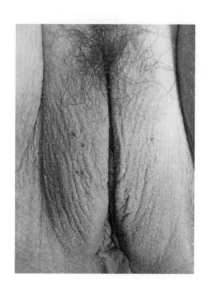

图 29-76-1　大阴唇有少数小圆形血管性丘疹

Figure 29-76-1　A few small vascular papules on the vulva

77. 卡波西样血管内皮细胞瘤
Kaposiform hemangioendothelioma

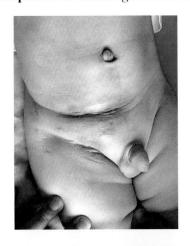

图 29-77-1　右下腹和腹股沟有暗红色斑块

Figure 29-77-1　Brown red plaques on the right lower abdomen and groin area

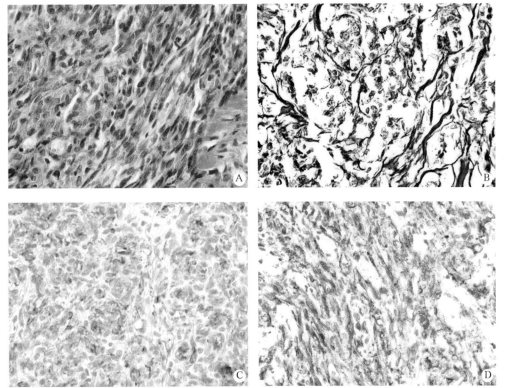

图 29-77-2　A. 真皮内有梭形细胞和椭圆形细胞结节中有血管腔隙含红细胞和铁血黄素沉积（HE 染色，× 400）；B. 真皮内肿瘤被黑色网状纤维包绕（网状纤维染色，× 400）；C. CD31 阳性（Vision 二步法，× 400）；D. CD34 阳性（Vision 二步法，× 400）

Figure 29-77-2　A. Nodular aggregates of spindled cells and ovoid cells associated with vascular spaces, blood red cell and hemosiderin in the dermis (HE stain, × 400); B. Tumor is surrounded by dark reticular fibers in the dermis (Reticular fiber stain, × 400); C. CD31 positive (Vision, × 400); D. CD34 positive (Vision, × 400)

78. 恶性血管内皮细胞瘤
Malignant endothelioma

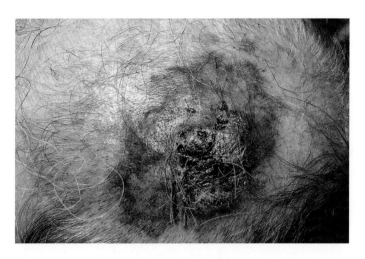

图 29-78-1　头顶有一个大的紫红色弥漫性浸润块,表面有坏死和结痂

Figure 29-78-1　A big purple red diffuse infiltrating mass covered necrotic and crusts on the scalp

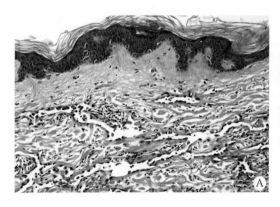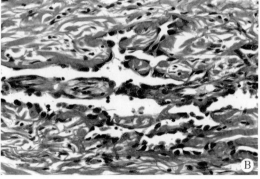

图 29-78-2　A. 真皮有多数大小不一管腔(HE 染色,×100);B. 衬有不典型内皮细胞的血管腔大小形态不一(HE 染色,×200)

Figure 29-78-2　A. The number of vascular lumina varies in the dermis (HE stain,×100);B. The vascular lumina lined by atypical endothelial cells are irregular in size and shape(HE stain,×200)

79. 恶性血管内皮瘤合并疱疹样天疱疮

Malignant hemangioendothelioma associated with herpetiform pemphigus

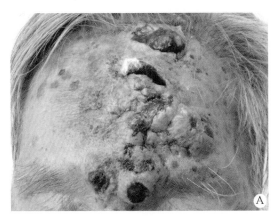
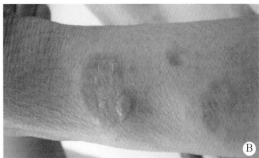

图 29-79-1　前额部数个溃疡出血性的暗红色斑块、结节；B. 躯干及四肢伸侧环状红斑的边缘可见小的及中等大小的水疱,尼氏征(一)

Figure 29-79-1　A. Purpuric papulonodular lesions with dotted ulceration and bleeding on the forehead; B. Numerous erythematous and edematous lesions in an annular arrangement, associated with small-medium-sized blisters on the trunk and extensor aspects of the extremities, Nikolsky sign was negative

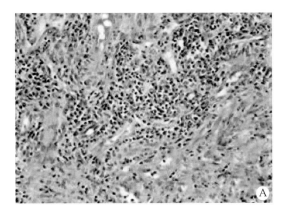
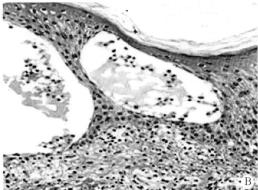

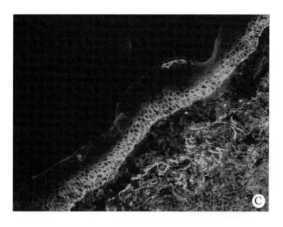

图 29-79-2　A. 血管增生,散在的非典型内皮细胞及中等量的单核细胞浸润,不规则的血管形成,红细胞渗出至血管外(HE 染色,×200);B. 多个表皮内水疱,疱内有嗜酸细胞、中性粒细胞浸润(HE 染色,×200);C. IgG 在表皮细胞间阳性表达,呈网状沉积(直接免疫荧光,×100)

Figure 29-79-2　A. Vascular hyperplasia, sporadic atypical endothelial cells and moderate dense mononuclear infiltrate with irregular vascular channel formation and extravasation of erythrocytes (HE stain, ×200); B. Intraepidermal acantholysis and blisters located in the mid to lower epidermis with mixed infiltration of eosinophils and neutrophils (HE stain, ×200); C. Direct immunofluorescence study showed intraepidermal deposition of immunoglobulin G localized to the lower upper epidermis (DIF, ×100)

80. 经典型 Kaposi 肉瘤
Classic Kaposi's sarcoma

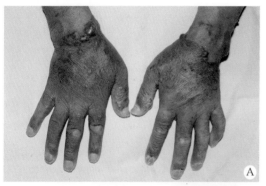

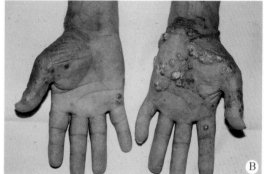

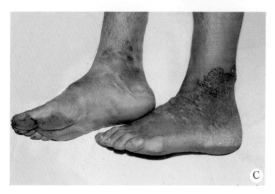

图 29-80-1　分布于手背(A)、手掌(B)和足(C)的三种 KS 主要皮损包括结节、斑块和斑片

Fig 29-80-1　three main lesions of KS including nodules, plaques and patches distributed on the extremites: on the dorsum of hands(A), on the palms(B); on the feet(C)

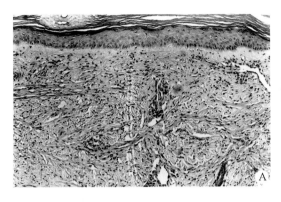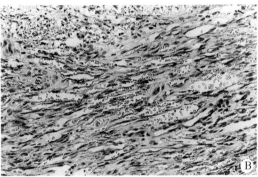

图 29-80-2 皮损的组织病理学特点:A. 斑片性损害为慢性非特异性炎症(HE 染色,×100);B. 组织中红细胞渗出及大量含铁血黄素沉积(HE 染色,×200)

Fig 29-80-2 Histological characteristics of the lesions. A. chronic nonspecific inflammation appeared in patch lesions (HE stain,×100); B. RBC extravation and abundant deposition of hemosiderin in the tissue (HE stain, ×200)

81. 实体型血管球瘤

Solid glomus tumor

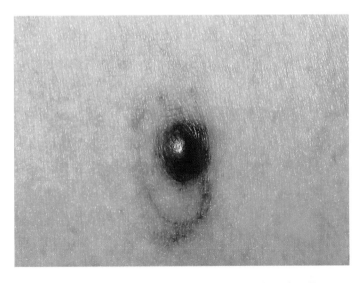

图 29-81-1 左大腿后内侧一黄豆大紫红色结节,周边淡红晕

Figure 29-81-1 A soybean in size purplish nodule with damask halation on the inboard of left thigh

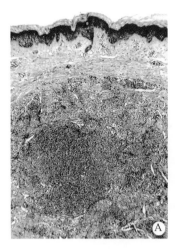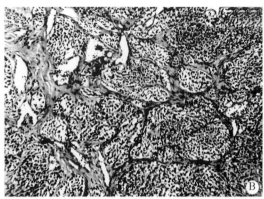

图 29-81-2　A. 真皮内可见肿瘤细胞团,与周围组织界限清楚,并可见少许裂隙状血管腔(HE 染色,×40);B. 肿瘤细胞的胞质淡染,细胞核位于中央,圆形或卵圆形,肿瘤团块之间有结缔组织间隔和少量裂隙状血管腔(HE 染色,×100)

Figure 29-81-2　A. Circumscribed glomus tumors with a few vascular spaces in the dermis(HE stain,×40);B. The glomus cells have a faintly eosinophilic cytoplasm,and round to oval nuclei in the centre,the glomus tumors surrounded by a fibrous capsule and a few vascular spaces (HE stain,×100)

82. 局限性多发性血管球瘤
Localized multiple glomus tumors

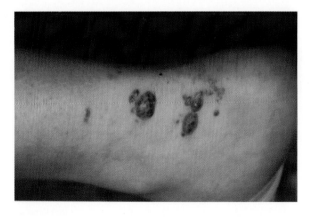

图 29-82-1　右内踝后 30 余个暗紫红色丘疹和结节,粟粒至花生米大

Figure 29-82-1　More than thirty purplish red papulas or nodules with tender on the right ankle

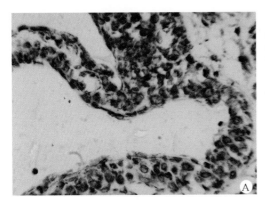
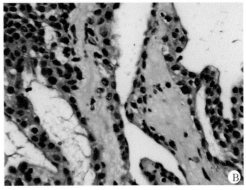

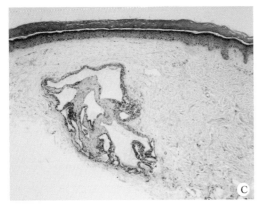

图 29-82-2　A. 真皮可见许多不规则管腔组成的肿瘤团块(HE 染色,×40); B. 血管壁由一至数层胞质轻度嗜伊红的血管球细胞组成(HE 染色,×400); C. 血管球细胞 Vimentin 阳性(免疫组化,×400)

Figure 29-82-2　A. There are several narrow vascular luminal in masses of tumor cells (HE stain, × 40); B. The vascular luminal lined by a single or many layers of glomas cells (HE stain, × 400);C. Vimentin positive in glomus cells(immunohistologic techniques, × 400)

83. 获得性渐进性淋巴管瘤
Acguired progressive lymphangioma

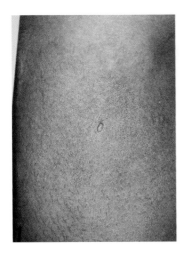

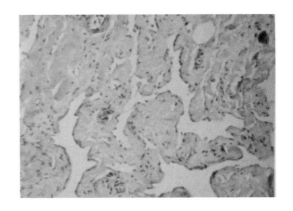

图 29-83-1　右小腿有色素沉着轻度硬结的不规则斑块

Figure 29-83-1　Hyperpigmented, slightly indurated, irreular patch on the right calf

图 29-83-2　真皮内有交织的内衬血管内皮细胞的腔隙,外有胶原纤维包绕(HE 染色,×200)

Figure 29-83-2　Interlacing channels in the dermis, lined by vascular endothelinm, that tend to coat collagen bundles(HE stain, × 200)

84. 额面部出血性淋巴管瘤
Bleeding lymphangioma on frontal plane

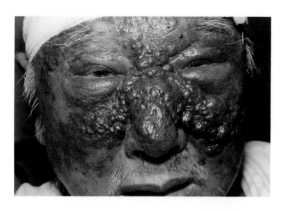

图 29-84-1　额部、双侧面颊、鼻梁及眶周可见大片对称性呈蝶形的暗紫红色瘀斑、丘疹及肿块,表面可见大小不等的血疱

Figure 29-84-1　A great soft tumor with ulcers and bleeding on the frontal plane

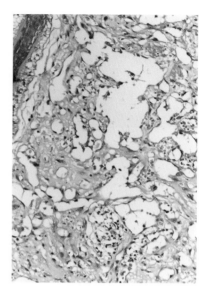

图 29-84-2　真皮见由单层内皮细胞构成的扩张性囊样管腔,似海绵状,间有少量淋巴细胞,内皮细胞肿胀(HE 染色,×400)

Figure 29-84-2　Dilated lymph tubes with endothelioid cell swelling, and a few lymphocytes infiltrate in the dermis(HE stain,×400)

85. 弥漫性海绵状淋巴管瘤
Cavernous lymphangioma

图 29-85-1　左胸、腹部弥漫分布的大小不一及形态各异的褐色丘疹,或疣状增生及厚壁水疱

Figure 29-85-1　Variously sized brown papules, verrucous and thick-walled vesicles in diffuse distribution on the left chest and abdomen

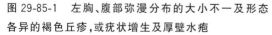

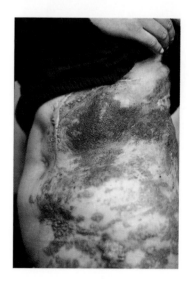

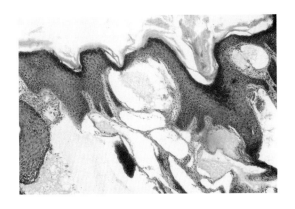

图 29-85-2　表皮角化过度,真皮内大而不规则扩张的增生淋巴管,管腔内衬以单层内皮细胞,真皮内毛细血管增生及淋巴细胞浸润(HE 染色,×100)

Figure 29-85-2　Hyperkeratosis and large irregular dilated lymph vessels lined by single-layer endothelioid cells associated with hyperplasia capillaries and lymphocytes infiltrate in the dermis (HE stain,×100)

五、脂肪、肌肉和骨组织肿瘤
Tumors of Fatty,Mascular and Osseus Tissue

86. 浅表脂肪瘤样痣
Nevus lipomatosus superficialis

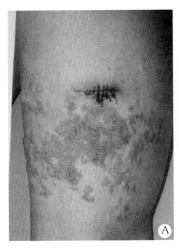
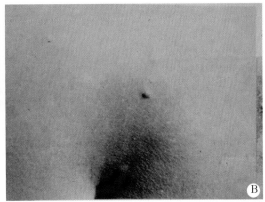

图 29-86-1　A. 左大腿有群集皮色丘疹和结节 ; B. 臀部有一个软皮色结节

Figure 29-86-1　Groups of soft skin color papules and nodules on the left thigh; B. A single soft skin color nodule located on the gluteal region

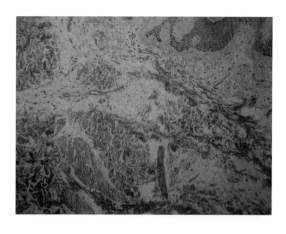

图 29-86-2　真皮胶原纤维束间有成团、束的成熟脂肪细胞(HE 染色，×100)

Figure 29-86-2　Groups and strands of mature fat cells are present embedded the collagen bundles of the dermis(HE stain ×100)

87. 硬化型浅表脂肪瘤样痣(伴脂肪组织增生的泛发型硬斑病)

Nevus lipomatosus superficialis

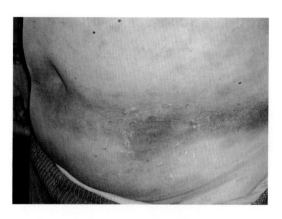

图 29-87-1　脐部两侧可见大小不规则的斑片，表面有色素沉着

Figure 29-87-1　Irregular hyperpigmentation on both aspect of umbilicus

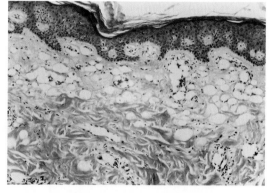

图 29-87-2　表皮角化过度，棘层肥厚，真皮浅层可见大量增生的脂肪组织，真皮内胶原纤维增粗，呈均质化改变(HE 染色，×100)

Figure 29-87-2　Hyperkeratosis and acanthosis, numerous fat tissues and collagen fiber in the upper dermis, like homogeneous change(HE stain, ×100)

88. 甲下外生骨疣和内生软骨瘤
Subungual exostosis and subungual enchondroma

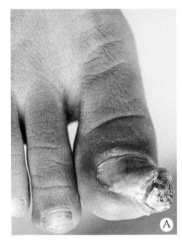
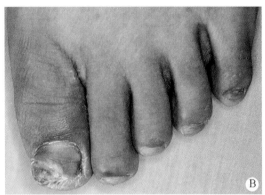

图 29-88-1　A. 右踇趾远端内侧甲板下半球形樱桃大结节,表面角化; B. 左踇趾远端甲板下一坚实结节,直径 0.8cm,部分甲板被破坏

Figure 29-88-1　A. Half ball nodule with hyperkeratosis on the right distal hallux subungual; B. A hard nodule 0.8cm in diameter on the left distal hallux subungual, part nail destroyed

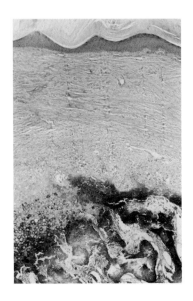

图 29-88-2　真皮浅中部结缔组织增生,中下部见软骨和成熟骨组织(HE 染色, × 100)

Figure 29-88-2　The tumors consisted of a proliferative fibrocartilaginous cap that merged into mature trabecular bone at its base (HE stain, × 100)

89. 多发性皮肤平滑肌瘤
Multiple leiomyoma

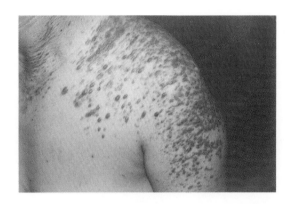

图 29-89-1　左颈、胸、肩及上臂散在大量粟粒到黄豆大小暗紫红色丘疹、结节,部分皮损相互融合

Figure 29-89-1　Numerous amaranth papules and nodules on the left of neck, chest, shoulder, and the upper of arm, and some of them confluent

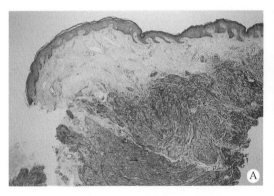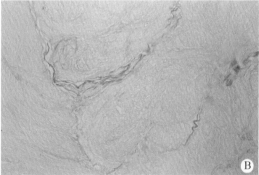

图 29-89-2　A. 真皮内可见肿瘤细胞团块,主要由平滑肌细胞组成,肿瘤团块周围无包膜(HE 染色,×40);B. 肿瘤团块由大量呈黄色的平滑肌纤维组成,其间有少量红色的胶原纤维(Van Giesson 染色,×100)

Figure 29-89-2　A. Tumor is composed of smooth muscle fibers without encapsulated in the dermis (HE stain, ×40); B. Tumor is composed of massive yellow smooth muscle fibres and a few red collagen in the midst of them (Van Giesson Stain, ×100)

90. 皮肤平滑肌肉瘤
Cutaneous leiomyosarcoma

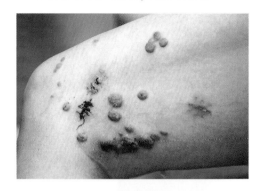

图 29-90-1　左大腿外侧至膝关节处散在分布数十个黄豆至蚕豆大的鲜红色孤立性结节,高出皮面

Figure 29-90-1　Numerous, turkey red nodules on the outside of left thigh

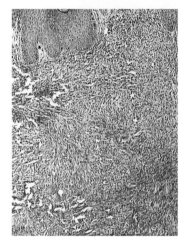

图 29-90-2　真皮内见许多梭形细胞,核呈杆状,两端钝圆,可见病理性核分裂象及灶状坏死,间质中有少量淋巴细胞及中性粒细胞浸润(HE 染色,×40);梭形肿瘤细胞胞质呈棕黄色,Vimtin 呈强阳性反应

Figure 29-90-2　Numerous pleomorphic elongated cells with atypical nuclei mitotic figures in the dermis (HE stain,×40); The tumor cells are Vimtin strong positive

91. 甲下外生骨疣
Subungual exostosis

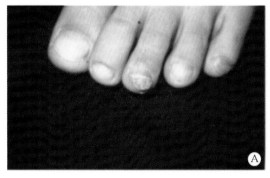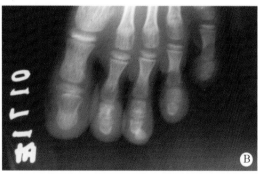

图 29-91-1　A. 左中趾甲前缘有一玉米粒大结节;B. X 线检查示左中趾骨末端见一黄豆大小高密度阴影

Figure 29-91-1　A. A nodule on the nail edge of the left third toe; B. X-rays exhibited a bone mass protruding from the third distal phalanx

92. 皮肤子宫内膜异位
Cutaneous endometriosis

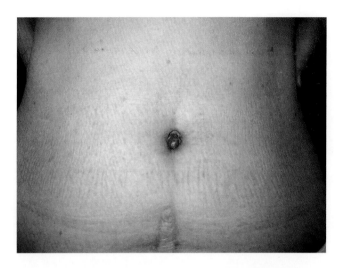

图 29-92-1   脐窝下半部见一圆形隆起性包块,呈棕褐色

Figure 29-92-1   A brown tumor on lower part of umbilical

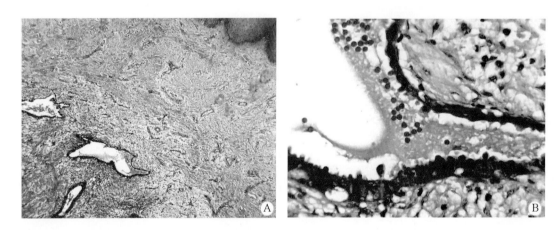

图 29-92-2   A. 真皮内大小不一的腺样管腔,周围由间质细胞和血管组成(HE 染色,×40);B. 腺样腔内见断头分泌(HE 染色,×400)

Figure 29-92-2   A. Varying size glandular luminal around cellular and vascular stroma in the dermis (HE stain, ×40); B. Decapitation secretion at their luminal surface(HE stain, ×400)

六、神经组织肿瘤 Tumors of Nerve Tissue

93. 皮肤 Merkel 细胞癌
Skin Merkel cell carcinoma

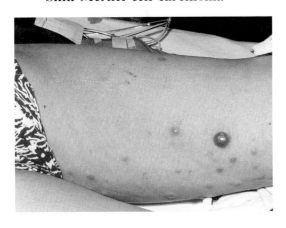

图 29-93-1　左大腿见紫红色结节,表面光滑

Figure 29-93-1　Red violet nodules with smooth surface on the left thigh

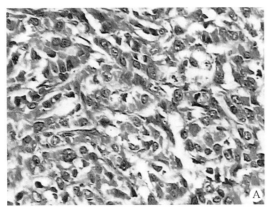

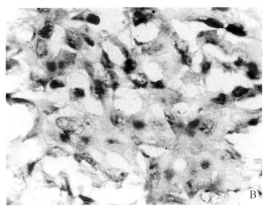

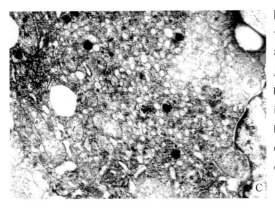

图 29-93-2　A. 癌细胞团片状排列,细胞核大(HE 染色,×200);B. 部分癌细胞胞质嗜铬素 A 阳性表达,呈棕黄色(链霉卵白素-过氧化物酶,×400);C. 癌细胞胞质见散在密电子神经分泌颗粒(透射电镜,×20 000)

Figure 29-93-2　A. The carcinoma cells with large nuclear in corium with the manner of mass (HE stain × 200); B. Chromogranin A positive in cytoplasm of the carcinoma cells (SP method, × 400); C. Nerve secretion granules in cytoplasm of the carcinoma cells (TEM, × 20 000)

94. 神经鞘瘤

Neurilemmoma（Schwannomatosis）

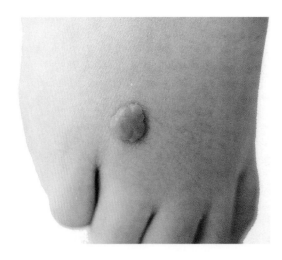

图 29-94-1　右足背一个粉红色软结节
Figure 29-94-1　A pink-grey and soft nodule on the dorsum of right foot

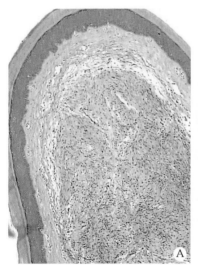
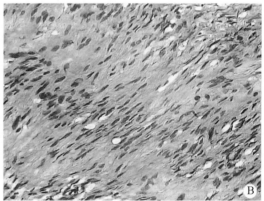

图 29-94-2　A. 真皮内有一境界清楚的无包膜肿瘤（HE 染色，×100）；B. 梭形细胞中嗜碱性核呈长圆形，胞质不清楚，核呈栅状排列或平行排列，在嗜伊红胞质中，称为 Verocay 小体（HE 染色，×400）

Figure 29-94-2　A. A circumscribe and encapsulated tumor is situated in the dermis with fissures around them（HE stain，×100）；B. The cells are sindle shaped with poorly defined cytoplasm and elongated basophilic nuclei，which are arranged in bands，which stream and interweave，the nuclei display palisading and are arranged in parallel rows with intervening eosinophilic cytoplasm in a typical appearance known as Verocay bodies （HE stain，×400）

95. 多发性神经鞘瘤
Multiple neurilemmoma

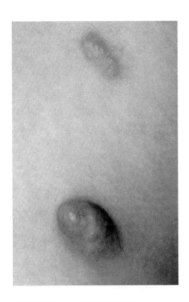

图 29-95-1 躯干部结节
Figure 29-95-1 The noduledis-
tributed on the trunk

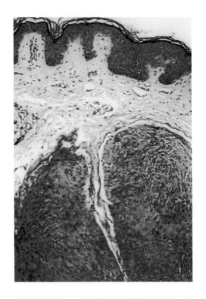

图 29-95-2 细胞排列成栅栏状,其
核排列成行(HE 染色,×200)
Figure 29-95-2 The pathology shows
the cells are arranged in palisades with
their nuclei aligned in paralled rows (HE
stain, ×200)

96. 多发性栅栏状神经鞘瘤
Multiple palisaded neurolemmoma

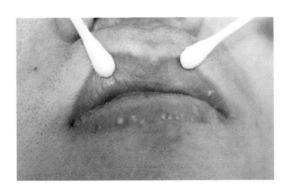

图 29-96-1 下唇粟粒大小米白色丘疹,多个散在分
布
Figure 29-96-1 Multiple creamy white papules in the
size of corn diffused on the lower lip

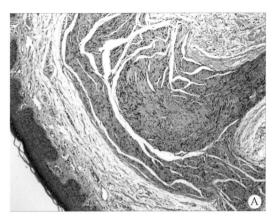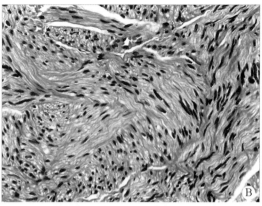

图 29-96-2　A. 表皮基本正常,真皮可见细胞团块样组织,形态不规则,界限清(HE 染色 ×200);B. 施万细胞核排列成不规则栅栏状和漩涡状(HE 染色,×400)

Figure 29-96-2　A. The epidermis was normal. Some irregular cell masses with well-defined margin appeared in the dermis. (HE stain ×200);B. The nucleus of Schwann cells arranged in an irregular palisading and whirling pattern(HE stain,×400)

七、色素痣和恶性黑素瘤
Pigmented Nevi and Malignant Melanoma

97. 甲母痣恶变
Malignant transformation of nail matrix nevi

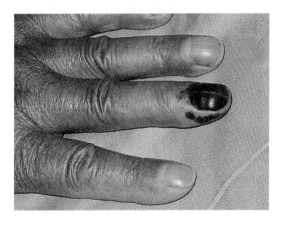

图 29-97-1　左中指甲板巾部条状墨黑色斑,周围有边缘不规则、颜色深浅不一的棕黑色斑

Figure 29-97-1　Striated jet black on the left middle finger nail, irregular, varying color dark brown macula around it

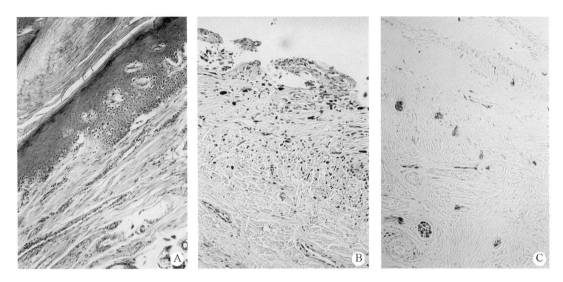

图 29-97-2　A. 表皮内可见成巢分布的黑素细胞(HE 染色)；B. 真皮浅层散在分布的黑素瘤细胞,血管周围中等密度淋巴细胞浸润(HE 染色,×100)；C. 真皮内可见散在 S-100 阳性黑素瘤细胞(S-100 染色,×100)

Figure 29-97-2　A. Nest melanocytes in the epidermis(HE stain)；B. Melanoma cells in the upper dermis,moderately perivascular lymphocytes infiltrate(HE stain,×100)；C. Tumor cell S-100 positive in dermis (S-100 stain,×100)

98. 肢端原位恶性黑素瘤
Acral lentiginous melanoma

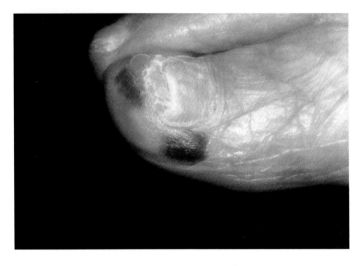

图 29-98-1　右足踇趾内侧缘有一个黑色结节

Figure 29-98-1　A black nodule on the periungual region of right first toe

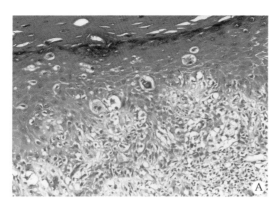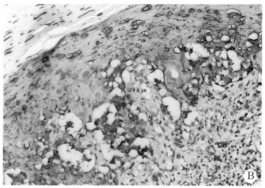

图 29-98-2　A. 表皮内有异形性黑素瘤细胞（HE 染色，×200）；B. 表皮内异形黑素瘤细胞 S-100 蛋白染色阳性（DAB 染色，×200）

Figure 29-98-2　A. Many atypical nevus cells in the epidermis（HE stain，×200）；B. S-100 positive of atypical nevus cells in the epidermis（DAB stain，×200）

99. 气球状细胞恶性黑素瘤
Balloon cell melanoma

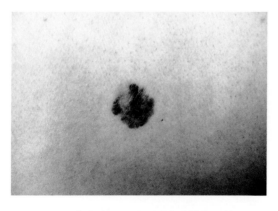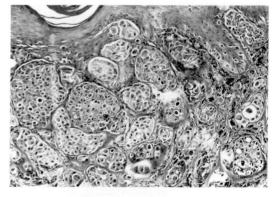

图 29-99-1　背部有一 5 分硬币大暗褐色斑块

Figure 29-99-1　A jitney size brownish red plaque on the back

图 29-99-2　肿瘤细胞体积大，胞质丰富，呈气球状（HE 染色，×200）

Figure 29-99-2　Balloon cells constitute the tumor（HE stain，×200）

100. 口唇恶性黑素瘤
Lip malignant melanoma

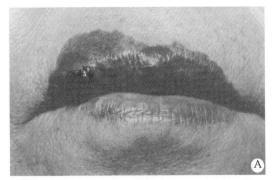
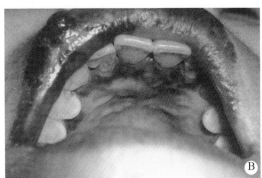

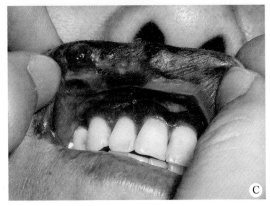

图 29-100-1　上唇(A)、上齿龈(B)、下齿龈(C)及上腭可见边界清楚的棕褐色、黑色斑片,形状不规则、颜色深浅不一,右上唇可见一直径 0.6cm 的紫红色肿物,表面有血痂

Figure 29-100-1　Extensive, black-pigmented and irregularly bordered macules on the upper lip(A), gingiva (B) and the palate(C), an amaranth mass 0.6cm in diameter with blood crust on the right upper lip

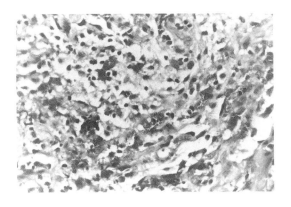

图 29-100-2　黏膜上皮的基底层被破坏,固有层和黏膜下层内密集分布大量肿瘤细胞,部分成巢状,瘤细胞多呈梭形,部分梭形细胞核大、深染,有明显的异形性(HE 染色,×400)

Figure 29-100-2　Rounded collections or nests of melanocytes fill the connective tissue, Tumor cells show cellular pleomorphism and smudged nuclei (HE stain, ×400)

101. 巨大先天性色素痣伴软脑膜恶性黑素瘤
Giant congenital pigmented nevus with malignant melanoma on the pia mater encephali

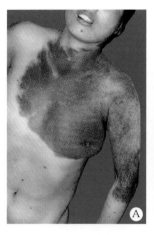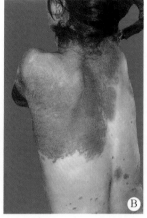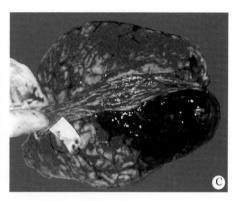

图 29-101-1　A. 左胸、颈、肩部、上臂；B. 左背、项部黑色斑片，形态不规则，表面有黑毛，部分皮损呈疣状增生，周边皮肤有卫星状皮损；C. 软脑膜大片黑色斑块，形态不规则

Figure 29-101-1　A. Large black patches with black hair on the left chest；B. neck, shoulder and the upper arm and the left nape；C. Large black, irregular plaques on the pia mater encephali

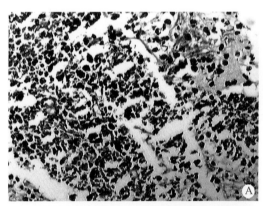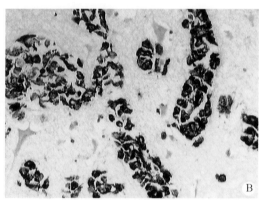

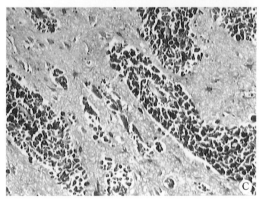

图 29-101-2　A. 蛛网膜下隙有大量异形肿瘤细胞，瘤细胞中有大量黑素颗粒沉着，细胞结构不清（HE 染色，×100）；B. 瘤细胞 HMB45 表达阳性，胞质见棕黄色颗粒沉着（SP 法，×400）；C. 瘤细胞 S-100 蛋白表达阳性，胞质见棕黄色颗粒沉着（SP 法，×100）

Figure 29-101-2　A. Large numbers of atypical tumor cells with multiple melanin granules in the subarachnoid space（HE stain, ×100）；B. HMB45 positive in tumor cells, brown granules in cytoplast（SP stain, ×400）；C. S-100 positive in tumor cells, brown granules in cytoplast（SP stain, ×100）

102. 肢端无色素性黑素瘤
Acral amelanotic melanoma

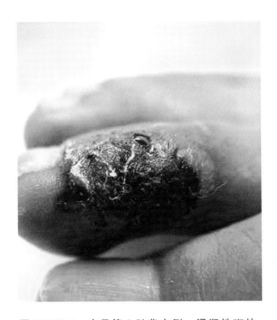

图 29-102-1 右足第 2 趾背内侧一浸润性斑块，呈暗红色，浅表糜烂，边界较清

Figure 29-102-1 An infiltrating plaque with superficial erosion at the dorsal side of the second toe of right foot

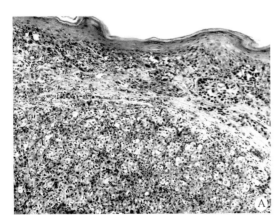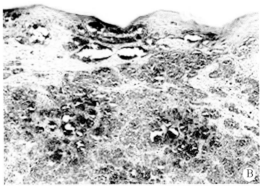

图 29-102-2 A. 真皮网状层一肿瘤细胞团块，肿瘤细胞核大深染，异形性明显，呈巢状或条索状分布（HE 染色，×100）；B. 真皮内肿瘤细胞胞质 S-100 阳性（SP 法，×100）

Figure 29-102-2 A. A mass of infiltrating tumor cells with large irregularly shaped and hyperchromatic nuclei in the reticular dermis (HE stain, ×100); B. S-100 positive in the cytoplasm of tumor cells (SP stain, ×100)

103. 簇发性斯皮茨痣
Agminated Spitz nevus

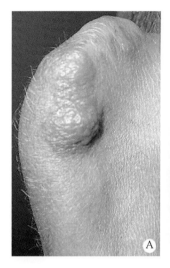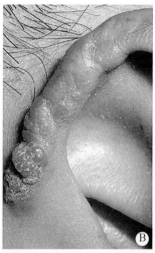

图 29-103-1　A. 左耳郭多发性淡红色小丘疹,融合成片；B. 部分皮损呈乳头瘤样外观

Figure 29-103-1　A. Multiple pink, small papules confluenting to plaques on the left auricle；B. Part papillary

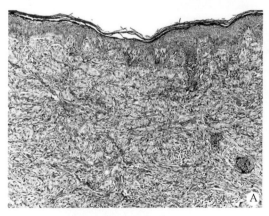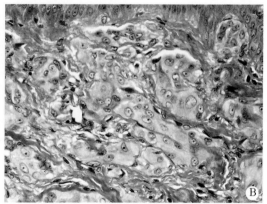

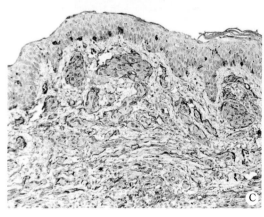

图 29-103-2　A. 真皮内有大量增生的上皮样细胞,呈明显的条索状或巢状分布(HE 染色,×100)；B. 肿瘤细胞为上皮样,部分细胞融合,与周围组织有明显裂隙(HE 染色,×400)；C. 肿瘤细胞 S-100 蛋白强阳性,细胞膜和细胞核明显着色(PV 二步法,×100)

Figure 29-103-2　A. Large amount of epithelioid cells arranged in nests or funicular in the dermis(HE stain, ×100)；B. Epithelioid tumor cells part confluenting, artifactual clefts between the nests of nevus cells and the epidermis (HE stain, ×400)；C. S-100 strong positive in the membrane of tumor cells and nuclei (PV double stain, ×100)

八、淋巴瘤和其他皮肤肿瘤
Lymphoma and other Skin Tumors

104. 单发性肥大细胞瘤
Solitary mastocytoma

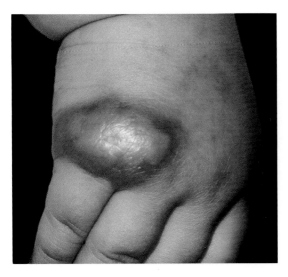

图 29-104-1 右手背有一个大的肤色结节,周围有棕红色晕

Figure 29-104-1 A Large skin color nodule with brown red ring on the dorsum of right hand

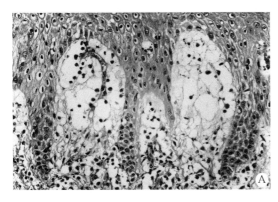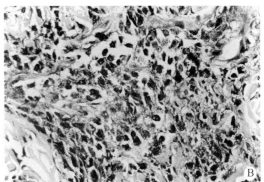

图 29-104-2 真皮内有许多胞质内含有紫红色异染颗粒的肥大细胞浸润(A:HE 染色,×100;B:吉姆萨染色,×400)

Figure 29-104-2 Lots of mast cells contained purple granules in the cytoplasm in the dermis(A:HE stain,×100;B:Giemsa stain,×400)

105. 以泛发性丘疹为表现的成人肥大细胞增生病
Adult mastocytosis with generalized papules on the trunk and extremeties

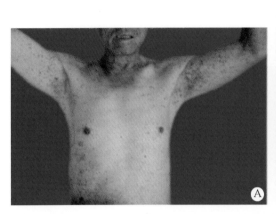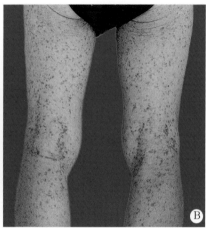

图 29-105-1　A. 躯干、四肢泛发红色丘疹，以褶皱部位明显；B. 部分皮损呈出血性改变
Figure 29-105-1　A. Generalized red papules on the trunk and extremities; B. Part bleeding lesions

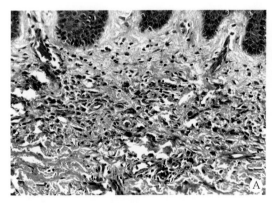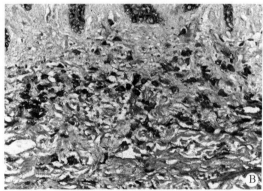

图 29-105-2　A. 真皮浅层较弥漫的单一核细胞浸润，细胞体积大，胞质丰富，部分胞质中细颗粒，部分浸润细胞明显核异形（HE 染色，×200）；B. Giemsa 染色为异染性紫红色颗粒（Giemsa stain，×200）
Figure 29-105-2　A. Moderate infiltration of mast cells in the upper dermis, some of which showed an abnormal morphology (HE stain, ×200); B. Violaceous, metachromatic granules are found (Giemsa stain, ×200)

106. 色素性荨麻疹
Urticaria pigmentosa

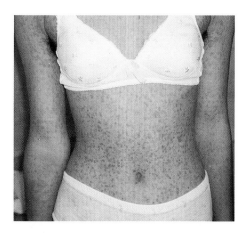

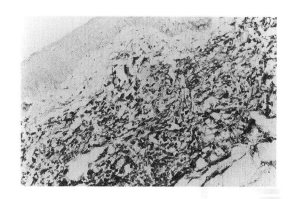

图 29-106-1　胸腹部密集分布褐色丘疹

Figure 29-106-1　Multiple brown papules on the trunk

图 29-106-2　真皮浅层肥大细胞浸润(吉氏染色,× 200)

Figure 29-106-2　Mast cell infiltration in the upper dermis (Giemsa stain,×200)

107. Jessner 皮肤淋巴细胞浸润症
Jessner's lymphocytic infiltration of the skin

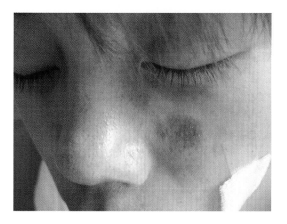

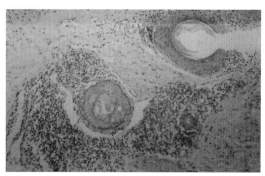

图 29-107-1　左颊部有一个持久的红色斑块

Figure 29-107-1　A persistent plaque-like erythema on the left chin

图 29-107-2　真皮上部血管周围有弥漫性淋巴细胞浸润

Figure 29-107-2　Dense perivascular and diffuse lyphocytic infiltrate in the upper dermis

108. 皮肤淋巴细胞瘤
Cutaneous lymphocytoma

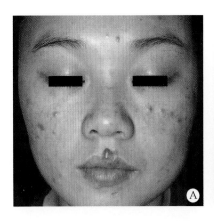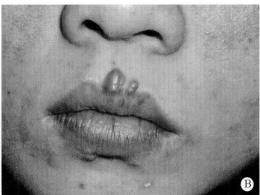

图 29-108-1　两侧颊部出现多个圆形丘疹,上唇数个暗红色丘疹,表面光滑

Figure 29-108-1　Multiple round papules on the cheeks,several brownish red papule on the upper lip

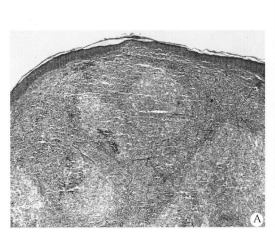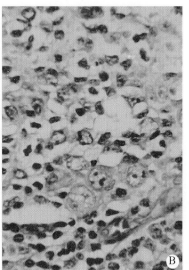

图 29-108-2　A. 表皮轻度萎缩,真皮内有多个淋巴滤泡形成(HE 染色,×100);B. 滤泡中心细胞呈多形性,有淋巴细胞、浆细胞、组织细胞及嗜酸粒细胞,可见核分裂象(HE 染色,×400)

Figure 29-108-2　A. Slight atrophy epidermis,many follical formation in the dermis (HE stain,×100);B. Lymphocytes,histocytes,eosinophils and atypical,mitotic figures are present in the follicles (HE stain,×400)

109. 皮肤白血病
Leukemia cutis

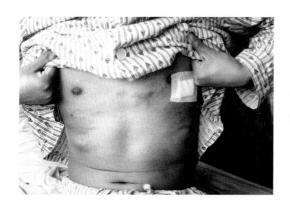

图 29-109-1　前胸紫红色结节、斑块

Figure 29-109-1　Erythematous-to-violaceous nodules and plaques on the chest

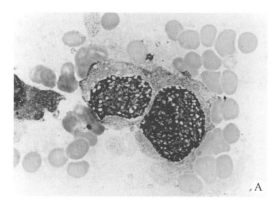

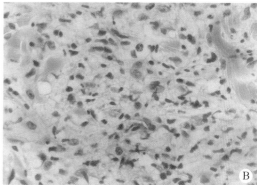

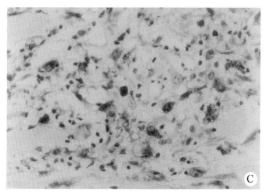

图 29-109-2　A. 大量幼稚单核细胞存在于骨髓中(Wright 染色,×1000);B. 血管周围及结缔组织间大量异形组织细胞样的细胞浸润(HE 染色,×40);C. 瘤细胞显示 CD68(kp-1)阳性(SP 染色,×40)

Figure 29-109-2　A. Large infantility monocytes in the bone marrow (Wright stain,×1000); B. Lots of small-to-medium-sized histiocytes with hyperchromatic nuclei infiltrate in perivascular (HE stain,×40); C. CD68 positive in tumor cells (SP stain,×40)

110. 真性红细胞增多症
Polycythemia vera

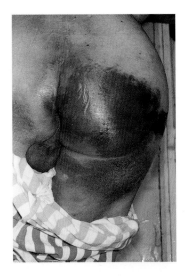

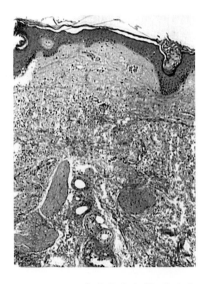

图 29-110-1　右臀部、右下肢近端屈侧及右阴囊部可见紫红色水肿性红斑，界限清晰

Figure 29-110-1　Violet macule with well-circumscribed on the right buttocks, lower limbs and scrotum

图 29-110-2　表皮轻度变薄，真皮水肿，可见大量红细胞外溢，血管周围少许炎性细胞浸润（HE 染色，×40）

Figure 29-110-2　Slight atrophy of epidermis, edematous with many e-rythrocytes effusion, and perivascular inflammation infiltrate in the dermis (HE stain, ×40)

111. 原发性皮肤浆细胞瘤
Primary cutaneous plasmacytoma

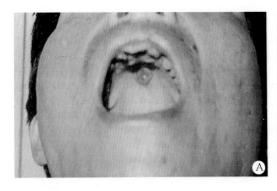

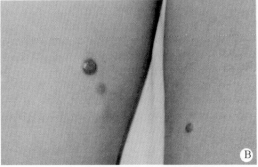

图 29-111-1　A. 上腭正中孤立性红色结节，中央溃疡；B. 两大腿内侧多发性紫红色或肤色结节
Figure 29-111-1　A. A solitary red nodules with ulcers in the center of palate；B. Numerous violaceous, skin-colored nodules on the internal aspect of both thighs

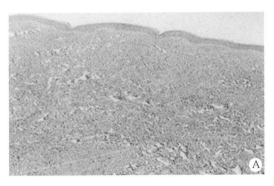 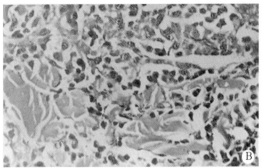

图 29-111-2　A. 真皮及皮下组织内致密浆细胞样细胞呈弥漫性浸润(HE 染色,×40);B. 浆细胞样细胞大小及形状不一,核染色深浅不等,见不典型的核分裂象(HE 染色,×400)

Figure 29-111-2　A. Diffuse infiltrates of plasma cells in the dermis and subcutaneous tissue (HE stain, × 40); B. The plasmacytes vary from size to clumping of chromatin associated with atypical mitotic figures (HE stain, × 400)

112. 继发性皮肤浆细胞瘤
Secondary cutaneous plasmacytoma

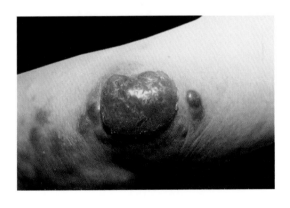

图 29-112-1　左上臂有一个巨大暗红色肿块和许多结节

Figure 29-112-1　A big dark red mass and many nodules on the left arm

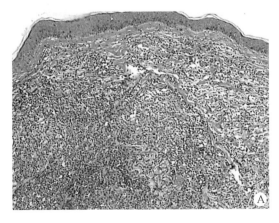 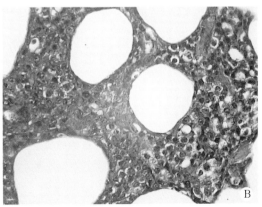

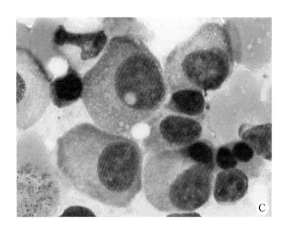

图 29-112-2　A. 真皮内有许多肿瘤细胞(HE 染色,×100);B. 肿瘤细胞核不规则,染色质浓,有不典型核分裂(HE 染色,×400);C. 骨髓涂片,见多个原始浆细胞、幼浆细胞及双核浆细胞(瑞氏染色,×1000)

Figure 29-112-2　A. Lots of tumor cell in the dermis (HE stain,×100);B. Tumor cells have hyperchromatic,irregularly shaped nuclei and atypical mitotic figures (HE Stain,×400);C. The bone marrow smear shows many plasmablasts,proplasmacytes binucleated plasmacytes (Wright's stain,×1000)

113. 皮下脂膜炎样 T 细胞淋巴瘤

Subcutaneous panniculitis-like T-cell lymphoma

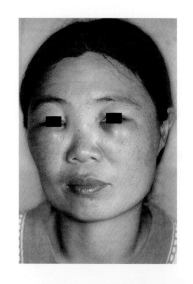

图 29-113-1　面部结节性损害
Figure 29-113-1　Nodules on the face

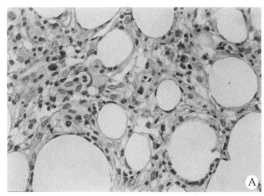

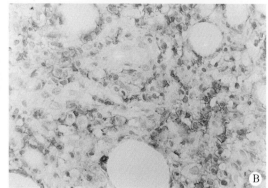

图 29-113-2　A. 脂肪层的异形淋巴细胞和组织细胞浸润,其中淋巴细胞有核丝分裂(HE 染色,×125);B. CD45RO 阳性(免疫组化,×125)

Figure 29-113-2　A. The infiltration of small or medium size lymphocytes in subcutaneous panniculus adiposus (HE stain,×125);B. CD45RO positive (SP stain,×125)

114. 红皮病型皮肤 T 细胞淋巴瘤
Erythrodermic cutaneous T-cell lymphoma

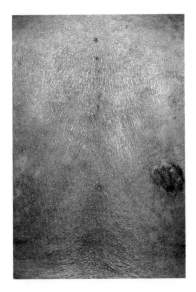

图 29-114-1　全身皮肤弥漫性潮红

Figure 29-114-1　Diffuse erythema on all over body

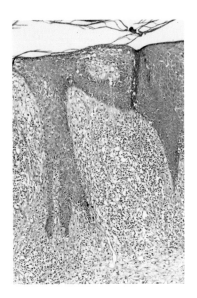

图 29-114-2　表皮内单个或少数聚集的淋巴细胞浸润,伴大的细胞核(HE 染色,×150)

Figure 29-114-2　A few masses of lymphocyte infiltrate with large nuclei in the epidermis (HE stain, × 150)

115. 牛痘样水疱病样皮肤 T 细胞淋巴瘤
Hydroa vacciniforme-like cutaneous T cell lymphoma

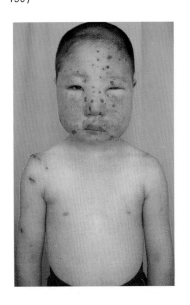

图 29-115-1　面部弥漫性潮红水肿,其上见散在水疱、结痂及痘疮样萎缩性瘢痕

Figure 29-115-1　Diffuse flushing edema, with some scattered blisters, crusts, and variola likeatrophic scars, resembling hydroa vacciniforme on the face

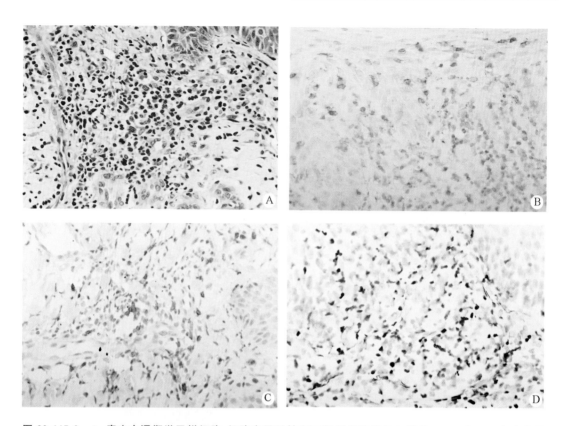

图 29-115-2　A. 真皮内浸润淋巴样细胞,细胞有异形性和不规则细胞核(HE 染色,×100);B. 真皮内浸润细胞 CD45RO(＋);C. 真皮内浸润细胞 CD8(＋);D. 真皮浸润细胞 EB 病毒原位杂交(＋)

Figure 29-115-2　A. Dermal lymphoid cell infiltration; atypical cells with irregular nuclei were noted. (HE stain,×100);B. Dermal infiltrating lymphoid cells showed postive for CD45RO;C. Dermal infiltrating lymphoid cells showed postive for CD8;D. By in situ hybridization,the majority of dermal lymphoid cells were positive for Epstein-Barr virus

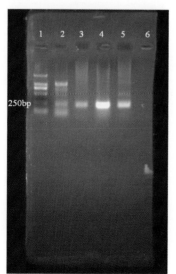

图 29-115-3　TCRγ 基因重排电泳图(250bp)

Figure 29-115-3　Electropheresis TCR-γ gene rearrangment (250bp band)

116. 鼻部 NK/T 细胞淋巴瘤
Nasal natural killer/T cell lymphoma

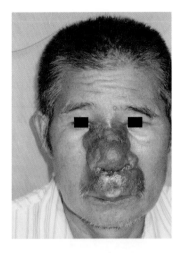

图 29-116-1 鼻背、鼻两侧暗红色斑块、结节,界限清楚

Figure 29-116-1 Well-circumscribed plaques and nodules on the sides and the bridge of the nose

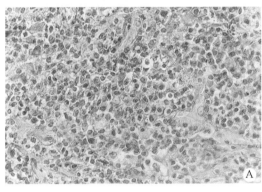

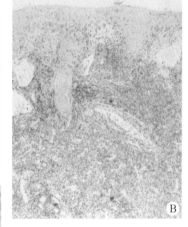

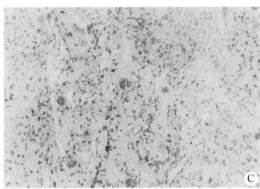

图 29-116-2 A. 真皮致密淋巴样细胞浸润,部分细胞有异形性(HE 染色,×100);
B. CD56(+)细胞(ABC 染色,×100);C. 浸润细胞 CD45RO(+)(ABC 染色,×100)
Figure 29-116-2 A. Lymphoid cells with part atypical infiltrate in the dermis(HE stain,×100);B. Positive CD56(ABC stain,×100);C. Positive CD45RO(ABC stain,×100)

117. 小腿皮肤血管内 NK/T 细胞淋巴瘤
Cutaneous intravascular NK/T cell lymphoma on legs

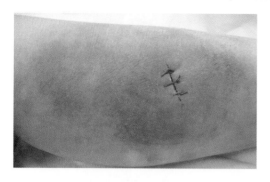

图 29-117-1　左小腿内后侧弥漫性水肿性暗红斑

Figure 29-117-1　Diffuse dark red erythema on the posterior regions of left calf

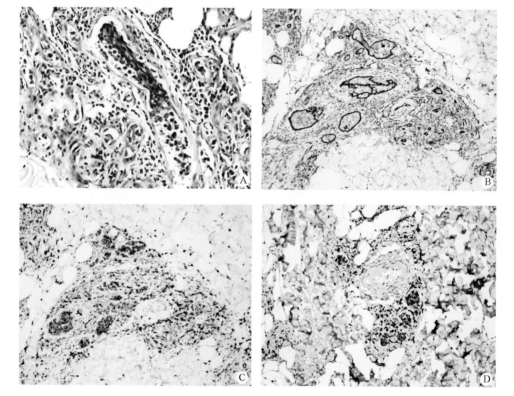

图 29-117-2　A. 真皮内及皮下血管周围淋巴样细胞浸润,多处血管壁坏死及血管闭塞,部分血管内可见成团的淋巴细胞,其中可见较多核大浓染异型细胞及病理性核分裂(HE 染色,×400);B. 血管呈 CD34 阳性反应,肿瘤细胞位于血管内(SP 法,×200);C. 血管内肿瘤细胞呈 CD3 强阳性反应(SP 法,×200);D. 血管内肿瘤细胞呈 CD3ε 强阳性反应(SP 法,×200)

Figure 29-117-2　A. Perivascular atypical lymphoid cellinfiltration in the dermis and subcutis;multiple necrosis of vascular walls and vascular occlusion; Intravascular clusters of lymphocytes with large,hyperchromatic nuclei and pathologic mitosis (HE stain,×400); B. The tumor cells with positve for CD34,are inside of the blood vessels (SP,×200); C. strongly postive for CD3 (SP,×200); D. strongly postive for CD3ε(SP,×200)

118. 非霍奇金淋巴瘤
Non-Hodgkin's lymphoma

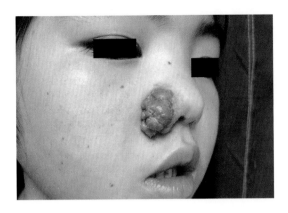

图 29-118-1　右侧鼻翼见一大肿块,表面凹凸不平,基底宽,无破溃,边缘可见成群、大小不一的结节,呈暗红色

Figure 29-118-1　The varying size and red-brown nodules grouped over the right nasal wing

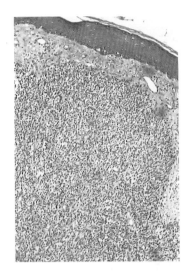

图 29-118-2　表皮轻度不规则增生,真皮肿瘤细胞弥漫浸润,并累及血管及表皮基底层(HE 染色,×100)

Figure 29-118-2　Tumor cells diffuse infiltrate and involve the vessels in the dermis with slight irregular hyperplasia epidermis (HE stain, ×100)

119. 蕈样肉芽肿误诊为蛎壳状银屑病
Mycosis fungoides misdiagnosed as psoriasis rupioides

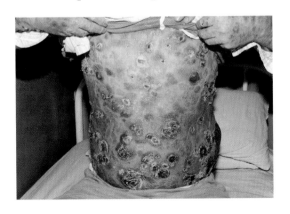

图 29-119-1　胸腹部银白色鳞屑、蛎壳状疹及其脱落后遗留的浸润性斑片

Figure 29-119-1　Erythematous, scaling patches and rupioid eruptions on the trunk

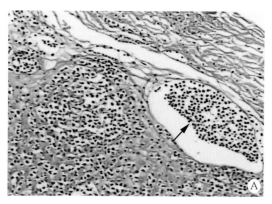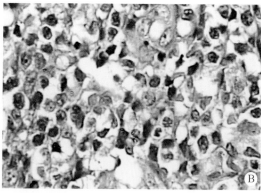

图 29-119-2 A. MF 细胞侵犯表皮、真皮并形成 Pautrier 脓肿(HE 染色,×40); B. 真皮内瘤细胞弥漫分布 (HE 染色,×400)

Figure 29-119-2 A. MF cells infiltrate within the epidermis and dermis, Pautrier microabscesses present in the epidermis (HE stain,×40); B. Diffuse tumor cells in the dermis (HE stain,×400)

120. 以四肢色素沉着为主要表现的蕈样肉芽肿
Mycosis fungoides with hyperpigmentation on limbs

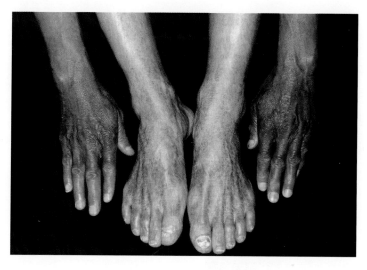

图 29-120-1 手足伸侧呈黑褐色斑片,境界不清

Figure 29-120-1 Dark brown patches on dorsa of hands and feet, border of the lesions was unclear

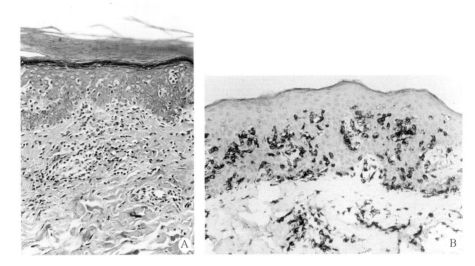

图 29-120-2　A. 表皮内可见 Pautrier 微脓肿，真皮内淋巴细胞带状浸润（HE 染色，×100）；B. 表皮及真皮内 LCA 在淋巴细胞呈阳性表达（ABC 法，×200）

Figure 29-120-2　A. Pautrier microabscesses within the epidermis, a bandlike lymphocytes infiltrate in the dermis (HE stain, ×100); B. LCA positive in the lymphocytes of the epidermis and dermis (ABC stain, ×200)

121. 蕈样肉芽肿继发皮肤 CD30 阳性大细胞淋巴瘤

Mycosis fungoides associated with cutaneous CD30 positive large T-cell lymphoma

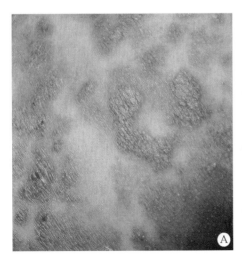
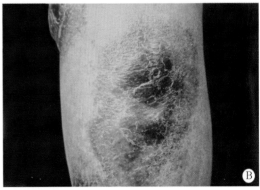

图 29-121-1　A. 臀部苔藓样斑块；B. 左小腿伸面暗红色结节

Figure 29-121-1　A. Lichenoid plaques on the buttocks; B. Brownish red nodules on the extensor of left calf

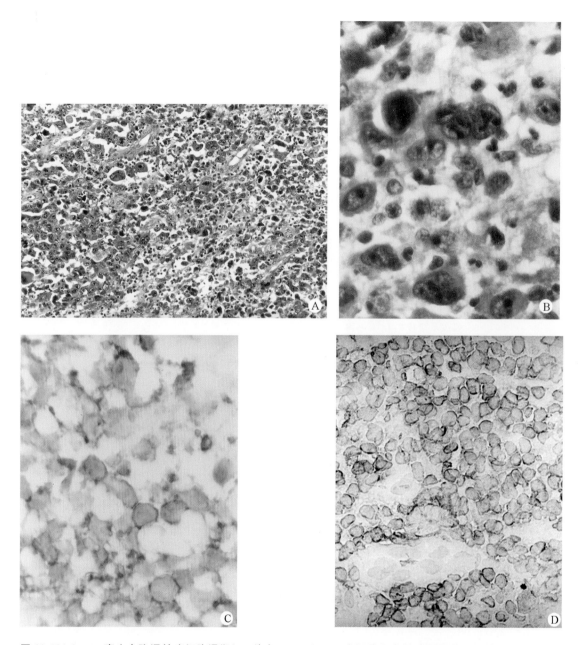

图 29-121-2　A. 真皮内弥漫性瘤细胞浸润(HE 染色,×100)；B. 瘤细胞和多核瘤巨细胞(HE 染色,×1000)；
C. 瘤细胞表达 CD45RO(ABC 法,×400)；D. 瘤细胞表达 CD30(ABC 法,×400)

Figure 29-121-2　A. Diffuse tumor cells infiltrate in the dermis (HE stain,×100)；B. Tumor cell and multinucleated tumor giant cells (HE stain,×1000)；C. CD45RO positive tumor cells (ABC method,×400)；D. CD30 positive tumor cells (ABC method,×400)

122. 具有多种表现的蕈样肉芽肿
Several variants of mycosis fungoides in one patient

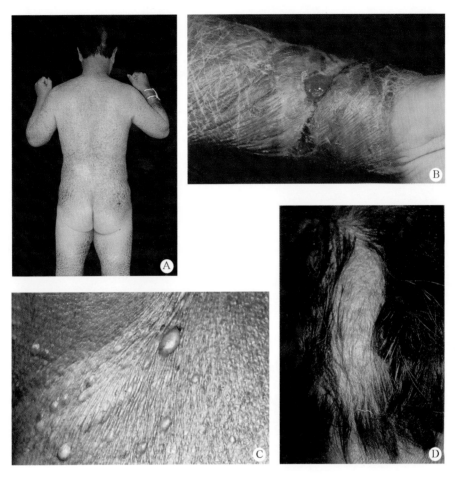

图 29-122-1 A. 全身皮肤干燥, 上有多量粗糙的灰白色大片状鱼鳞样鳞屑、痂皮; B. 右前臂明显肿胀, 中央有一直径约 6cm 的溃疡; C. 腋窝可见数十个豆粒大的丘疹, 结节, 呈白色半透明状; D. 枕部有条片状的秃发斑块, 上有多个毛囊性丘疹, 覆少量黏着性鳞屑

Figure 29-122-1　A. Dry skin in the whole body, covered with multiple coarse, whitish, large scales and crusts; B. Marked swelling with a ulcer 6 cm in diameter in the center on the right forearm; C. Numerous bean in size, translucent, white papules and nodules on the axilla; D. Strip and sheet bald plaques on the occiput, several hair follicle papules on the plaques, covered with a few adherent scales

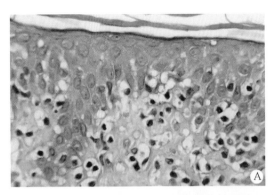
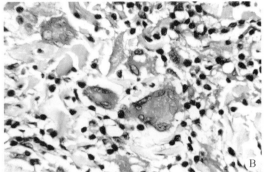
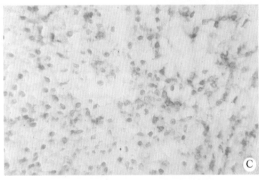

图 29-122-2 A. 表皮萎缩,表皮内单一核细胞浸润,呈不典型的 Pautrier 微脓肿(HE 染色,×400);B. 真皮内可见较多的多核巨细胞(HE 染色,×400);C. 免疫组化示 CD45RO(＋)(ABC 染色,×400)

Figure 29-122-2 A. Epidermal atrophy had mononuclear cells infiltration presenting atypical Pautrier microabscess (HE stain,×400); B. Multiple multinucleated giant cells in the dermis (HE stain,×400); C. CD45RO positive (ABC stain,×400)

123. 以皮肤斑块浸润和肿瘤表现为主的 B 细胞淋巴瘤
Tumorous and infiltrated plaque variant of cutaneous B-cell lymphoma

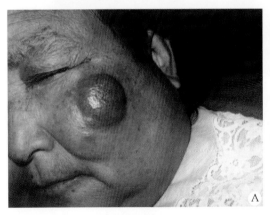
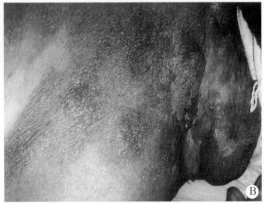

图 29-123-1 A. 面部肿块,鸽蛋大,半球形,色暗红;B. 腋下弥漫性红斑及浸润性斑块

Figure 29-123-1 A. Pigeon egg sized, half ball, brownish red tumor on the face; B. Diffuse erythema and infiltrate plaques on the axilla

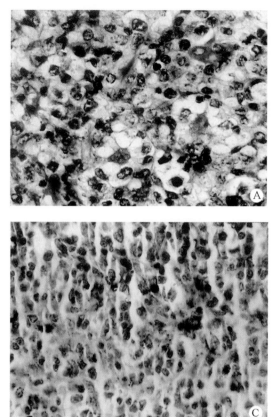

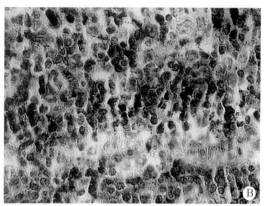

图 29-123-2　A. 大量异形瘤细胞；B. 大量棕黄色 CD20⁺ 细胞；C. 少量 CD68⁺ 细胞

Figure 29-123-2　A. Numerous atypical tumor cells; B. Numerous CD20 positive cells; C. A few CD68 positive cells

124. 皮肤假性淋巴瘤
Cutaneous pseudolymphoma

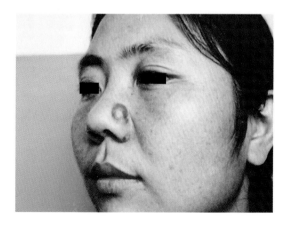

图 29-124-1　左侧鼻翼暗红色半球形结节

Figure 29-124-1　A brownish red nodular on the nose

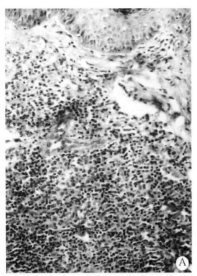

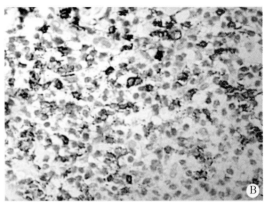

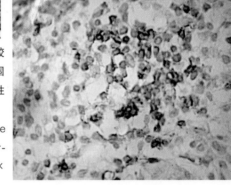

图 29-124-2　A. 真皮浅层，浸润细胞与表皮间有一较窄的正常胶原带，真皮中下部、皮下组织和附属器周围淋巴样细胞浸润（HE 染色，×100）；B. CD45RO 阳性（SP 染色，×400）；C. CD20 阳性（SP 染色，×400）

Figure 29-124-2　A. Below epidermis a narrow free zone, an infiltration of lymphocytes in the superficial dermis（HE stain, ×400）；B. CD45RO positive（SP, ×400）；C. CD20 positive（SP, ×400）

125. 皮肤窦性组织细胞增生症

Cutaneous Rossai-Dorfman disease, or Cutaneous sinus histocytosis

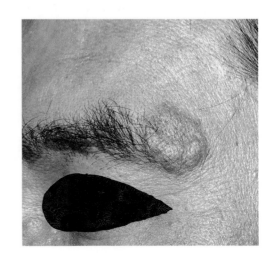

图 29-125-1　左眼眶外上方有一红色浸润斑块

Figure 29-125-1　A red infiltrate plague on the left orbita

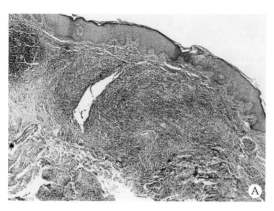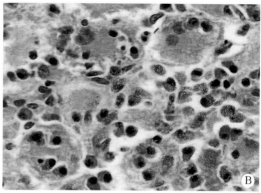

图 29-125-2　A. 真皮内有大量组织细胞和炎症细胞浸润（HE 染色，×20）；B. 组织细胞胞质中有淋巴细胞、浆细胞或中性粒细胞（HE 染色，×400）

Figure 29-125-2　A. Lots of histocytes and inflammatory cells in the dermis（HE stain，×20）；B. Lymphocytes plasma cells and neutrophils are present in the cytoplasm of histocytoses（HE stain，×400）

126. 皮肤原发性窦性组织细胞增生症

Cutaneous primary sinus histiocytosis with massive lymphadenopathy

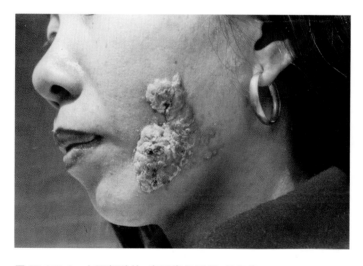

图 29-126-1　左面颊肿块，表面高低不平，呈红色

Figure 29-126-1　Two red tumours on left face

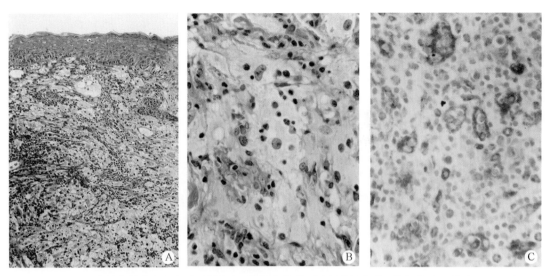

图 29-126-2   A. 真皮内许多组织细胞,胞体大,核呈空泡状,间有淋巴细胞、浆细胞(HE 染色,×100); B. 真皮内见体积大、蜘蛛样的组织细胞,胞质内有少量中性粒细胞和淋巴细胞(HE 染色,×400); C. 组织细胞 CD68 染色阳性,胞质内见淋巴细胞(Envision 法,×400)

Figure 29-126-2   A. Multiple histiocytes with cytoplastic and vacuole nuclei in dermis, some lymphocytes and plasma cells(HE stain, ×100); B. Large histiocytes exhibiting emperipolesis with phagocytized lymphocytes, neutrophils, and plasma cells within the cytoplasm(HE stain, ×400); C. CD68 positive histocytes, lymphocyte in the histocyte cytoplasm (Envision method × 400)

127. 皮肤型 Rosai-Dorfman 病
Cutaneous Rosai-Dorfman disease

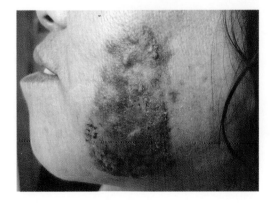

图 29-127-1   左面颊可见 4.5 cm×7.1 cm 紫红色斑块

Figure 29-127-1   A brown-red plaque in 4.5 cm to 7.1 cm size on the left check

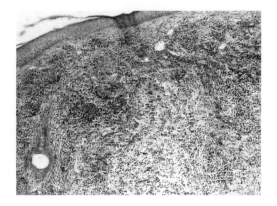

图 29-127-2   表皮萎缩,真皮密集组织细胞、淋巴细胞和浆细胞浸润,有淋巴滤泡样结构(HE 染色,×100)

Figure 29-127-2   Epidermal atrophy and many histocytes, lymphocytes and plasma cells associated with lymph follicular structure were present in the dermis (HE stain, ×100)

348

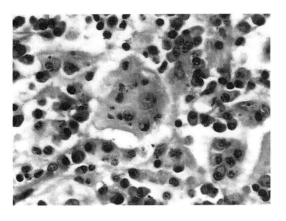

图 29-127-3 大组织细胞吞噬淋巴细胞、浆细胞和碎核,周围有较多浆细胞(HE 染色,×400)
Figure 29-127-3 The lymphocyte, plasma cell and nuclear debris were phagocytosed in a big histocyte around many plasma cells(HE stain,×400)

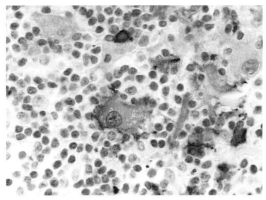

图 29-127-4 组织细胞 S100 阳性(Envision 法,×400)
Figure 29-127-4 S100 positive in histiocyte (Envision method,×400)

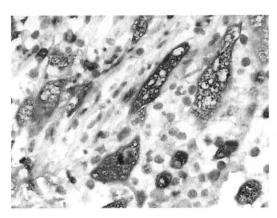

图 29-127-5 组织细胞 CD68 阳性 (Envision 法,×400)
Figure 29-127-5 CD68 positive in histiocyte (Envision method,×400)

128. 淋巴瘤样丘疹病

Lymphomatoid papulosis

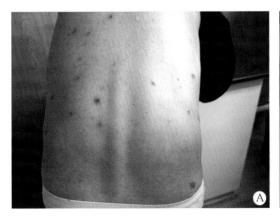

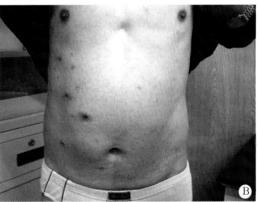

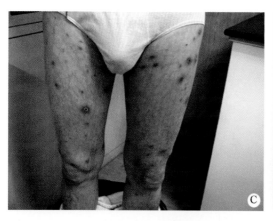
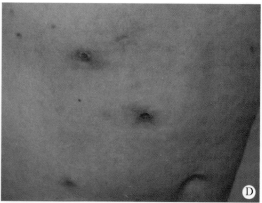

图 29-128-1 　在四肢和躯干有多数结节,表面有溃疡和结痂

Figure 29-128-1 　There are many nodules with ulceration and crusting on the extremities and trunk

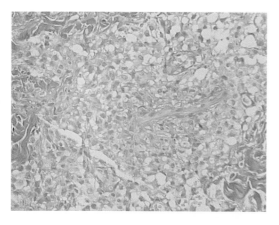
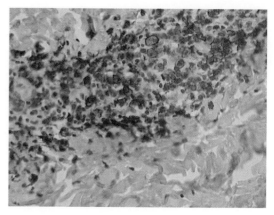

图 29-128-2 　真皮内有大量核淡染的组织细胞,核仁明显(HE 染色,×400)

Figure 29-128-2 　There are many large histiocytic cells with a pale-staining nucleus and a prominent nucleolus in the dermis (HE stain,×400)

图 29-128-3 　CD30RO 阳性 Figure 29-128-2 CD30RO positiue

129. 肺癌皮肤转移

Lung cancer with skin metastasis

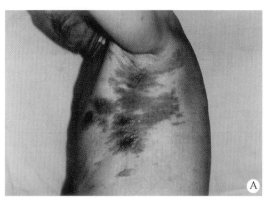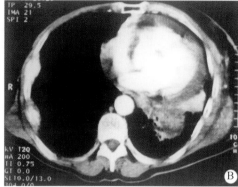

图 29-129-1　A. 左腋下、胸背部及季肋部皮损；B. CT 示：左肺下叶见 4.5 cm×4.0 cm 肿块影,呈分叶状,不均匀强化

Figure 29-129-1　A. The left axilla,chest,back and hypochondrium lesions；B. A 4.5 cm×4.0 cm tumour in left lower lung

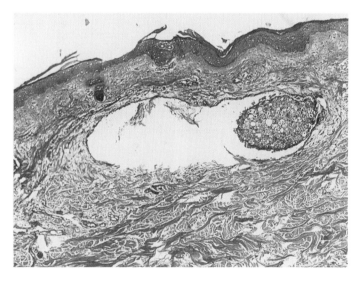

图 29-129-2　真皮内癌栓形成(HE 染色,×160)

Figure 29-129-2　Tumor embolism in the dermis(HE stain,×160)

130. 胃癌皮肤转移
Stomach cancer with skin metastasis

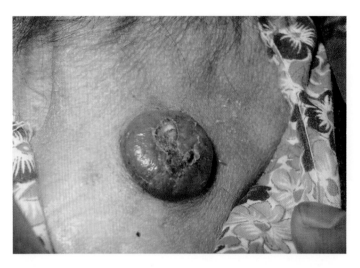

图 29-130-1 颈后部有一 2cm×2cm×1cm 的肿块,隆起于皮肤表面,中央凹陷

Figure 29-130-1 A 2cm×2cm×1cm tumor with depressed center on the back of neck

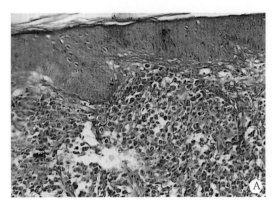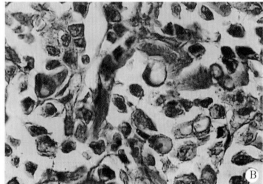

图 29-130-2 A. 真皮内可见大量密集分布的癌细胞,呈巢状分布(HE 染色,×100);B. 多数印戒细胞,细胞大小、形态不一(HE 染色,×400)

Figure 29-130-2 A. Numerous tumor cells nest in the dermis(HE stain,×100);B. Numerous signet ring cells with varying size and shape(HE stain,×400)

131. 来源于脐尿管低分化腺癌
Low differentiated adenocacinoma from umbilco-urethral canal

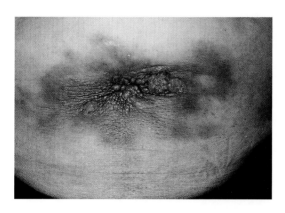

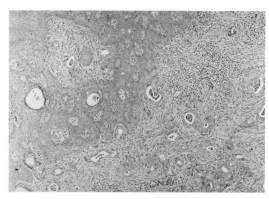

图 29-131-1　脐周有一 9cm×10cm 椭圆形斑块,边界清,质硬,浸润较深,表面皮肤有色素沉着,脐窝及脐周可见较多米粒至黄豆大丘疹,部分呈乳头瘤状,脐窝消失

Figure 29-131-1　A oval well-circumscribed plaque 9 cm × 10 cm in diameter with hyperpigmentation, and papules with papillomatous surface

图 29-131-2　低分化腺癌,多系来自脐尿管残件(HE 染色,×88)

Figure 29-131-2　Low differentiated adenocacinoma from umbilical-urethral canal remnant (HE stain, × 88)

132. 铠甲癌
Carcinoma en cuirasse

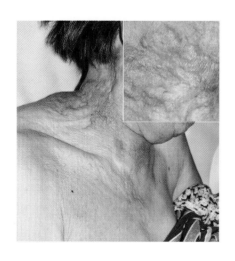

图 29-132-1　右上胸由许多细小皮下结节融合成的 20cm×15 cm 皮下斑块,向上累及颈部约 20cm×10cm 皮肤,皮肤表面严重变形成脑回形。皮肤似木头样硬度不能被捏起

Figure 29-132-1　Indurated plaque was found on the right side of the upper anterior chest wall measuring 20cm×15 cm in size, and it extended upward to the right part of the neck over an area of 20cm×10cm, which was grossly distorted and convolutional in shape. The underlying skin was wood hard and un-pinchable

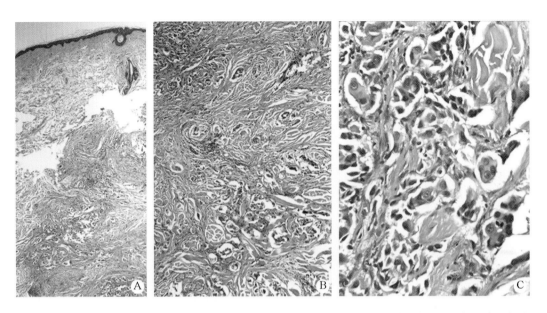

图 29-132-2　真皮内广泛性瘤团,其胞质丰富,细胞核大小不一,明显异形且染色较深,分布于胶原纤维束间(A:HE 染色,×40;B:HE 染色,×100;C:HE 染色,×400;)

Figure 29-132-2　Monomorphous tumor cells with a rich cytoplasm in vacuoles,presented singly or in small clusters between dense collagen bundles in the dermis(A:HE stain,×40;B:HE stain,×100;C:HE stain,×400)

第30章
与皮肤病有关的综合征
Cutaneous Syndromes in Dermatology

1. Ascher 综合征
Ascher syndrome

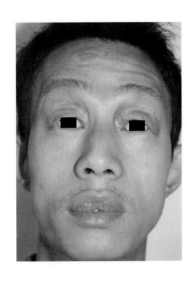

图 30-1-1　双上睑松弛下垂,皮肤萎缩变薄,边缘轻度水肿,上唇明显肿胀,呈双唇表现

Figure 30-1-1　Relaxation and ptosis of the both upper eyelids with atrophy and slight edema; Markedly swollen upper lip and double upper lip

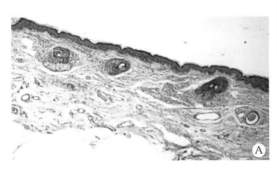
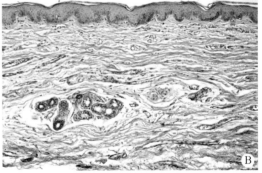

图 30-1-2　表皮大致正常,真皮明显萎缩变薄,真皮内毛细血管扩张、增生(HE 染色,×40);B. 真皮弹性纤维明显减少(Verhoff 染色,×100)

Figure 30-1-2　A. Obvious dermal atrophy and associated with telangiectasia and capillary proliferation (HE stain, ×40); B. Reduced elastic fibers in the dermis (Verhoff stain, ×100)

2. 狒狒综合征
Baboon syndrome

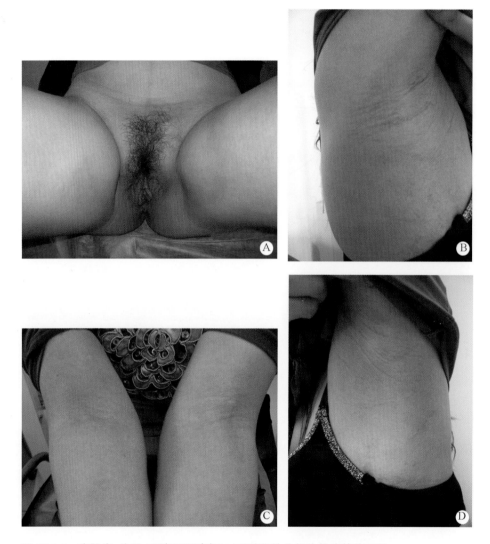

图 30-2-1　腹股沟、外阴、双腋下及肘窝（A-D）对称性分部边界清楚的红斑

Figure 30-2-1　Circumscribed erythema symmetrically on the gluteal, perianeal and other major intertriginous（A-D）

3. Bloom 综合征
Bloom's syndrome

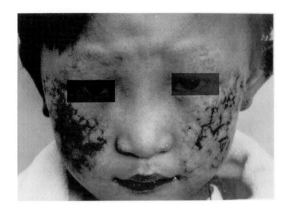

图 30-3-1 双面颊毛细血管扩张,呈网状
Figure 30-3-1 Telangiectatic erythema in the butterfly area of the face

4. 蓝色橡皮-大疱性痣综合征
Blue rubber-bled nevus syndrome

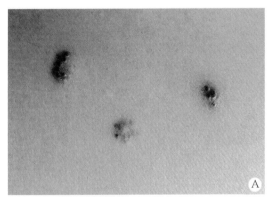

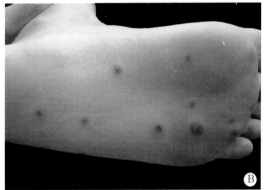

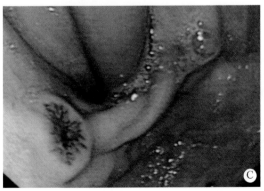

图 30-4-1 A、B. 躯干和足跖多数紫色斑、丘疹和结节;C. 胃体、胃窦有数个 0.5~1 cm 直径的血管瘤
Figure 30-4-1 A、B. Multiple blue macules,papules and nodules with various sizes on the trank and feet; C. Several angioma-like tumors 0.5 cm to 1 cm in diameter on the stomach

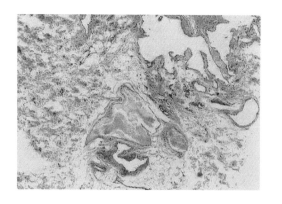

图 30-4-2　真皮下方有大小不规则充满血液的血管，内衬以单层内皮细胞（HE 染色）

Figure 30-4-2　Large irregular spaces filled with blood in the lower dermis，which lined by a single layer of endothelial cells（HE stain）

5. 息肉-色素沉着-脱发-甲营养不良综合征

Cronkhite-Canada syndrome

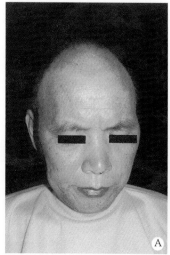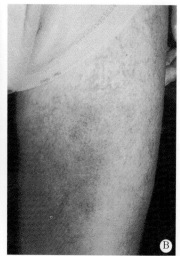

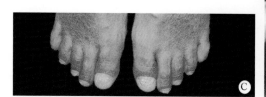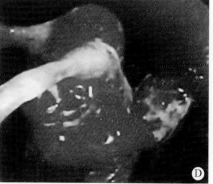

图 30-5-1　A. 头顶发稀疏细小；B. 右大腿有弥漫性点状色素沉着斑；C. 趾甲破坏脱落，甲床凹凸不平；D. 结肠脾曲有许多大小不等的息肉

Figure 30-5-1　A. Sparse and thin hairs on the scalp；B. Diffuse and spotty hyperpigmentation on the right thigh；C. Nail destrophy with triangular nail plate；D. Lots of various size polyposis in the splenic flexure of colon

6. 局灶性真皮发育不全综合征
Focal dermal hypoplasia syndrome

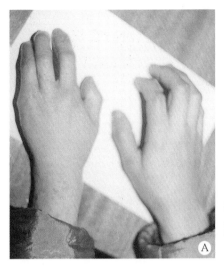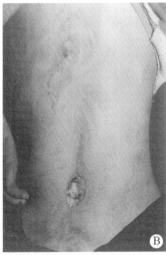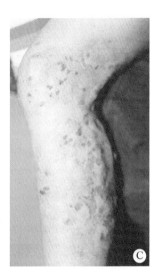

图 30-6-1　A. 右手发育正常,左手 3、4 并指已行分指术,第 5 指已截指;B. 背部两处萎缩性瘢痕,网状色素沉着,毛细血管扩张,脊柱纵行凹陷;C. 右下肢萎缩性瘢痕,脂肪疝,色素沉着及减退

Figure 30-6-1　A. The right hand is normal, the left third and forth finger are split with syndactyly and the fifth finger amputation; B. Two cicatricial atrophy on the back, reticular pigmentation, telangiectasis, longitudinal cupped on the spinal column; C. Cicatricial atrophy, fatty herniation, hypo-and hyperpigmented patches on the right lower limb

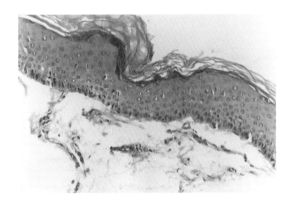

图 30-6-2　表皮突消失,真皮胶原纤维减少且发育不良,脂肪组织增生(HE 染色,×200)

Figure 30-6-2　Marked dermal atrophy with thin collagen fibers consistent hypoplasia and fat hyperplasia (HE stain, ×200)

7. Favre-Racouchot 综合征合并眼睑乳头状瘤

Favre-Racouchot syndrome associated with eyelid papilloma

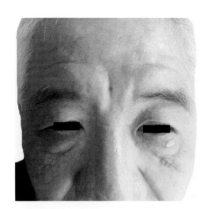

图 30-7-1　开放性粉刺位于患者的双侧眶下区沿着斜行的皱纹，皮损呈对称分布。患者左下眼睑，花生粒大小肉色增生物

Figure 30-7-1　Several open comedones located at two obliquely linear furrows in his both infraorbital regions. The distribution of these lesions is bilaterally symmetrical. A flesh-colored nipple-like growth, approximately in the size of groundnut kernels on the patient's left lower eyelid

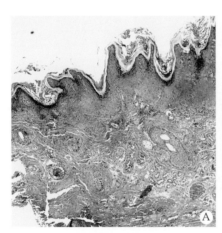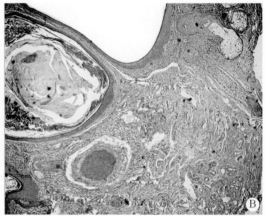

图 30-7-2　A. 眼睑乳头瘤的病理：角化过度，颗粒层增厚和多个毛囊角栓的棘层增厚，表皮突增长，似乳头瘤样向上增生(HE 染色，×100)；B. 开放性粉刺的病理：狭长的漏斗扩张，充满角化和角化不全的物质。粉刺的上部包含酵母样微生物(糠秕孢子菌)和细菌(HE 染色，×200)

Figure 30-7-2　A. The pathology of papilloma revealed that hyperkeratosis, hypergranulosis andacnthosis with multiple follicular keratinous plugs. (HE stain, ×100)；B. The pathological findings of open comedones showed dilated elongated infundibula filled with keratosic and parakeratotic materials. The upper part of the comedo contained nests yeast-like organisms (pityrosporum) and bacteria(HE stain, ×200)

8. Gorham 综合征
Gorham syndrome

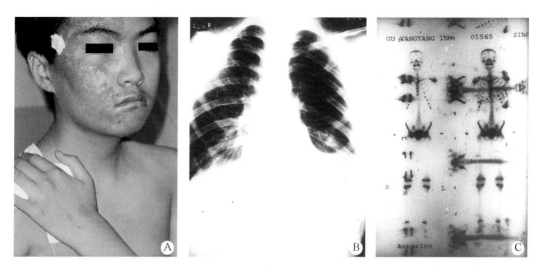

图 30-8-1　A. 右侧颜面部密集白色、粟米状、厚壁疱疹,外观油腻;B. 双侧胸腔积液,右锁骨发育畸形;
C. 全身 SPECT 示:左肱骨上端呈放射性异常浓聚

Figure 30-8-1　A. White, millet-like vesicles with greasy appearance in the right face; B. Bilateral pleuro-
clysis effusions, right clavicle deformity; C. Increased signal intensity in the proximal aspect of left humerus
by SPECT

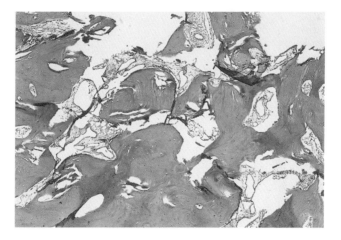

图 30-8-2　右锁骨活检示纤维化和淋巴管增生(HE 染色,×
40)
Figure 30-8-2　The fibrosis and lymphangial hyperplasia in right
clavicle biopsy (HE stain, ×40)

9. 先天性额顶部皮下脂肪瘤-胼胝体发育不良-颅内脂肪瘤综合征

Innate frontoparietal subcutaneous fat oncoma-callosal dysplasia-intracranial fat oncoma syndrome

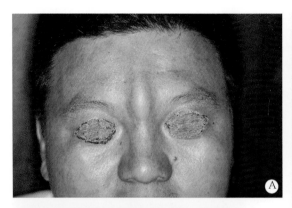
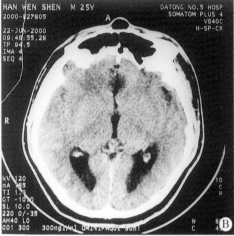
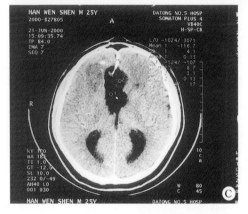

图 30-9-1　A. 额正中皮下脂肪瘤；B. 额顶部大脑镰下脂肪瘤；C. 胼脂体发育不良

Figure 30-9-1　A. Innate frontoparietal subcutaneous fat oncoma; B. A fat oncoma of cerebral falx; C. Callosal dysplasia

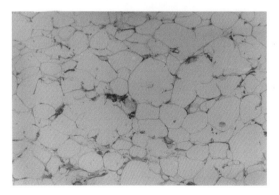

图 30-9-2　棕色脂肪细胞，分化良好（HE 染色，× 300）

Figure 30-9-2　Brown fat cell with differential well (HE stain, × 300)

10. 角膜炎-鱼鳞病-耳聋综合征
Keratitis-ichthyosis-deafness syndrome

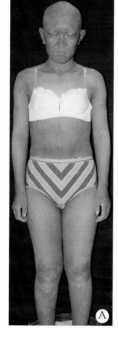
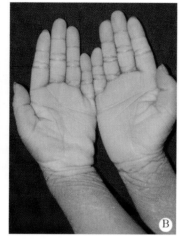
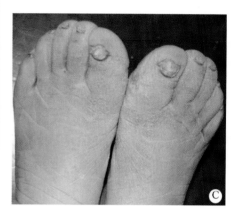

图 30-10-1　A. 全身皮肤干燥,无毛发,无汗,面部,双耳,颈部,红斑,粗糙,四肢腋下,腹股沟,腘窝角化,增厚,脱屑;B、C. 指、趾呈颗粒样或皮革样角化,有较多的棘状赘生物,甲肥厚,变白

Figure 30-10-1　A. Generalized dry skin; atrichia and anhydrosis; rough erythemas on the face, ears and neck; hyperkeratosis and desquamation on armpits, inguinal grooves and popliteal fossa; B, C. Grain or leather-like hyperkeratosis with acanthoid neoplasms on the fingers and toes; pachyonychia and whitening

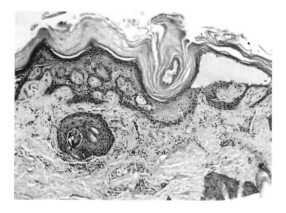

图 30-10-2　角质层显著增厚伴有角化不全,棘层增厚,轻度乳头瘤样增生,可见毛囊角栓,真皮浅层血管周围少量的淋巴细胞和组织细胞浸润(HE 染色,×100)

Figure 30-10-2　Hyperkeratosis with parakeratosis and acanthosis; slight papillomatous hyperplasia and keratotic follicular plugs, mild lymphocyte and histocyte infiltration around the vessels in the upper dermis (HE stain, ×100)

11. 外阴-阴道-牙龈综合征型扁平苔藓

Lichen planus-vulvo-vaginal-gingival syndrome

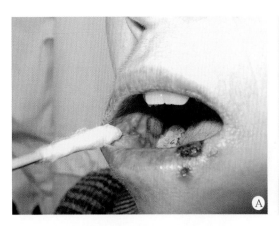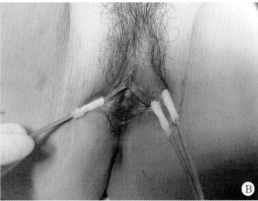

图 30-11-1　A. 右颊膜和上、下牙龈有糜烂；B. 阴道口及小阴唇下方有糜烂面

Figure 30-11-1　A. The erosions are present in right buccal mucosa, and on the upper and lower gingival; B. The erosions are present on the aditus vaginae, and the lower part of labium minus

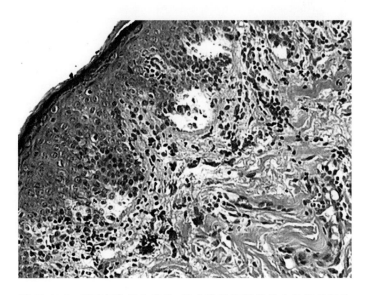

图 30-11-2　基底细胞液化变性，真皮浅层有带状分布的淋巴细胞和组织细胞浸润(HE 染色，×200)

Figure 30-11-2　There are hydropic degeneration of basal cells and a bandlike infiltrate composed of lymphocytes and histocytes beneth the epidermis(HE stain, ×200)

12. Jackson-Lawler 综合征
Jackson-Lawler syndrome

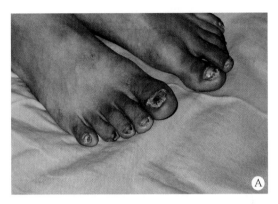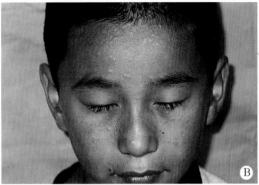

图 30-12-1　A. 趾甲板增厚,部分呈污褐色；B. 前额见绿豆至黄豆大淡黄色结节

Figure 30-12-1　A. Hypertrophic nails of all toenails, part of them with brownish appearance; B. The yellow nodules from mung bean to soybean size on the forehead

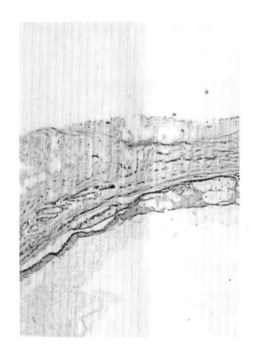

图 30-12-2　真皮内囊肿,皮脂腺小叶与囊壁相连,囊壁的一部分由皮脂腺小叶构成(HE 染色,×40)

Figure 30-12-2　The part wall of cysts was composed of sebaceous gland lobule in the dermis (HE stain, ×40)

13. Laugier-Hunziker 综合征
Laugier-Hunziker syndrome

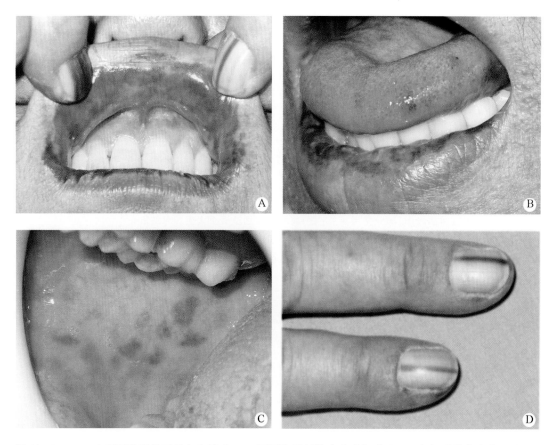

图 30-13-1　A. 上下唇弥漫性不均匀色素斑；B. 下唇和舌侧缘有色素沉着斑；C 右颊黏膜有色素沉着斑；D. 右手指间关节伸侧深褐色斑，指甲有深褐色纵条

Figure 30-13-1　A. Lentiginous pigmentation of the upper and lower lip; B. Lentiginous pigmentation of the lower lip and tonque; C. Lentiginous pigmentation of the right buccal mucosa; D. Lentiginous pigmentation of aspect of finger joint of right hand, Dark brow stripes of the fingernail

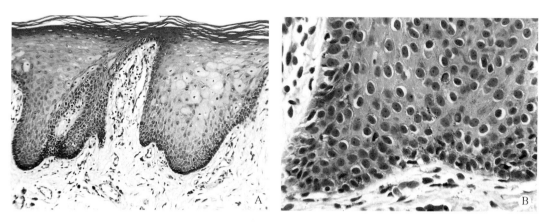

图 30-13-2　A. 基底层色素增加(HE 染色,×100);B. 基底细胞内有较多黑素颗粒(HE 染色,×400)
Figure 30-13-2　A. Hyperpigmintation in basal cell layer (HE stain,×100);B. Neumerous melanin granules in basal cells (HE stain,×400)

14. Madelung 综合征
Madelung syndrome

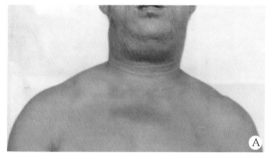
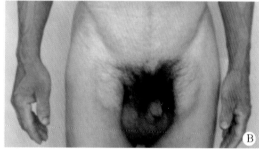

图 30-14-1　A. 多发性脂肪瘤肿块围绕颈部;B. 多发性脂肪瘤肿块在双侧腹股沟
Figure 30-14-1　A. Multiple massive lipomas are around neck;B. Multiple massive lipomas are symmetrical in both groin

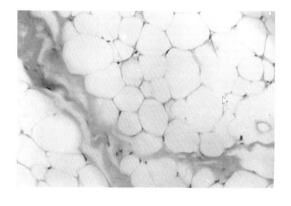

图 30-14-2　脂肪瘤由和正常脂肪细胞一样的细胞组成(HE 染色,×400)
Figure 30-14-2　Lipoma composed of fat cells which do not differ from normal fat cells(HE stain,×400)

15. Marshall-White 综合征
Marshall-White syndrome（Bier's Spot）

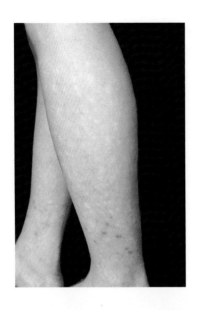

图 30-15-1　双小腿多数 0.2～2.0 cm 直径大的小白斑，散在夹杂在淡红和暗红斑中

Figure 30-15-1　Neumerous small pales macules 0.2 to 2.0 cm in diameter scattered within pink or red erythema on the both legs

16. 甲、髌、肘发育不良综合征
Nail-whirlbone-elbow syndrome（Nail-patella-elbow syndrome）

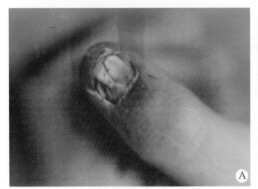

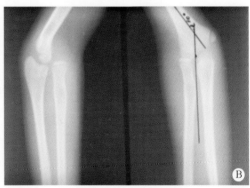

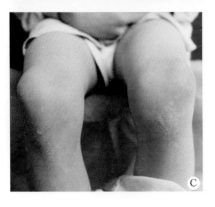

图 30-16-1　A. 拇指甲萎缩为正常甲 2/3 大小，有纵嵴，薄而脆易折断，甲半月呈 V 形；B. X 线下左桡骨小头发育不良，不全性联结伴尺桡交叉畸形；右桡小头发育尚可，但尺桡间宽，呈尺桡小头分离畸形；C. 髌骨小，屈曲位时向外侧半滑脱，外观隆凸呈"方膝"状

Figure 30-16-1　A. Severe dysplasia on the ulnar border of the thumbnail, ridged longitudinallyor horizontally, separated into two halvesby a longitudinal cleft or ridge of skin, triangular lunula; B. X ray of elbow showing a dysplastic, dislocated radial head and hypoplasia of the left capitellum; C. The patellae small and subluxed patellae on knee flexion, flattened profile

17. Netherton 综合征
Netherton's syndrome

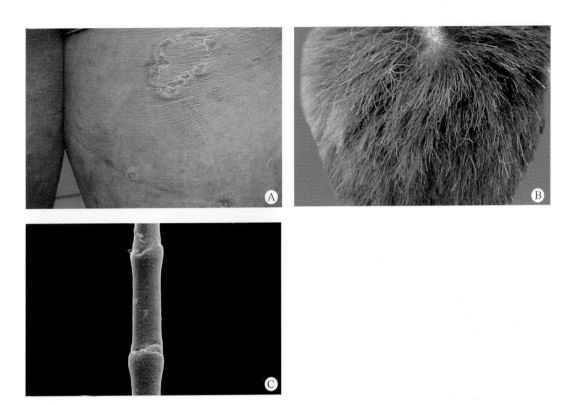

图 30-17-1 A. 左侧股部内侧环状皮损,周边有小片灰白色"双边"鳞屑;B. 头发粗糙、干燥无光泽;C. 病发在扫描电镜下呈竹节状

Figure 30-17-1 A. Annular lesions on the left thigh's inner side、and small gray"double border"scaling aroundit;B. Hairs are coarse,dry and lusterless; C. Sick hair looked like "bamboo node" observed by scanning electron microscopy

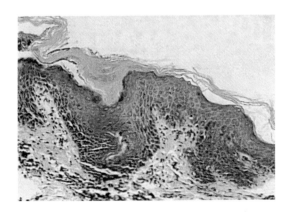

图 30-17-2 角化过度伴灶性角化不全,棘细胞间可见细胞间水肿(HE 染色,×160)

Figure 30-17-2 Hyperkeratosis and local parakeratosis,intercellular edema(HE stain,×160)

18. Olmsted 综合征
Olmsted syndrome

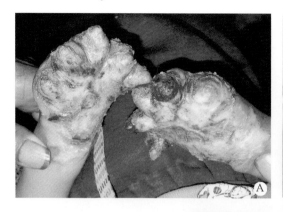
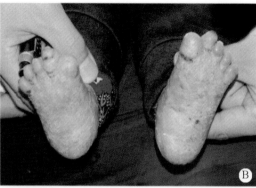
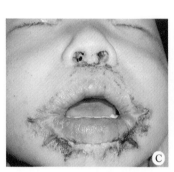
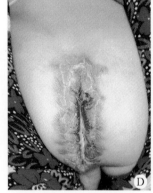
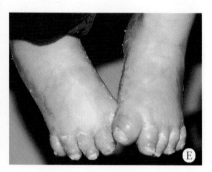

图 30-18-1　A. 双手掌明显角化过度,大部分手指残缺;B. 双足跖弥漫性角化增厚,有皲裂,出血;C. 口周有红斑,角化,其上有放射状皲裂;D. 骶尾部和肛周边界清楚的角化性斑块,上覆痂,周围有红斑;E. 双足趾甲增厚、混浊,部分有横沟

Figure 30-18-1　A. Both severe palmar keratoderma and digital spontaneous amputation;B. Both severe plantar keratoderma with fissure and bloody;C. Hyperkeratotic erythematous plaques around the mouth with radial fissures;D. Hyperkeratotic plaques with crusts around the sacrococcyx and anus;E. Thick toe nails of feet with lateral groove

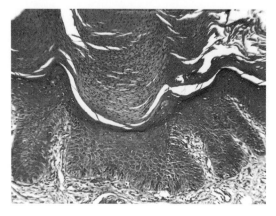

图 30-18-2　表皮角化过度伴角化不全,棘层肥厚,真皮浅层有少量淋巴细胞浸润(HE 染色,×100)

Figure 30-18-2　Epidermal hyperkeratosis with parakeratosis and acanthosis are associated with a few lymphocyte infiltration in the upper dermis (HE stain, ×100)

19. Papillon-Lefèvre 综合征伴沟纹舌
Papillon-Lefèvre syndrome with fissured tongue

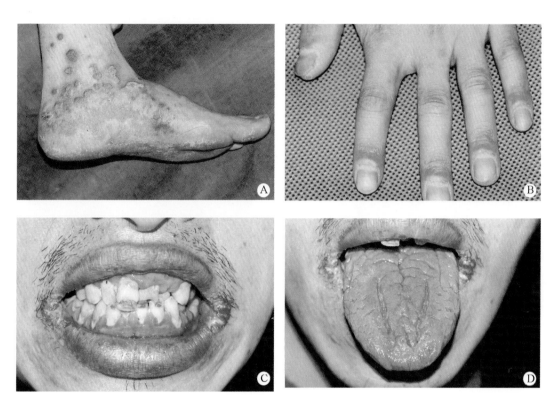

图 30-19-1　A. 左足内侧至踝部有许多丘疹,部分融合,足跖见黄色角化性斑块,表面许多鳞屑;B. 手指末节背侧甲小皮周围皮肤增生,甲小皮皱缩,指甲正常;C. 口周糜烂,牙龈红肿,可见牙周袋;D. 舌体见2 条较深纵行沟纹和许多横行沟纹

Figure 30-19-1　A. Many papules partly confluent on the inboard of left ankle, yellowish, scaly, keratotic plaques over the soles; B. Thickened skin around crimp eponychium and the extensor surface of distal interphalangeal joint; C. Erosion around the mouth, gingival inflammation and periodontal pocket; D. Numerous deep grooves or furrows on the dorsal surface of the tongue

20. 面部单侧萎缩合并颅脑病变
Parry-Romberg syndrome with subclinical cerebral involvement

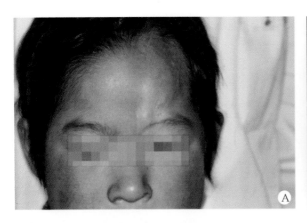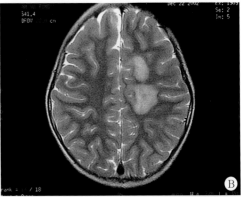

图 30-20-1　A. 前额中线略偏左侧见一纵行刀砍状凹痕，长约 10cm，左侧额部明显凹陷，正常肤色，静脉显露，同侧鼻翼皮肤较对侧略变薄；B. 左侧顶、枕、颞叶皮质下白质不规则病灶，左侧额顶区皮下脂肪缺如，颅骨变薄

Figure 30-20-1　A. Parasagittally on the left forehead, about 10 cm in length, sunken on the left forehead; B. Foci in white matter of the left occipital, temporal lobe under cortical, fat scarcity and skull attenuation in the left forehead

21. 先天性环状缩窄带综合征
Pseudo-Ainhum syndrome

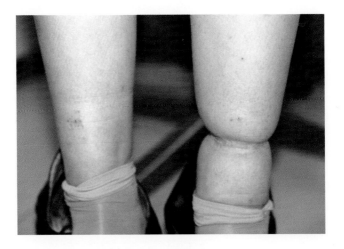

图 30-21-1　左小腿下段肢体环状凹陷如束带状

Figure 30-21-1　Ringy hollow caused by linear constriction on the left calf

22. Proteus 综合征

Proteus syndrome

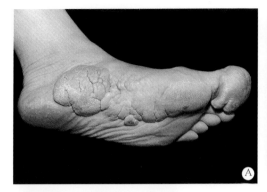
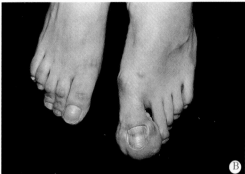
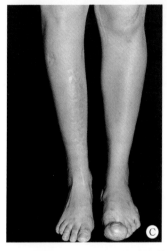
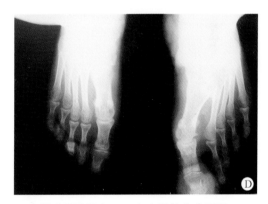

图 30-22-1　A. 左足弓有脑回状皮肤斑块和结节；B. 左踇趾明显粗大；C. 左小腿较右小腿粗；D. X
线检查示左侧第 1 趾骨头的外侧有外生骨疣

Figure 30-22-1　A. Cerebriform hyperplasie mass and nodules on the left sole；B. Macrodactyly of the
left thumb；C. Hemihypertrophy of the left lower extremity；D. Roentgenogram demonstrated on exostosis on the lateral side of left first metatarsal caput

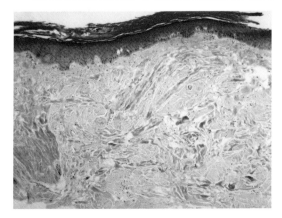

图 30-22-2　表皮角化过度,真皮胶原纤维致密、增粗
(HE 染色,×40)

Figure 30-22-2　Hyperkeratosis of epidermis and
dense and thick of collagen fibers in the dermis (HE
stain,×40)

23. 色素沉着-息肉综合征
Pigmentation-polyposis syndrome

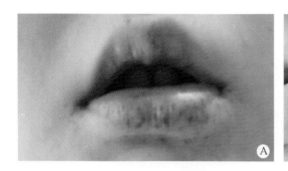 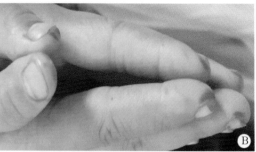

图 30-23-1　下唇(A)和指部(B)有黑色斑

Figure 30-23-1　Dark maculae on the lower lip(A) and fingers(B)

24. 梅干腹综合征
Prune-belly syndrome

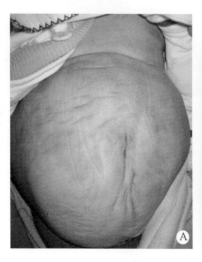 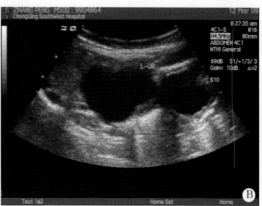

图 30-24-1　A. 腹部皮肤增厚,凹凸不平；B. 腹部超声:双侧肾积水,左侧巨输尿管,右肾肾窦分离,膀胱分离,膀胱壁增厚,壁上有钙化

Figure 30-24-1　A. Wrinkly folds of skin covering the abdomen；B. Abdominal ultrasonography：hydronephrosis in both kidneys,large left ureter,right renal sinus and bladder separation, thickened bladder wall with calcification

25. Rapp-Hodgkin 综合征
Rapp-Hodgkin like syndrome

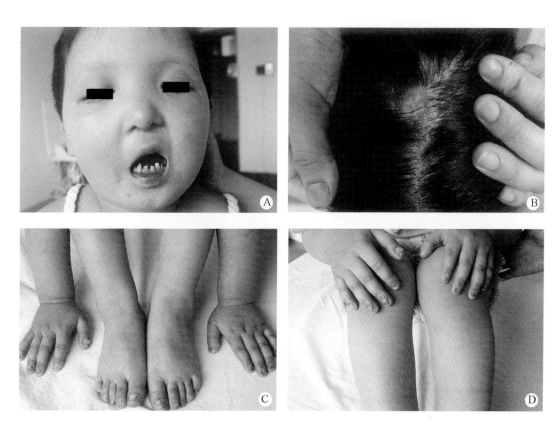

图 30-25-1　A. 牙齿稀疏、不齐,切齿呈锥形和不规则形;B. 头顶部斑块状脱发;C. 指、趾甲增厚,呈锥状,甲质变脆,部分剥脱;D. 两小腿皮肤干燥、粗糙,毛周角化

Figure 30-25-1　A. Sparse teeth, irregular and cone-shaped incisor teeth; B. Sheet alopecia on the scalp; C. Cone-shaped thickened nails nad toenails; D. Dryness and coarse skin with keratosis perifollicular on the calf

26. Rombo 综合征

Rombo syndrome

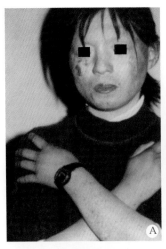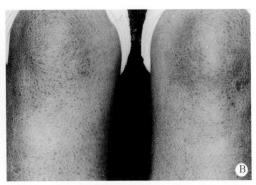

图 30-26-1　A. 上、下唇及眶周多个白斑及多发性粟丘疹及虫蚀斑,睫毛脱失,仅内侧有少许稀疏的眉毛,上、下眼睑外翻,以下眼睑为著,面及手部红斑和毛细血管扩张;B. 膝部红色毛囊性丘疹,小腿有细小鳞屑

Figure 30-26-1　A. Multiple whitish macules, numerous milia, atrophoderma vermiculatum, loss of lashes of eye the upper and lower lids, only several eyebrows very thinly implanted on the interior sides, and ectropion of both upper and lower eyelids, especially the lower ones, erythema and telangiectases on the face and hands; B. Red follicular papules on the knees, and fine scales on the calfs

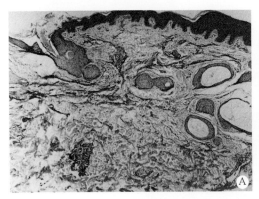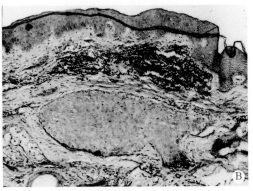

图 30-26-2　A. 真皮中上部有三个囊状结构,囊内被覆正常鳞状上皮。囊内可见毳毛及角化物。可见小血管增生及扩张,伴淋巴细胞浸润(HE 染色,×40);B. 部分区域高度不规则的块状弹性纤维,而其他区域无弹性纤维 (Verhoeff 染色,×40)

Figure 30-26-2　A. Three cystic structures located in the upper and middle dermis, covered on the inside with normal-appearing squamous epithelium. Inside the cysts, multiple vellus hairs and horny material were seen. Some proliferation and dilation of small vessels were noted, accompanied by a lymphocytic infiltration (HE stain, ×40); B. Highly irregular distribution of elastin, with clumping in some areas, whereas other skin areas appeared no elastin (Verhoeff stain, ×40)

27. Rothmund-Thomson 综合征

Rothmund-Thomson syndrome

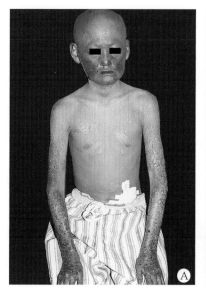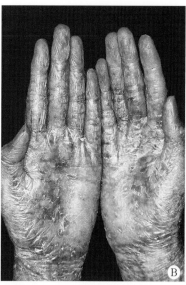

图 30-27-1　A. 面、臀部和四肢有泛发性皮肤异色症，网状红斑，毛细血管扩张，色素沉着和色素减退；B. 双手掌红斑角化

Figure 30-27-1　A. Generalized poikiloderma: reticulated erythema, telangiectasias, hyperpigmentation, and hyporpigmentation on face, buttock and extremities; B. Erythematous and hyperkeratosis of both palms

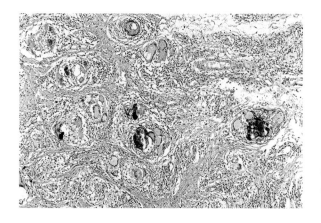

图 30-27-2　真皮中有钙和类脂质沉积，伴有泡沫细胞、多核巨细胞和肉芽肿样结构（HE 染色，×25）

Figure 30-27-2　The deposition of calcium and lipoid associated with foamy cells, multinucleated macrophages and granulomatous structure in the dermis (HE stain, ×25)

28. 僵硬皮肤综合征

Stiff skin syndrome

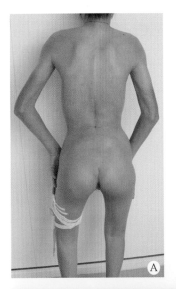

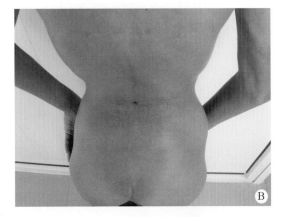

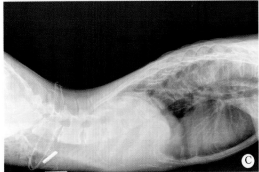

图 30-28-1　A、B. 双侧肩、肘、髋、膝关节活动受限,膝内翻;颈项部、躯干部、双上臂、臀部及大腿皮肤僵硬如石,腰部多毛; C. X 线检查见胸、腰椎生理曲度增大,骨盆呈类猿型

Figure 30-28-1　A、B. Limitation of large joint（shoulder,elbow,hip and knee）mobility,and genu varum; Stony hard skin on the neck,trunk,upper limbs,thighs and buttocks,Hirsutism on the lumbar area;C、D. X-ray image：Abnormal physiological curvature of the thoracic and lumbar spine,Ape-like pelvis

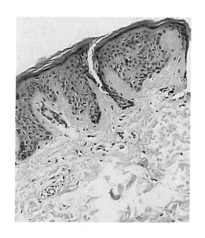

图 30-28-2　表皮大致正常,基底层色素增加,真皮层增厚,胶原纤维增粗,皮肤附属器存在

Figures 30-28-2　Normal epidermis,and thickened dermis with increased number of fibroblasts and well-preserved appendages

29. 毛发-鼻-指趾综合征

Tricho-rhino-phalangeal syndrome

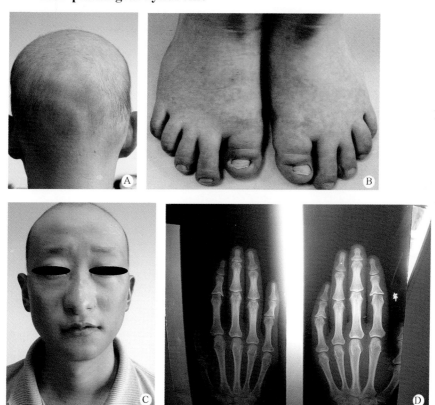

图 30-29-1　A. 毛发稀疏细软,尤以颞顶部明显;B. 踇趾短,第 4、5 趾甲内收,趾甲薄;C. 眉毛外侧稀疏,梨形鼻,上唇薄,无胡须;D. 部分指骨骺呈锥形

Figure 30-29-1　A. Sparse and brittle hairs on the scalp,prominent feature on the temple; B. Spare hairs of eyebrow,pear-shaped broad nose, thin upper lip and no beard; C. Short thumb and thin toe nails; D. Radiological features showed cone-shaped epiphyses

30. Waardenbury 综合征

Waardenbury syndrome

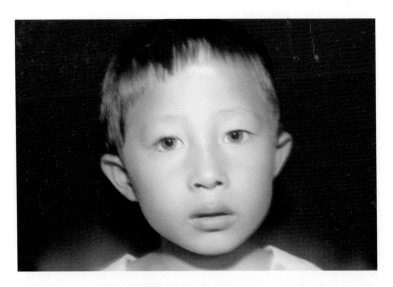

图 30-30-1　先天性感觉神经性聋,蓝色虹膜,前额白斑和白发

Figure 30-30-1　The case with congenital sensorineural hearing loss, blue irises, white forelock and depigmentation of hair and skin

参考文献(或图片提供者)

第1章

[1] 陈仁贵,钱黎华,张定国,庄寅,邓艳.新生儿单纯疱疹病毒感染1例.临床皮肤科杂志,2003,32(11):659-660.

[2] 李萍,冯建军,李增杰.双侧带状疱疹1例.临床皮肤科杂志,2006,35(2):127.

[3] 汪晨,相广财,王纪英,等.巨大寻常疣并发皮疹[J].临床皮肤科杂志,2008,37(2):84-87.

[4] Xia MY,Zhu WY,Lu Ju,Lu Q,Chen L. Ultrastructure and human papillomavirus DNA in papillomatosis of external auditory canal.Int J Dermatol 1996;35(5):337-339

[5] 陈思远,夏颖,杨珍等.浅表肉芽肿性脓皮病.临床皮肤科杂志,2013,42(1):26-28.

[6] 吴信峰,方方,胡兹嘉.鲍恩样丘疹病.临床皮肤科杂志,2006,35(1):1-2.

[7] 谭城,朱文元,闵仲生,等.成人非对称性近屈曲部疹2例.临床皮肤科杂志,2010(012):765-767.

第2章

[1] 韦应波,叶庆佾,郝飞,向明明,邓军,张琬,尹锐,郝进,张晖.严重Fournier坏疽1例.临床皮肤科杂志,2005,34(2):102-103.

[2] 陈思远,夏颖,杨珍等.浅表肉芽肿性脓皮病.临床皮肤科杂志,2013,42(1):26-28.

第3章

[1] 姜薇,乌日娜,沈丽玉,涂平,朱学骏.界线类偏结核样型麻风.临床皮肤科杂志,2003,32(10):565-566.

[2] 陶晓苹,伍友成,刘林,杨为.增殖性寻常狼疮.临床皮肤科杂志,2004,33(8):455-456.

[3] 戚丽华,张怀亮,曾学思.疣状皮肤结核.临床皮肤科杂志,2000,29(5):图谱.

[4] 张建中,赵亭,金江,邵勇,贾军,朱铁君,丁北川.游泳池肉芽肿2例报告.临床皮肤科杂志,2002,31(1):34-36.

[5] 曹发龙,来身德,董世珍.皮肤炭疽病1例.临床皮肤科杂志,2006,35(1):37.

[6] 朱文元,夏明玉,黄立,芦勤.窝状角质松解症皮损的扫描电镜观察.临床皮肤科杂志,1983,12(4):190.

第4章

[1] 王铃艳,谢红付,施为,李吉.Reiter综合征.临床皮肤科杂志,2005,34(11):791-792.

第5章

[1] 成人不典型黄癣 朱文元供图.

[2] Zhu WY,Xia MY,Li H,Wu SX,Zhong Q,Zhao B.Electron microscope observation on infected hairs of kerion caused by M.anum.Int J Dermatol,1987,26(10):641-645.

[3] 李雪,朱文元,鲁严,朱丰.红色毛癣菌致股癣合并龟头癣1例.中国麻风皮肤病杂志,2014;30(5):310-312.

[4] 吴绍熙.名医病例分析.临床皮肤科杂志,2002,31(11):737-738.

[5] Yang XY,Liu WD,Chen ZQ,Lin L.Diffused dermatophytosis resulting from Trichophyton rubrum treated with itraconazole pulse regimen. Journal Clinical Dermatology, 2003, 32(suppl):S112-114.

[6] 戴迅毅,张海平.掌黑癣1例.临床皮肤科杂志,2004,33(5):290-291.

[7] Tan C,Zhu W Y,Min Z S.Blaschkoid pityriasis versicolor.Mycoses,2010,53(4):366-368.

[8] 杨淑欣,赵娟,黄静.皮肤念珠菌性肉芽肿合并念珠菌性颈淋巴结炎1例.临床皮肤科杂志,2003(12):724-725.

[9] 陈征,李薇,熊琳,周光平,汪盛,代亚林,冉玉平,郭在培.慢性皮肤黏膜念珠菌病.临床皮肤

科杂志,2004,33(5):288-289.

[10] 廖万清.原发性皮肤隐球菌病.临床皮肤科杂志,2004,33(4):259-260.

[11] 林自华,阎国富,何云志,张国威,何威.皮肤隐球菌病1例.临床皮肤科杂志,2004,33(1):25.

[12] 张超英,方栩,李莉,怀有为.传染性软疣样皮损表现的播散性隐球菌病2例.临床皮肤科杂志,2002,31(7):452-453.

[13] Ran YP,Xiong L,Li W,Luo Q,Li ZY,Yuan CT,Peng XM,Lu YH,Liao WQ,Dai YL,Du XP,Zhou GP. A case of disseminated crypto-coccosis with multiple cutaneous lesions and osteomyelitis. Journal Clinical Dermatology,2003,32(suppl):S48-51.

[14] 陈颖,施秀明.多发结节表现的孢子丝菌病1例.临床皮肤科杂志,2002,31(10):654-655.

[15] 李莉,徐浩生,王家俊.淋巴管型着色芽生菌病1例.临床皮肤科杂志,2002,31(7):450-451.

[16] Xue ZY,Luo D,Cheng BG,Yu ML,Mei YL. Basidiobolomycosis.Journal Clinical Dermatology,2003,32(suppl):S85-90.

[17] 赖声正,王芳乾.手部放线菌病1例.临床皮肤科杂志,2003,32(1):30.

[18] 张金松,刘志梅,张信江,罗显华,张更建,郑庭铭.皮肤中型原藻病.临床皮肤科杂志,2006,35(11):705-706.

[19] 钱坚革,沈昃,余爱如,孙建方,吕桂霞.奴卡氏菌性足菌肿1例.临床皮肤科杂志,2002,31(5):312-313.

[20] 李春阳,李颖,胡志敏.多变根毛霉引起原发皮肤毛霉病1例.临床皮肤科杂志,2004,33(3):158-159.

[21] 尤海燕,尤刚,李晓杰,刘冰梅,张美莲,王敬.皮肤链格孢霉病1例.临床皮肤科杂志,2005,34(2):82-84.

[22] 赵娟,杨淑欣,赵安成,李霞.镰刀菌皮肤肉芽肿1例.临床皮肤科杂志,2006,35(6):385-386.

[23] 夏明玉,朱文元,黄立,芦勤.腋毛菌病扫描电镜观察.中华皮肤科杂志,1981,14(2):70-71(腋毛菌病 朱文元供图).

第6章

[1] 霍亚兰,李凡,徐萍,齐雪玲.皮肤利什曼病(东

方疖型)误诊1例.临床皮肤科杂志,2005,34(9):614.

[2] 孔庆云,张铮章,吴炽昌,张建平.皮肤并殖吸虫病1例.临床皮肤科杂志,1999,28(2):137-139.

[3] 李利.匐行疹1例.临床皮肤科杂志,2004,33(9):555.

[4] 王迎林,刘淑华,王泽民,董其斌.皮肤、脑猪囊虫病.临床皮肤科杂志,1997,26(6):图谱.

[5] 张浩,何晓丹,冉玉平,等.牛皮蝇幼虫所致皮肤蝇蛆病1例.临床皮肤科杂志,2007,36(5):320-320.

[6] 郑优优,范卫新,朱文元.3岁女童眼睑睫毛阴虱感染一例及文献复习.临床皮肤科杂志,2012,41(12):24-26.

[7] 朱文元,夏明玉:蜱叮咬一例(附扫描电镜观察).中华皮肤科杂志,1989,22(1):45-46.

[8] 马东来,方凯,刘芳.挪威疥.临床皮肤科杂志,2002,31(4):205-206.

[9] 周冼苡,于娜沙.婴儿蒲螨皮炎1例.临床皮肤科杂志,2003,32(7):405-406.

[10] 水母皮炎 陆原供图.

第7章

[1] 周春丽,叶庆佾.多发性硬下疳1例.临床皮肤科杂志,2004,33(11):675.

[2] 刘升云,李澄,郝燕萍,陆金文.环形疹、扁平湿疣共存的二期梅毒1例.临床皮肤科杂志,2002,31(3):183.

[3] 杨健,杨文林,刘丹蓉.结节性二期梅毒疹5例.临床皮肤科杂志,2002,31(9):591-593.

[4] 童燕芳.环状红斑样二期梅毒疹1例.临床皮肤科杂志,2004,33(11):691-692.

[5] 于娜沙,周冼苡,李建华.梅毒性脱发4例.临床皮肤科杂志,2004,33(9):552-553.

[6] 鲁严,朱文元.扁平型生殖器疣1例.临床皮肤科杂志,2003,32(5):279-280.

第8章

[1] 马东来,方凯,张晓红.火激红斑.临床皮肤科杂志,2002,31(3):135-136.

[2] 李波,李久宏,宋芳吉.光线性扁平苔藓1例.临

床皮肤科杂志,2004,33(3):176-177.

[3] 李澄,李燕.植物光皮炎1例.临床皮肤科杂志,
2005,34(8):536.

[4] 李峰,马东来,晋红中,等.植物光皮炎伴手指
坏疽.临床皮肤科杂志,2007,36(6):375-376.

[5] Zhang RZ,Zhu WY.Phytophotodermatitis due
to wild carrot decoction.Indian J Dermatol Venereol Leprol,2011,77(6):731-2.

[6] 朱文元.中草药煎液引起植物光皮炎3例和文
献复习.临床皮肤科杂志,2010,39(8):495-
497.Zhang RZ,Zhu WY.Phytophotodermatitis
due to Chinese herbal medicine decoction.Indi-
an J Dermatol,2011,56(3):329-31.

[7] 杨敏,张秀春,常建春.胶样粟丘疹1例.临床皮
肤科杂志,2005,34(11):760.

[8] 陈坚,梁尚清.人为皮炎1例.临床皮肤科杂志,
2006,35(8):527.

第9章

[1] 范光明,郑占才.形态罕见的刺激性接触性皮
炎1例.临床皮肤科杂志,2002,31(2):119.

[2] 芒果皮炎　陆原供图

[3] 袁华刚.水芹菜致刺激性接触性皮炎1例.中国
皮肤性病学杂志,2012,26(11):1045-1045.

[4] 谭城,朱文元,刘岩.Blaschko皮炎.临床皮肤科
杂志,2010(010):643-645.

[5] 创伤后湿疹　谭诚供图.

[6] 谭城,朱文元,司海鹏.继发脂溢性角化上晕皮
炎一例.

[7] 谭城,朱文元,闵仲生等.记忆性荨麻疹.临床皮
肤科杂志,2008,37(6):361-362.

[8] 岳学状,朱文元.大疱性荨麻疹1例.临床皮肤
科杂志,2006,35(10):671.

[9] 妊娠瘙痒性荨麻疹性丘疹斑块　侯麦花供图.

[10] 刘春平,陈强,赵淑肖.泛发性固定性药疹1例.
临床皮肤科杂志,2004,33(8):497.

[11] Tan C,Zhu W Y.Annular fixed drug eruption.
JDDG:Journal der Deutschen Dermatologisch-
en Gesellschaft,2010,8(10):823-824.

[12] Tan C,Zhu WY.Furazolidone induced nonpig-
menting fixed drug eruptions affecting the
palms and soles.J Clin Dermatol,2003(suppl):
S107-109.

[13] Li L,Zhu XJ.Dapsone hypersensitivity syn-
drome.J Clin Dermatol,2003(suppl):S115-
117.

第10章

[1] 刘玉峰,刘仲荣,高天文.职业性疣赘.临床皮肤
科杂志,2003,32(2):117-118.

第11章

[1] 苏向阳,顾有守,陆春.环状红斑型亚急性皮肤
型红斑狼疮.临床皮肤科杂志,2004,33(1):65-
66.

[2] 顾有守,陆春,刘毅.大疱性系统性红斑狼疮.临
床皮肤科杂志,2003,32(3):177-178.

[3] 马东来,方凯,王定邦.肿胀性红斑狼疮1例.临
床皮肤科杂志,2003,32(3):124-126.

[4] 马东来,何志新,刘方.新生儿红斑狼疮.临床皮
肤科杂志,2003,32(7):371-372.

[5] 严淑贤,郑捷.抗磷脂抗体综合征1例.临床皮
肤科杂志,2003,32(7):399-400.

[6] 渠涛,田亚萍,方凯,苑勰,张保如.结节性硬皮
病.临床皮肤科杂志,2006,35(5):294-295.

[7] Zhang RZ,Zhu WY.Two uncommon cases of
idiopathic atrophoderma of pasini and pierini:
Multiple and giant.Indian Journal of Dermatology,Venereology,and Leprology,2011,77(3):
402.

[8] 萎缩性肢端皮炎　康定华供图.

[9] 马立文,朱文元,骆丹等.Moulin线状皮肤萎
缩.临床皮肤科杂志,2013,42(12):747-748.

[10] 带状分布的皮肤萎缩症　郑云燕供图.

[11] 谭城,朱文元,闵仲生等.类风湿嗜中性皮炎
[J].临床皮肤科杂志,2010,39(1):17-18.

[12] 马东来,方凯.结节性皮肤狼疮性黏蛋白病.临
床皮肤科杂志,2006,35(7):427-429.

第12章

[1] 胡瑾,刘晓雁,马东来.先天性胸腺发育不良1
例.临床皮肤科杂志,2005,34(6):351-353.

[2] 移植物抗宿主病　朱文元供图.

第13章

[1] 马东来,方凯,王洪琛.显著角化过度型汗孔角

化症.临床皮肤科杂志,2002,31(12):741-742.

[2] 曹碧兰,陈晓红,郑庭铭.偏侧性汗孔角化症1例.临床皮肤科杂志,2003,32(10):597-598.

[3] 张勇枚,刘跃华,甘戈.汗孔角化症合并假性阿洪病1例.临床皮肤科杂志,2004,33(9):550-551.

[4] 李雪,朱文元,鲁严.卡泊三醇治疗播散性浅表性光线性汗孔角化症(1例并文献复习)临床皮肤科杂志,2014,43(1):53-55.

[5] 李明,杨森,李诚让,葛宏松,张学军.点状掌跖角皮症家系报道1例.临床皮肤科杂志,2003,32(1):23-24.

[6] 马东来,方凯,刘平.条纹状掌跖角皮症1例.临床皮肤科杂志,2005,34(5):314.

[7] 刘跃华,李远,方凯,马东来.棘状角皮症.临床皮肤科杂志,2005,34(10):647-649.

[8] 刘建军,郭淑兰.表皮松解性掌跖角化病1例.临床皮肤科杂志,2006,35(2):98-99.

[9] 黎兆军,李顺凡.疣状肢端角化症1例.临床皮肤科杂志,2004,33(9):558.

[10] 肖尹,关杨,纪华安,薛丑文.疣状角化不良瘤2例.临床皮肤科杂志,2005,34(4):242.

[11] 曹鸿玮,晋红中,刘跃华.进行性对称性红斑角皮症1例.临床皮肤科杂志,2002,31(10):655.

[12] 姜薇,段周英,朱学骏.砷角化病3例.临床皮肤科杂志,2002,31(11):716-717.

[13] 乳头乳晕角化过度症 朱文元供图.

[14] Tan C,Zhu W Y.An adult case of waxy keratosis[J].International Journal of Dermatology,2012.

[15] 朱铁山,马东来,王宝玺,方凯.肢端角化性类弹性纤维病.临床皮肤科杂志,2002,31(9):541-542.

[16] 马东来,方凯,刘芳.扁平苔藓样角化病1例.临床皮肤科杂志,2002,31(11):724-725.

[17] Zhang RZ,Zhu WY,Yu YH.Aquagenic acrokeratoderma in a 5-year-old boy.Eur J Pediat Dermatol,2009,19(4):203-6.

第 14 章

[1] 李丽,王宝玺,方凯.匐形性回状红斑.临床皮肤科杂志,2005,34(10):641-642.

[2] 谭城,朱文元,闵仲生等.可触及游走性弧形红斑.临床皮肤科杂志,2010,39(6):337-339.

[3] 刘跃华,王家璧,高晶,陆菁菁,方凯,王宏伟.以掌跖疼痛性红斑为首发表现的左心房黏液瘤1例.临床皮肤科杂志,2004,33(1):26-27.

[4] 张淑环,边鹊桥,崔雄桦,陈鸣皋.复发性疼痛性红斑1例.临床皮肤科杂志,2006,35(5):324.

[5] Song Z,Chen W,Zhong H,et al.Erythema Papulosa Semicircularis Recidivans:A New Reactive Dermatitis? Dermatitis,2012,23(1):44-47.

[6] 侯麦花,卢新政,朱文元,等.红色阴囊综合征.临床皮肤科杂志,2013,42(11):668-669.

第 15 章

[1] 狄梅.掌跖银屑病4例.临床皮肤科杂志,2006,35(5):318.

[2] 万东芳,马东来,方凯.反向银屑病1例.临床皮肤科杂志,2003,32(2):98.

[3] 徐素芹,丁政云,高顺强,林元珠,张增强,李彦群.急性痘疮样苔藓状糠疹.临床皮肤科杂志,2004,33(5):261-262.

[4] 鲁严,朱文元.紫癜型玫瑰糠疹1例.临床皮肤科杂志,2003,32(2):95-96.

[5] 沈剑鸣.泛发性丘疹型玫瑰糠疹.临床皮肤科杂志,2003,32(10):627-628.

[6] 色素性玫瑰糠疹 朱文元供图.

[7] Zhu WY,Fang QG.Unusually case of follcular keratosis squamousa of Dohi.Int J Dermatol,1988,27:276-277(鳞状毛囊角化症 朱文元供图).

[8] Lu Y,Zhang MH,Zhu WY.A case of facial keratosis follicularis squamosa resembling atrophic acne scarring,successfully treated with topical pimecrolimus.Indian J Dermatol Venereol Leprol,2011,77(1):69-70.

[9] 肥厚性扁平苔藓 朱文元供图.

[10] 毛发扁平苔藓 朱文元供图.

[11] 张汝芝,朱文元.色素性扁平苔藓1例.临床皮肤科杂志,2003,32(4):208-209.

[12] 谭城,朱文元,赖仁胜,闵仲生.褶皱部色素性扁平苔藓.临床皮肤科杂志,2006,35(9):585-586.

[13] Zhang RZ, Zhu WY. Lichen planus pigmentosus over superficial leg veins. J Dtsh Dermatol Ges, 2011, 9(7):540-541.

[14] Zhang RZ, Zhu WY. One case of unilateral linear lichen planus pigmentosus. Open Dermatol J, 2012, 6:25-28.

[15] 龙福泉, 周晓鸿, 冒长峙, 李学平, 邓丹琪, 樊应俊. 20 甲扁平苔藓 1 例. 临床皮肤科杂志, 2003, 32(12):729.

[16] 张卉, 朱文元, 范卫新. 扁平苔藓并发白癜风 1 例. 临床皮肤科杂志, 2007, 36(3):169.

[17] 常建民, 付裕, 金祖余. 急性泛发性扁平苔藓 1 例. 临床皮肤科杂志, 2006, 35(5):315-316.

[18] 王磊, 朱文元, 曹蕾等. 黑色丘疹性皮病. 临床皮肤科杂志, 2009, 38(2):99-100.

[19] 硬化性苔藓 朱文元供图.

[20] 曹扬, 车敦发, 沈东, 倪容之. 非生殖器部位特殊形态硬化性萎缩性苔藓 1 例. 临床皮肤科杂志, 2002, 31(8):522-523.

[21] 面颈部毛囊性红斑黑变病 朱文元供图.

[22] 李诚让, 朱文元. 金色苔藓 1 例. 临床皮肤科杂志, 2005, 34(9):592-593.

[23] 朱文元, 鲁严. 名医病例分析. 临床皮肤科杂志, 2002, 31(10):673-674.

[24] 闫洁, 王宝玺, 刘跃华, 方凯. 连圈状秕糠疹 2 例. 临床皮肤科杂志, 2005, 34(4):235-236.

第 16 章

[1] 雷山川, 胡平. 寻常型天疱疮患者娩出一天疱疮患儿. 临床皮肤科杂志, 2005, 34(5):300-301.

[2] 杨希川, 刘荣卿, 郝飞, 钟白玉. 毛囊角化病样天疱疮 1 例. 临床皮肤科杂志, 2004, 33(7):419-420.

[3] 朱学骏, 陈喜雪, 涂平, 李丽, 王爱平, 杨海珍, 杨淑霞, 谢忠. 伴限局性 Castleman 病的副肿瘤性天疱疮临床及实验室研究. 临床皮肤科杂志, 2003, 32(1):7-10.

[4] 李颂, 王京, 朱学骏. 副肿瘤性天疱疮. 临床皮肤科杂志, 2004, 33(8):519-520.

[5] 谢作刚, 吴凤, 钱悦等. 结节性类天疱疮 1 例. 临床皮肤科杂志, 2012, 41(1):51-52.

[6] 谭琦, 王华, 欧阳莹等. 儿童线状 IgA 大疱性皮病. 临床皮肤科杂志, 2010, 39(10):607-608.

[7] 郭生红, 李薇. 成人线状 IgA 大疱性皮病 1 例. 中国皮肤性病学杂志, 2011, 25(9):709-710.

[8] 姜一化, 陈龙. 复发性线状棘层松解皮病. 临床皮肤科杂志, 2006, 35(6):366-367.

[9] 万川, 胡国红, 罗来华. 外生殖器部位的棘层松解性皮病 1 例. 临床皮肤科杂志, 2013, 42(5):295-296.

[10] 郝进, 阎衡, 邓军, 郝飞, 叶庆佾, 邹锋. 获得性大疱性表皮松解症 1 例. 临床皮肤科杂志, 2004, 33(10):623-624.

[11] 樊平申, 李森, 高天文, 廖文俊, 陈必良. 疱疹样脓疱病并发妊娠期肝内胆汁淤积症 1 例. 临床皮肤科杂志, 2004, 33(10):620-621.

[12] 掌跖脓疱病合并前胸壁综合征 朱文元供图.

[13] 马东来, 方凯, 杜荣昕. 嗜酸性脓疱性毛囊炎. 临床皮肤科杂志, 2005, 34(4):203-204.

[14] 张峻岭, 李维云, 纪华安, 肖尹, 沈剑鸣. 婴儿肢端脓疱病 1 例. 临床皮肤科杂志, 2002, 31(7):469-4705.

[15] 泛发性连续性肢端皮炎 徐美萍供图.

第 17 章

[1] 闫洁, 叶庆佾, 郝飞, 杨希川. 播散型匐行性穿通性弹性纤维病 1 例. 临床皮肤科杂志, 2006, 35(3):160-161.

[2] 苗青. 先天性皮肤松弛症 1 例. 临床皮肤科杂志, 2004, 33(12):758.

[3] 刘玮, 赵广, 孟如松, 郑旭. 全身性皮肤松弛症 1 例. 临床皮肤科杂志, 1999, 28(5):插图.

[4] 马东来, 胡瑾, 方凯. 局限性皮肤松弛症. 临床皮肤科杂志, 2006, 35(7):417-418.

[5] 王刚. 眼睑松弛症 1 例. 临床皮肤科杂志, 2005, 34(9):621.

[6] 樊翌明, 王映芬, 李顺凡, 吴志华. 弹性纤维性假黄瘤 1 例. 临床皮肤科杂志, 2002, 31(8):528-529.

[7] 庞晓文, 赵广, 刘玮, 冯燕君, 吴卫红. 皮肤弹性过度伴免疫学检查异常 1 例. 临床皮肤科杂志, 2003, 32(12):720-721.

[8] 李卉, 雷鹏程, 刘洁. 巨大结缔组织痣伴发幼年类风湿关节炎 1 例. 临床皮肤科杂志, 2000, 29(2):117-118.

［9］ 鞠强,夏隆庆,孙建方,李仪芳,林彤.发疹性皮肤胶原瘤1例.临床皮肤科杂志,2005,34(10):669-670.

［10］ Wang DG,Zhu WY.White fibrous papulosis of the neck:a chinese case.J Clin Dermatol,2003,32(suppl):S102-S104.

［11］ 王大光,朱文元.颈部白色纤维丘疹病1例.临床皮肤科杂志,2004,33(5):296-297.

第18章

［1］ 膨胀纹和局限性萎缩　朱文元供图.

［2］ 郭生红,李薇.斑状萎缩.临床皮肤科杂志,2012,41(7):393-394.

［3］ 王大光,朱文元.包皮假性阿洪病1例.临床皮肤科杂志,2005,34(1):33-34.

第19章

［1］ 韩春雷,廖小玉,胡春梅.持久性隆起红斑1例.临床皮肤科杂志,2004,33(8):496.

［2］ 王鹰,叶庆佾,郝飞,杨希川,钟白玉.Sweet病1例.临床皮肤科杂志,2005,34(11):766.

［3］ 张春香,曲才杰,朱学骏.皮下型急性发热性嗜中性皮肤病1例.临床皮肤科杂志,2006,35(2):96-97.

［4］ 陈仁贵,庄寅,钱黎华,李敏.Wegener肉芽肿1例.临床皮肤科杂志,2003,32(12):722-723.

［5］ 孙国钧,吴荣荣,刘伦飞,蔡绥勃.坏疽性脓皮病.临床皮肤科杂志,2003,32(4):241-242.

［6］ 敖俊红,杨蓉娅,郝震锋,张洁,王文岭,宋克敏.恶性萎缩性丘疹病伴肠穿孔1例.临床皮肤科杂志,2004,33(10):611-613.

［7］ 常建民.青斑样血管炎.临床皮肤科杂志,2004,33(9):521-522.

［8］ 熊霞,周培媚,朱玉祥,陈德宇.血小板增多性紫癜.临床皮肤科杂志,2006,35(7):470.

［9］ 徐斌,康定华,张汝芝.播散性瘙痒性血管性皮炎1例.中国皮肤性病学杂志,2013,27(7):744-744.

第20章

［1］ 谭城,朱文元,闵仲生,赖仁胜.发疹性复发性色素沉着性毛细血管扩张症.临床皮肤科杂志

（待发表）.

［2］ 景红梅,曹鸿玮,俞宝田.持久性发疹性斑状毛细血管扩张症1例.临床皮肤科杂志,2002,31(5):308-309.

［3］ 朱文元,薛京华,陈希萍.单侧性皮肤浅表毛细血管扩张症(附一例报告).临床皮肤科杂志,1988,17(4):188-190.

［4］ Tan C,Zhu W Y.Unilateral nevoid telangiectasia superimposed on the Bier spots:another demonstration of vascular twin spotting.JDDG:Journal der Deutschen Dermatologischen Gesellschaft,2011,9(5):389-390.

［5］ 张理涛,纪华安,肖尹,王庆文.胸腹壁血栓性静脉炎.临床皮肤科杂志,2006,35(8):535-536.

［6］ 马东来,李国新,叶炜.闭塞性动脉硬化症.临床皮肤科杂志,2005,34(8):491-492.

［7］ 谭城,朱文元,闵仲生等.发疹性假性血管瘤病.临床皮肤科杂志,2010,39(2):97-98.

第21章

［1］ 阎衡,邓军,郝进,叶庆佾.组织细胞吞噬性脂膜炎1例.临床科杂志,2006,35(4):241-242.

［2］ 王大光,朱文元.硬化性脂膜炎.临床皮肤科杂志,2007,36(4):242-243.

［3］ 杨玲,何威,黄海,任莉.嗜酸细胞性脂膜炎1例.临床皮肤科杂志,2006,35(4):221-222.

［4］ 陈仁贵,陈戟,余红,姜媛芳.先天性全身性脂肪萎缩1例.临床皮肤科杂志,1998,27(1):50-52.

［5］ 高瑛瑛,朱文元,骆丹等.腹部离心性脂肪营养不良2例.临床皮肤科杂志,2009,38(10):674-675.

第22章

［1］ 环状肉芽肿　谭诚供图.

［2］ 杨岚,晋红中,方凯.儿童播散型环状肉芽肿1例.临床皮肤科杂志,2004,33(8):498-499.

［3］ 马东来,方凯,王定邦.穿通性环状肉芽肿.临床皮肤科杂志,2005,34(7):413-414.

［4］ 马慧军,朱文元.播散性环状肉芽肿合并乙型肝炎病毒感染.临床皮肤科杂志,2004,33(9):

535-537.

[5] 谭城,朱文元.多形性肉芽肿.临床皮肤科杂志,
2010,39(7):432-433.

[6] 马东来,方凯,郑和义,等.环状弹性纤维溶解
性巨细胞肉芽肿.临床皮肤科杂志,2008,37
(8):496-499.

[7] 侯麦花,朱文元,卢新政,叶宇达.皮肤硅石肉
芽肿.临床皮肤科杂志,2006,35(11):694-695.

[8] 常建民,鲍迎秋.反应性结节性增生.临床皮肤
科杂志,2012,41(8):455-456.

第23章

[1] 曹蕾,朱文元,王磊,等.鼻红粒病1例.临床皮
肤科杂志,2008,37(8):508-508.

[2] 石仁琳.Fox-Fordyce病1例.临床皮肤科杂志,
2005,34(6):397.

[3] 谭城,朱文元.蛇形斑秃2例报告.临床皮肤科
杂志,2002,31(7):454-455.

[4] 谭城,朱文元.全秃再生发呈马蹄形、蛇形嵌合
型分布1例.临床皮肤科杂志,2002,31(8):
520-521.

[5] 毕新岭,顾军,刘燕芳.Brocq假性斑秃1例.临
床皮肤科杂志,2004,33(9):557.

[6] 刘栋,朱文元.蛇形脱发和W形脱发嵌合分布
1例.临床皮肤科杂志,2003,32(6):342-343.

[7] 谭城,朱文元,闵仲生.未累及皮损内白发的斑
秃.临床皮肤科杂志,2008,37(8):521-522.

[8] Zhang RZ,Zhu WY,Zhou L.Coexistence of ac-
quired hypertrichosis and ophiasis in a patient
with infiltrating ductal carcinoma.Indian J Dermatol Venereol Leprol,2012,78(1):122.

[9] 陈柳青,石继海,孙建方.羊毛状发.临床皮肤科
杂志,2004,33(1):1-2.

[10] 袁姗,雷鹏程.念珠形发1例(附扫描电镜观
察).临床皮肤科杂志,1999,28(1):56-57.

[11] 马东来,胡瑾,方凯.环纹发.临床皮肤科杂志,
2009,38(6).

[12] Zhu WY,Xia MY.Trichonodosis.Pediatr Dermatol,1993,10(4):392-393.

[13] 张汝芝,朱文元.管型毛发合并牵拉性脱发.临
床皮肤科杂志,2004,33(5):292-293.
Zhang RZ,Zhu WY.Traction alopecia combined hair casts.J Clin Dermatol,2003,32(sup-

pl):S95-S97.

[14] 小棘毛壅症　朱文元供图.

[15] Xie H,Zhang RZ,Zhu WY.A new site of cutaneous pili migrans in a 6-month-old infant.In-
dian J Dermatol Venereol Leprol,2012,78
(4):498-9.

[16] 黄发　朱文元供图.

[17] Tan C,Zhu WY.Permanent poliosis following
repetitive plucking in an adolescent.Journal of
cutaneous medicine and surgery,2010,14(4):
193-194.

[18] Xu B,Zhang RZ,Zhu WY.Pachyonychia con-
genita associated with granulosis rubra nas:
Eur J Pediat Dermatol 2013,23:214-8.

[19] Li HJ,Feng Z,Wang JP,Fan JF,Ge P,Wen
HY.Congenital leukonychia totalis:a case of
report.J Clin Dermatol,2003(suppl):S118-
119.

[20] Zhu WY,Xia MY,Huang SD,Du DA.Hyper-
pigmentation of the nail from lead deposition.
Int J Dermatol,1989,273-275.

[21] 谭城,朱文元.纵行红甲.临床皮肤科杂志,
2010,39(10):638-639.

[22] Rigopoulos D,Prantsidis A.(张汝芝,朱文元
译).甲变色.临床皮肤科杂志,2005,34(1):56-
60.

[23] 谭城,朱文元.甲下裂片形出血.临床皮肤科杂
志,2007,36(11):702-703.

[24] 颈部皮脂腺增生　朱文元供图.

[25] 马慧军,朱文元.阴囊皮脂腺增生1例.临床皮
肤科杂志,2005,34(7):451-453.

[26] 朱文元,陈希萍.临床皮肤科杂志,1988,17
(2):老年皮脂腺过度增生(彩图).

[27] Yin Z Q,Xu J L,Luo D,et al.Sebaceous hyperplasia within epidermis after scald.Journal of
cutaneous pathology,2012,39(1):75-77.

第24章

[1] 李丽,王宝玺,刘跃华,方凯.胫前黏液性水肿.
临床皮肤科杂志,2002,31(11):675-676.

[2] 何弘,高效贤,岳新华.皮肤钙质沉着症1例.临
床皮肤科杂志,2002,31(11):717-718.

[3] 朱家洪,许定安.阴囊特发性皮肤钙沉着症.临

床皮肤科杂志,2003,32(3):119-120.

[4] 刘金耀,王玉坤,郭淑兰.单侧痣样黑棘皮病.临床皮肤科杂志,2003,32(7):431-432.

[5] 谭立恒,倪容之.恶性黑棘皮病.临床皮肤科杂志,2003,32(6):369-370.

[6] Yang YH,Zhang RZ,Kang DH,Zhu WY. Three paraneoplastic signs and wide spread vitiligo in the same patient with gastric adeno- carcinoma.Dermatol J Online,2013.

[7] 刘玉峰,樊建勇,夏汝山,沈柱,党育平,胡绍文.高雄激素血症-胰岛素抵抗-黑棘皮病综合征1例.临床皮肤科杂志,2005,34(6):378- 379.

[8] 虞瑞尧.坏死松解游走性红斑与胰高糖素瘤综合征.临床皮肤科杂志,2004,33(10):649-650.

第25章

[1] 赵娟,谭琦,颜兰香.结节性黄瘤病并发主动脉瓣狭窄1例.临床皮肤科杂志,2006,35(3): 140-141.

[2] 孙建方.名医病例析.临床皮肤科杂志,2002,31 (12):805-806.

[3] 谢勇,郑和义,方凯,刘跃华.类脂蛋白沉积症1例.临床皮肤科杂志,2002,31(1):43-44.

[4] 朱国兴,陆春,赖维,顾有守,苏向阳.类脂质渐进性坏死.临床皮肤科杂志,2006,35(7):483- 484.

[5] 林建华,王刚.幼年性黄色肉芽肿1例.临床皮肤科杂志,2004,33(11):673.

[6] 李雪,吴迪,苏忠兰,张美华,鲁严.面部苔藓样型幼年黄色肉芽肿.中华皮肤科杂志.2013,46 (10):67-68.

[7] 赵广,工毅侠,李东光,史飞,张红,孟如松.渐进性坏死性黄色肉芽肿1例.临床皮肤科杂志,2003,32(5):281-282.

[8] 杨敏,常建民.成人单发黄色肉芽肿.临床皮肤科杂志.2007,36(5):273.

[9] 沈征宇,廖康煌.先天性红细胞生成性卟啉病1例.临床皮肤科杂志,2003,32(12):718-719.

[10] 陈珺怡,汪蓓青,陈向东.皮肤异色病样淀粉样变病1例及家系调查.临床皮肤科杂志,2004,33(12):751-752.

[11] 袁小英,赵广.痒疹样结节型皮肤淀粉样变性1

例.临床皮肤科杂志,2006,35(11):740.

[12] 晋红中,方凯.黏液水肿性苔藓2例.临床皮肤科杂志,2005,34(7):457-459.

[13] 廖文俊,付萌,孙林潮,赵小东.硬化性黏液水肿性苔藓1例.临床皮肤科杂志,2006,35(4): 225-226.

[14] 张倩,王云,郭静,张宝元,沈力.毛囊黏蛋白病1例.临床皮肤科杂志,2003,32(1):27-28.

[15] 吴迪,葛以信.网状红斑黏蛋白病1例.临床皮肤科杂志,2004,33(8):483-484.

[16] 苏忠兰,岳学状,朱文元,陈斌.皮肤局灶性黏蛋白病.临床皮肤科杂志,2004,33(9):587- 588.

[17] 狄梅,任正忠.肢端持续性丘疹性黏蛋白沉积症.临床皮肤科杂志,2006,35(11):709-710.

[18] 马东来,郑和义,方凯.烟酸缺乏症.临床皮肤科杂志,2002,31(6):339-340.

[19] 武小红,郭利劲,陈雪,张建中.胡萝卜素血症1例.临床皮肤科杂志,2004,33(8):480.

[20] 朱小红.糖原累积病I型1例.临床皮肤科杂志,2004,33(12):747-748.

[21] 陈龙,朱林学,陈柳青等.褐黄病.临床皮肤科杂志,2007,36(6):359-361.

第26章

[1] (1).A型色素型分界线　朱文元供图.
(2).陈小娥,朱文元,骆丹.妊娠色素性分界线14例分析.临床皮肤科杂志,2008,37(12): 772-773.

[2] Xu.C,Zhang R,Zhu W Types E and C of Pig- mentary demarcation lines in two Chiness sisters. Eur J Pediat Dermatol,2014,24:71-73.

[3] Zang R,Zhu W. Coexistence of Pigmentary de- marcation lines tygpes C and E in one subject, Int J Dermatol,2011,50,863-865.

[4] 李丽,刘跃华,方凯.多发性黑子综合征.临床皮肤科杂志,2006,35(5):273-274.

[5] 张汝芝,朱文元.补骨脂素长波紫外线雀斑样痣1例.临床皮肤科杂志,2003,32(9):534- 535.

[6] 李雪,朱文元,鲁严.非典型阴茎雀斑样痣.临床皮肤科杂志,2013,42(8):480-482.

[7] 彭少文,杨希川,叶庆俏,钟华,郝飞.巨大先天

性黑素细胞痣1例.临床皮肤科杂志,2005,34(5):321.

[8] 太田痣 朱文元供图.

[9] 王宏伟,王家璧,姜国调.太田痣合并鲜红斑痣3例.临床皮肤科杂志,2002,31(12):787-788.

[10] 常建民.伊藤痣.临床皮肤科杂志,2006,35(8):485-486.

[11] 谭城,朱文元,司海鹏.伊藤痣上继发色素减退斑1例.临床皮肤科杂志,2007,36(11):685-687.

[12] 面部褐青色痣 张汝芝供图.

[13] Becker痣中并发痤疮 谭诚供图.

[14] 李敏,高洁,朱文元.双侧分布的Becker痣并发颈部白色纤维性丘疹病.临床皮肤科杂志,2008,37(4):213-215.

[15] Becker综合征 朱文元供图.

[16] 徐磊,曾维惠,耿松梅,等.神经皮肤黑变病.临床皮肤科杂志,2011,40(11):676-678.

[17] 潘敏,朱文元,骆丹.进行性肢端黑变病.临床皮肤科杂志,2008,37(11):729-731.

[18] 张汝芝,朱文元.家族性眶周色素沉着症1例.临床皮肤科杂志,2004,33(2):114.

[19] 田中华,谭兴友,牛长秀,辛莉,王养岭,孙心君,张仁亚.木村网状肢端色素沉着症一家系调查.临床皮肤科杂志,2006,35(2):101-102.

[20] 赵小东,高天文,张海龙,刘玉峰,范雪莉,党育平.伴大疱的先天性皮肤异色症1家3例报告.临床皮肤科杂志,2004,33(2):98-100.

[21] 张汝芝,朱文元.一家族中8例患屈侧网状色素沉着症.临床皮肤科杂志,2003,32(3):152-154.
Zhang RZ,Zhu WY.A study of immunohistochemical and electron microscopic changes in Dowling-Degos disease.J Dermatol,2005,32(1):12-18.

[22] 孙怡,王玉坤.遗传性对称性色素异常症并发掌跖角化病1例.临床皮肤科杂志,2006,35(2):109.

[23] Zhang RZ,Zhu WY.A variant case of Familial Progressive hyperpigmentation.Eur J Dermatol,2011,21(4):620-621.

[24] Zhang RZ,Zhu WY.Familial progressive hypo- and hyperpigmentation:a variant case.Indian J Dermatol Venereol Leprol,2012,78(3):350-353.

[25] 鲁严,朱文元.遗传性泛发性色素异常症1例.临床皮肤科杂志,2002,31(11):705-707.

[26] 伴巨大黑素小体表现的遗传性对称性色素异常症 谭诚供图.

[27] 邢有兰,李欢.线状和旋涡状痣样过度黑素沉着病.临床皮肤科杂志,2006,35(8):515-516.

[28] Cheng Tan;Wen-Yuan Zhu.Pointillist melanotic macules:a new clinical entity? Advances in Dermatology & Allergology,2012,29(6):475-479.

[29] 获得性真皮黑素细胞增生症 朱文元供图.

[30] 意外粉粒沉着病 朱文元供图.

[31] 波纹状融合性网状乳头瘤 谭诚供图.

[32] 郭志飞,劳力民,孙国钧.先天性巨大色素痣并发白癜风1例.临床皮肤科杂志,2003,32(2):89-90.

[33] 曹元华,崔盘根,林彤,贾虹,曾学思,林麟.三色白癜风20例临床分析.临床皮肤科杂志,2004,33(1):3-5.

[34] Zhang RZ,Zhu WY.Pentachrome vitiligo in a zosteriform pattern Photodermatology,Photoimmunology & Photomedicine,2013,29(2):100-102.

[35] 炎症性白癜风 朱文元供图.

[36] Xing H,Fu LB.Clinical features of nevus depigmentosus in 154 children.J Clin Dermatol,2003,32(suppl):S36-39.

[37] 常建民,鲍迎秋,杨敏.星状自发性假瘢.临床皮肤科杂志,2006,35(11):707-708.

第27章

[1] Jin HL,Zhang RZ,Zhou L,Jiang CJ,Zhu WY.Incontinentia pigmenti associated with unilateral complete cleft lip in a neonatal boy.Eur J Pediat Dermatol,2012,22(2):123-126.

[2] Zhang R Z,Zhu W Y,Zhou L.Unusual hyperpigmented patches,an undeveloped breast and a cataract in a female with incontinentia pigmenti.The Journal of Dermatology,2013.

[3] 黄淑琼.家族性慢性良性天疱疮一家系调查.临床皮肤科杂志,2005,34(12):844.

［4］鞠强,石继海,康晓静,姜祎群,夏隆庆.单纯型大疱性表皮松解症 Weber-Cockayne 亚型临床特征、诊断和治疗分析.临床皮肤科杂志,2003,32(10):579-581.

［5］孙莹,姜薇,陈喜雪,朱学骏.常染色体隐性遗传的 Hallopeau-Siemens 型营养不良型大疱性表皮松解症 1 例.临床皮肤科杂志,2005,34(8):526-527.

［6］孙建方,徐秀莲.胫前大疱性表皮松解症.临床皮肤科杂志,2004,33(11):712-714.

［7］翟立新,杜钦玲,孙可,翟一阳.痒疹样显性遗传营养不良型大疱性表皮松解症一家系调查.临床皮肤科杂志,2004,33(11):694-695.

［8］孙秀坤,关欣,朱学骏.Siemens 大疱性鱼鳞病基因突变国内首次报道.临床皮肤科杂志,2002,31(10):610-612.

［9］潘健楷,曾学思,陈爱英.表皮松解性角化过度型鱼鳞病 1 例.临床皮肤科杂志,2004,33(12):755-748.

［10］赵广,史飞,庞晓文,田燕.表皮松解性角化过度鱼鳞病伴侏儒 1 例.临床皮肤科杂志,2005,34(8):528-530.

［11］火棉胶婴儿　陆原供图.

［12］马东来,王家璧,王宏伟.先天性角化不良 6 例.临床皮肤科杂志,2002,31(11):712-714.

［13］廖文俊,胡雪慧,樊平申等.残留性多指症.临床皮肤科杂志,2007,36(2):92-93.

［14］李军,马东来,王定邦.骨膜增生厚皮症.临床皮肤科杂志,2003,32(1):1-2.

［15］Zhu WY,Wu JH.Congenital localized absence of skin associated with dystrophic epidermolysis bullosa.Pediatr Dermatol,1991,8(2):176-177.

［16］Zhu WY,Xia MY,Huang YE.Infantile digital fibromatosis:ultrastructural human papillomavirus and herpes simplex virus DNA observatio.Pediatr Dermatol,1991,8(2):137-139.

［17］钟桂书,史丙俊,熊霞.掌跖多发性皮肤纤维瘤 1 例.临床皮肤科杂志,2003,32(4):224.

［18］赵亮,曾同祥,张彦秀,王焱,曾学思.着色性干皮病继发恶性肿瘤 8 例临床及病理分析.临床皮肤科杂志,2005,34(5):295-296.

［19］马东来,石秀艳,方凯等.棘状秃发性毛发角化病.临床皮肤科杂志,2011,40(6):340-342.

［20］肖尹,关杨,纪华安,薛丑文,李鹏.幼年透明蛋白纤维瘤病.临床皮肤科杂志,2006,35(8):524-525.

［21］小斑片三色皮肤征　谭诚供图.

［22］Tan C,Zhu W Y,Min Z S.Papular elastorrhexis located on occipito-cervical and mandibular regions.European Journal of Dermatology,2009,19(4):399-400.

第 28 章

［1］梅尔克松－罗森塔尔综合征　贾雪松供图.

［2］孙青,侯建新,刘金耀.浆细胞性唇炎 1 例.临床皮肤科杂志,1999,28(3):192-193.

［3］王宏伟,乐嘉豫.阴茎硬化性淋巴管炎 6 例.临床皮肤科杂志,2003,32(3):163.

第 29 章

［1］肖尹,纪华安.棘层松解性角化不良表皮痣 1 例.临床皮肤科杂志,2002,31(2):118.

［2］蔡林,杜娟,张建中.棘层松解角化不良性表皮痣并发色素性毛表皮痣.临床皮肤科杂志,2006,35(7):436-437.

［3］张桂秀.泛发性表皮痣 1 例.临床皮肤科杂志,2003,32(3):140.

［4］祝永航.疣状痣.临床皮肤科杂志,2003,32(8):433-434.

［5］唐莉,刘凯,乔树芳,沈剑鸣,王庆文,肖尹,纪华安.表皮痣综合征 1 例.临床皮肤科杂志,2003,32(10):602-603.

［6］Zhu WY.Multiple small popular seborrehic keratosis.Chinese Medical Journal,1988,101(7):490-492.

［7］Li XJ,Zhu WY.A case of seborreic keratosis distributed along skin cleavage.The Journal of Dermatology,1998,25:272-274.

［8］Zhang RZ,Zhu WY.Seborrheic keratoses in five elderly patients:An appearance of raindrop and stream.Indian J Dermatol,2011,56(4):432-434.

［9］夏明王,朱文元,黄立,芦勤.脂溢性角化病表面孢子的扫描电镜观察.中华皮肤科杂志,

1982,15(3):164-165.

[10] 王雷,杨励,王刚,等.大细胞棘皮瘤9例临床及组织病理学分析.临床皮肤科杂志,2008,37(9):562-563.

[11] 任英,白秀荣.巨大皮角1例.临床皮肤科杂志,2004,33(9):531.

[12] 马东来,万东芳,方凯.发疹性毳毛囊肿1例.临床皮肤科杂志,2002,31(5):314-315.

[13] 张卉,朱文元,范卫新.Pinkus纤维上皮瘤1例.临床皮肤科杂志,2007,36(5):284-285.

[14] Pinkus纤维上皮瘤合并基底细胞癌 朱文元供图.

[15] 项力俭,吴能定,项晶晶.多发性角化棘皮瘤.临床皮肤科杂志,1998,27(4):图谱.

[16] 张武,李铮,谈英,王昕.鲍恩病1例.临床皮肤科杂志,2005,34(11):758.

[17] 周辉谱,林宝珠,李希清.多发性鲍温病1例.临床皮肤科杂志,2003,32(2):99-100.

[18] 潘德海,汪晨.生殖器Paget病的临床及组织病理分析.临床皮肤科杂志,2004,33(9):529.

[19] 郑艳红,马东来.疣状表皮发育不良继发基底鳞状细胞癌和多发性纤维毛囊瘤1例.临床皮肤科杂志,2003,32(9):530-531.

[20] 苏金发,李慧琼,岳青,等.浅表性基底细胞上皮瘤1例.临床皮肤科杂志,2007,36(7):473-473.21.

[21] 高洁,朱文元,骆丹.毛漏斗囊性基底细胞癌.临床皮肤科杂志,2007,36(9):572-573.

[22] 杜娟,刘海杰,张建中.慢性放射性皮炎继发鳞状细胞癌1例.临床皮肤科杂志,2005,34(2):116-117.

[23] 侯麦花,朱文元.皮肤透明细胞鳞状细胞癌.临床皮肤科杂志,2009,38(8):509-510.

[24] Zhang RZ,Zhu WY.Bilateral Milia en plaque in a 6-year-old Chinese boy.Pediatr Dermatol,2012,29(4):504-506.

[25] Zhang RZ,Zhu WY.A new site of milia en plaque.Indian J Dermatol Venereol Leprol,2012,78(1):122.

[26] Zhang RZ,Zhu WY,Zhou L.One case of multiple eruptive milia.G Ital Dermatol Venereol.2013 Jun,148(3):308-310.

[27] 吕淑琴,张益珠.黑头粉刺痣.临床皮肤科杂志,

2000,29(6):367-368.

[28] 四黑头扩张孔 朱文元供图.

[29] 杨希川,叶庆俏,郝飞,钟白玉.倒置性毛囊角化病1例.临床皮肤科杂志,2005,34(8):542.

[30] Zhang RZ,Zhu WY,Zhou L.Facial nevus sebaceous in six infants:bizarre appearance.Eur J Pediat Dermatol,2013,23(1)9-13.

[31] 吴艳,李家文,林能兴.皮脂腺痣合并大汗腺囊腺瘤1例.临床皮肤科杂志,2002,31(12):791-792.

[32] 张继玲,袁伟,瓦庆彪,曹碧兰.乳晕皮脂腺增生1例.临床皮肤科杂志,2006,35(10):655.

[33] 张红,刘兵,王玉颖,孟如松,江丽.线状皮脂腺痣综合征1例.临床皮肤科杂志,2004,33(11):679-681.

[34] 刘刚,帅海林,靖亚莎,郭海霞,李鹏远.大汗腺囊瘤1例.临床皮肤科杂志,2006,35(4):238.

[35] 肖尹,关杨,纪华安,薛丑文,李鹏.恶性小汗腺汗孔瘤1例.临床皮肤科杂志,2005,34(9):601-602.

[36] 闫洁,叶庆俏,杨希川,等.呈带状分布的小汗腺螺旋腺瘤.临床皮肤科杂志,2007,36(4):238-239.

[37] Zhu WY.Syringoma associated with milium-like lesions.J Am Acad Dermatol,1988,19(2):360-361.

[38] 宫立民,于智明.发疹型汗管瘤.临床皮肤科杂志,2003,32(5):243-244.

[39] 杨岚,马东来,方凯.粟丘疹样表现的外阴汗管瘤.临床皮肤科杂志,2004,33(10):589-590.

[40] 侯麦花,朱文元.泛发性发疹性透明细胞汗管瘤.临床皮肤科杂志,2008,37(3):172-173.

[41] 关杨,肖尹,纪华安,薛丑文,李鹏.乳头状汗管囊腺瘤1例.临床皮肤科杂志,2005,34(9):594-595.

[42] 林挺,罗中权.鼻翼部毛囊瘤1例.临床皮肤科杂志,2003,32(2):93.

[43] 闫言,刘跃华,王宝玺,王宏伟.微囊肿性附属器癌1例.临床皮肤科杂志,2003,32(10):591-592.

[44] 彭少文,杨希川,叶庆俏,郝飞.孤立性毛发上皮瘤1例.临床皮肤科杂志,2005,34(6):395.

[45] 孙志平,邱实,石文植.多发性毛发上皮瘤.临床

皮肤科杂志,2003,32(11);629-630.

[46] 谭城,朱文元.水疱型钙化上皮瘤 1 例.临床皮肤科杂志,2002,31(10);648-649.

[47] 杨励,王雷,高天文.结缔组织增生性毛发上皮瘤 1 例.临床皮肤科杂志,2006,35(6);368-369.

[48] 李葆春,董兵卫,张江安,谭升顺,孔春艳.小汗腺血管错构瘤 1 例.临床皮肤科杂志,2003,32(12);727.

[49] 关杨,肖尹,纪华安,薛丑文.透明细胞汗腺瘤 1 例.临床皮肤科杂志,2005,34(5);318.

[50] 李顺凡,吴国凤,吴志华.乳头状汗管囊腺瘤.临床皮肤科杂志,2006,35(3);131-132.

[51] 方木平,刘汉忠,刘倩萍,胡友红,龙峰.乳头状汗管囊腺瘤并发基底细胞上皮瘤 1 例.临床皮肤科杂志,2006,35(3);162-163.

[52] 王雷,杨励,高天文.上皮样组织细胞瘤.临床皮肤科杂志,2006,35(8);492-493.

[53] 唐珊,雷鹏程,袁姗,钟延丰.全身性发疹性组织细胞瘤 1 例.临床皮肤科杂志,1999,28(5);314-315.

[54] 张晓梅,池凤好,范瑞强.多中心网状组织细胞增生症 1 例.临床皮肤科杂志,2004,33(8);493.

[55] 周建华,漆军,李恒进,吕勇,王京生,虞瑞尧.以多发残毁性关节炎为显著表现的多中心网状组织细胞增生症 1 例.临床皮肤科杂志,2002,31(4);244-245.

[56] 孙建方,林敏乐.勒-雪病.临床皮肤科杂志,2003,32(2);59-60.

[57] 杨慧兰,林挺,杨军,陈晓东,关蕾,刘仲荣.发疹性朗格汉斯细胞组织细胞增生症 1 例.临床皮肤科杂志,2005,34(9);589-590.

[58] 崔炳南,渠涛,赵岩松,等.播散型 Paget 样网状细胞增生病国内首报.临床皮肤科杂志,2007,36(2);67-70.

[59] 吴艳,郑丽端,李家文,王椿森.上皮样肉瘤的临床与病理分析.临床皮肤科杂志,2005,34(5);273-275.

[60] 谢忠,李楠,涂平.结节性(假肉瘤性)筋膜炎 1 例.临床皮肤科杂志,2004,33(6);364-365.

[61] 李顺凡,吴国凤,吴志华.先天性隆突性皮肤纤维肉瘤.临床皮肤科杂志,2006,35(2);65-66.

[62] 吴凤,朱里,钱悦,等.萎缩斑块样隆突性皮肤纤维肉瘤 1 例.临床皮肤科杂志,2012,41(3);170.

[63] 翟志芳,杨希川,郝飞,钟白玉.获得性指(趾)部纤维角化瘤 1 例.临床皮肤科杂志,2006,35(6);391-392.

[64] 李文海,张建中.色素血管性斑痣性错构瘤病.临床皮肤科杂志,2002,31(1);1-2.

[65] 马东来,何志新,方凯,刘克英.匍行性血管瘤 2 例.临床皮肤科杂志,2002,31(11);718-719.

[66] 谭城,朱文元,赖仁胜等.反应性血管内皮细胞瘤病.临床皮肤科杂志,2010,39(8);486-488.

[67] 马东来,李峰,方凯.微静脉性血管瘤.临床皮肤科杂志,2009,38(10);637-638.

[68] 姜红浩,吴凤,朱里,等.梭形细胞血管瘤.临床皮肤科杂志,2011,40(11);679-680.

[69] 张春敏,侯建新,袁奎封,史永俭,魏国,王蘋,刘金耀.上皮样血管瘤 1 例.临床皮肤科杂志,2003,32(11);661-662.

[70] 王刚,李春英,高天文.疣状血管瘤.临床皮肤科杂志,2004,33(7);393-394.

[71] 张贤.丛状血管瘤 1 例.临床皮肤科杂志,2005,34(10);687.

[72] 侯麦花,朱文元.浅表性血管黏液瘤.临床皮肤科杂志,2006,35(7);446-447.

[73] 谭城,朱文元,赖仁胜,等.靶样含铁血黄素沉积性血管瘤.临床皮肤科杂志,2006,35(9);591-592.

[74] 蔡梅,冒长峙,周晓鸿,袁志伟.弥漫性躯体血管角皮瘤 1 例.临床皮肤科杂志,2000,29(1);54-55.

[75] 单侧阴囊血管角皮瘤   侯麦花供图.

[76] 女阴血管角皮瘤   朱文元供图.

[77] 金江,陈雪,张建中.卡波西样血管内皮细胞瘤 1 例.临床皮肤科杂志,2005,34(1);35-37.

[78] 常建民.恶性血管肿瘤.临床皮肤科杂志,2006,35(1);62-64.

[79] Lu Y,Zhang M.Pemphigus herpetiformis in a patient with well-differentiated cutaneous angiosarcoma:case report and review of the published work.J Dermatol,2012,39(1);89-91.

[80] Pu XM,Wu WD,Kang XJ,Shi DR,Shen DW. Clinical and experimental study on thirty-eight

patients with classic Kaposis'sarcoma in Xin-jiang Uighar Autonomous region. J Clin Dermatol,2003,32(suppl):S25-31.

[81] 马东来,刘平,方凯.实体型血管球瘤.临床皮肤科杂志,2006,35(9):555-556.

[82] 马东来,孙秋宁,方凯等.局限性多发性血管球瘤.临床皮肤科杂志,2007,36(10):609-610.

[83] Zhu WY,Penneys NS,Reyesm B,Khatib Z,Schachner L.Acquired progressive lymphangioma.J Am Acad Dermatol,1991,24(5 Pt 2):813-815.

[84] 朱晓浚,刘次伟,刘小珍.额面部出血性淋巴管瘤1例.临床皮肤科杂志,2003,32(11):657-658.

[85] 周存才,邢红斌,王丽冰.弥漫性海绵状淋巴管瘤1例.临床皮肤科杂志,2005,34(3):178.

[86] 吴建华,朱文元.浅表脂肪瘤样痣6例报告.临床皮肤科杂志,1988,17(6):312-313.
朱文元,吴建华,陈希萍.浅表脂肪瘤样痣.临床皮肤科杂志,1989,18:1.

[87] 乔树芳,张玉环,纪华安,肖尹,薛丑文,毛舒和.伴脂肪组织增生的泛发型硬斑病1例.临床皮肤科杂志,2003,32(11):671.

[88] 彭军,孙则胜.甲下外生骨疣1例.临床皮肤科杂志,2007,36(7):473.

[89] 吴黎明,孙建方,赵亮.甲下外生骨疣和内生软骨瘤3例.临床皮肤科杂志,2003,32:593-594.

[90] 马东来,何志新,王定邦.多发性皮肤平滑肌瘤4例.临床皮肤科杂志,2002,31(5):310-311.

[91] 徐益明,居哈尔,普雄明,刘玉琴.皮肤平滑肌肉瘤1例.临床皮肤科杂志,2005,34(12):831-832.

[92] 晋红中,刘跃华,方凯.皮肤子宫内膜异位1例.临床皮肤科杂志,2005,34(9):596-598.

[93] 邢传平,曹晓哲,李宁,钱震.皮肤Merkel细胞癌3例.临床皮肤科杂志,2003,32(6):338-339.

[94] 方晶,朱文元,张美华等.神经鞘瘤.临床皮肤科杂志,2007,36(12):743-744.

[95] Zuo YG,Wang JB,Wang HW,Fang K.Multiple neurilemmoma.J Clin Dermatol,2003,32(suppl):S105-106.

[96] 多发性栅栏状神经鞘瘤　徐春兴供图.

[97] 皮肖冰,张建中.甲母痣恶变1例.临床皮肤科杂志,2003,32(8):466-467.

[98] 王家璧,王宏伟.肢端原位恶性黑素瘤.临床皮肤科杂志,2004,33(3):195-196.

[99] 肖尹,关杨,纪华安,薛丑文,李鹏.气球状细胞恶性黑素瘤1例.临床皮肤科杂志,2005,34(9):622.

[100] 曾建英,马东来,方凯,王宝玺.口唇恶性黑素瘤.临床皮肤科杂志,2002,31(2):67-68.

[101] 庄殿英,郑永雄.巨大先天性色素痣伴软脑膜恶性黑素瘤1例.临床皮肤科杂志,2006,35(2):90-91.

[102] 黄敏,杨帆,曾学思,王立阳.肢端无色素性黑素瘤.临床皮肤科杂志,2006,35(9):587-588.

[103] 王雷,杨励,范雪莉,高天文.簇发性斯皮茨痣.临床皮肤科杂志,2006,35(9):593-594.

[104] 胡瑾,刘晓雁,马东来.单发性肥大细胞瘤.临床皮肤科杂志,2004,33(3):137-138.

[105] 郑敏,李蜀华.皮肤肥大细胞增生症1例.临床皮肤科杂志,2004,33(9):569.

[106] 姜祎群,宋琳毅,郭晓光,冯素英,孙建方,曾学思,崔盘根.以泛发性丘疹为表现的成人肥大细胞增生病.临床皮肤科杂志,2006,35(8):521-523.

[107] Jessner皮肤淋巴细胞浸润症　朱文元供图.

[108] 刘方,刘跃华,方凯,王家璧,晋红中,王宝玺.皮肤淋巴细胞瘤1例.临床皮肤科杂志,2003,32(8):463-464.

[109] 蔡林,杜娟,何炎玲,张文娟,朱铁君.皮肤白血病1例.临床皮肤科杂志,2002,31(3):186-187.

[110] 陈敬,李振英,翟成,李景云.真性红细胞增多症皮肤表现1例.临床皮肤科杂志,2004,33(7):433.

[111] 杨光河,程春林,赵长秀.原发性皮肤浆细胞瘤1例.临床皮肤科杂志,2003,32(2):94-95.

[112] 葛峥,陆化,张建富,李建勇.继发性皮肤浆细胞瘤.临床皮肤科杂志,2004,33(6):346-348.

[113] 宋佩华,宣红梅,庞亦红,汪晨.皮下脂膜炎样T细胞淋巴瘤1例.临床皮肤科杂志,2003,32(4):210-212.

[114] 朱学骏,李航,涂平.红皮病型皮肤T细胞淋巴瘤.临床皮肤科杂志,2004,33(7):453-454.

[115] 相广才,宋楠萌,桑建利,等.牛痘样水疱病样皮肤 T 细胞淋巴瘤.临床皮肤科杂志,2009,38(8):483-486.

[116] 刘广仁,李会申,张建中.鼻部 NK/T 细胞淋巴瘤 1 例.临床皮肤科杂志,2003,32(8):465-466.

[117] 陈思远,郑丽端,吴艳,等.皮肤血管内 NK/T 细胞淋巴瘤一例.中华皮肤科杂志,2012,45(003):151-154.

[118] 陈晓红,袁伟,张信江.非霍奇金淋巴瘤 1 例.临床皮肤科杂志,2005,34(10):677-678.

[119] 郭小艳,齐凤琴,韩凤艳,富学东,李淑萍,曹海鹏,朱桢.蕈样肉芽肿误诊为蛎壳状银屑病 1 例.临床皮肤科杂志,2004,33(11):676-677.

[120] 林彤,孙建方,曾学思,桑红桂,李阿梅,姜祎群.以四肢色素沉着为主要表现的蕈样肉芽肿 1 例.临床皮肤科杂志,2004,33(9):543-544.

[121] 邱丙森.蕈样肉芽肿继发皮肤 CD30 阳性大细胞淋巴瘤.临床皮肤科杂志,2003,32(8):495-496.

[122] 宿斌,渠涛,王宝玺,王宏伟,方凯,钟定荣,凌庆.具有多种表现的蕈样肉芽肿 1 例.临床皮肤科杂志,2006,35(7):419-422.

[123] 谭升顺,江惟苏,付勇,冯义国,袁景奕,张磐谏.以皮肤斑块性浸润和肿瘤表现为主的 B 细胞淋巴瘤.临床皮肤科杂志,2003,32(9):563-564.

[124] 李春阳,孙青,王玉坤,郭淑兰.皮肤假性淋巴瘤 9 例临床与组织病理分析.临床皮肤科杂志,2004,33(12):732-734.

[125] 傅志宜,车雅敏,周之海,邢卫斌.皮肤窦性组织细胞增生症.临床皮肤科杂志,2004,33(5):327-328.

[126] 肖家诚,金晓龙,夏群力.皮肤原发性窦性组织细胞增生症 1 例.临床皮肤科杂志,2003,32(9):527-529.

[127] 杜娟,蔡林,沈丹华等.皮肤巨淋巴结病性窦组织细胞增生症.临床皮肤科杂志,2007,36(2):80-82.

[128] 朱文元,赵辨.淋巴瘤样丘疹病一例报告.皮肤病防治研究通讯,1977,4:273-275.

[129] 汪盛,李薇,赵廷方,郭在培.肺癌皮肤转移 1 例.临床皮肤科杂志,2003,32(9):537-538.

[130] 刘安,谭升顺,张江安,冯义国,任小蓉,雷小兵,文京华.胃癌皮肤转移 1 例.临床皮肤科杂志,2003,32(12):730.

[131] 蒋献,汪盛,熊心猜,吴蕊,郭在培,周光平.来源于脐尿管低分化腺癌 1 例.临床皮肤科杂志,2002,31(12):779-780.

[132] 铠甲癌　谭诚供图.

第 30 章

[1] 翟志芳,钟华,杨希川,等.Ascher 综合征伴睑黄瘤一例.中华皮肤科杂志,2012,45(003):214-214.

[2] 谭城,朱文元,闵仲生等.狒狒综合征.临床皮肤科杂志,2007,36(12):765-766.

[3] 王宏伟,夏维波,左亚刚,刘跃华.姐妹同患 Bloom 综合征 2 例.临床皮肤科杂志,2003,32(2):84-86.

[4] 宋志强,叶庆佾,郝飞.蓝色橡皮-大疱性痣综合征.临床皮肤科杂志,2004,33(4):213-215.

[5] 甘戈,许焱,王宝玺.息肉-色素沉着-脱发-甲营养不良综合征 1 例.临床皮肤科杂志,2006,35(3):158-159.

[6] 赵淑肖,陈强,孙惠琪,刘春平,马淑珍.局灶性真皮发育不全综合征 1 例.临床皮肤科杂志,2002,31(5):319-320.

[7] Zhang RZ, Zhu WY. Favre-Racouchot syndrome associated with eyelid papilloma:a case report.J Biomed Res,2012,26(6):474-477.

[8] 王文岭,杨蓉娅,敖俊红,苏有明,朱金良.Gorham 综合征 1 例.临床皮肤科杂志,2002,31(1):45-46.

[9] 梁建平,朱学骏.先天性额顶部皮下脂肪瘤-胼胝体发育不良-颅内脂肪瘤综合征 1 例.临床皮肤科杂志,2002,31(11):708-709.

[10] 王涛,付兰芹,刘跃华,等.角膜炎-鱼鳞病-耳聋综合征.临床皮肤科杂志,2009,38(12).

[11] 王惠琳,阎衡,向明明,叶庆佾,邓军,郝飞,杨希川.外阴-阴道-牙龈综合征型扁平苔藓 1 例.临床皮肤科杂志,2006,35(3):142-143.

[12] 李会申,张文娟,崔树岩,孙祎山,苏燕晨.Jackson-Lawler 综合征 1 例.临床皮肤科杂志,2004,33(1):28-29.

［13］ 马东来,刘克英,李军,方凯.Laugier-Hunziker 综合征.临床皮肤科杂志,2006,35(12):757-759.

［14］ 宋志新,李宝,贺长江,冯春余.Madelung 综合征.临床皮肤科杂志,2004,33(6):330.

［15］ 罗迪青,何定阳,黄应表,刘隽华.Marshall-White 综合征 12 例分析.临床皮肤科杂志,2006,35(3):133-134.

［16］ 甘吉洪.甲、髌、肘发育不良综合征一家系 3 例报告.临床皮肤科杂志,2002,31(7):467-468.

［17］ 袁肖海,王学民.Netherton 综合征 1 例.临床皮肤科杂志,2004,33(3):162-163.

［18］ 马东来,胡瑾,方凯.Olmsted 综合征国内首报.临床皮肤科杂志,2006,35(10):637-639.

［19］ 李颂,涂平,朱学骏.Papillon-Lefèvre 综合征伴沟纹舌 1 例.临床皮肤科杂志,2006,35(2):94-95.

［20］ 王娣,涂平,朱学骏.面部单侧萎缩合并颅脑病变 1 例.临床皮肤科杂志,2004,33(1):30-31.

［21］ 杨恩品,刘华济.先天性环状缩窄带综合征 1 例.临床皮肤科杂志,2005,34(9):579.

［22］ 马东来,左亚刚,郑和义,王宝玺.Proteus 综合征 1 例.临床皮肤科杂志,2005,34(4):205-207.

［23］ 色素沉着—息肉综合征 朱文元供图.

［24］ 翟志芳,王莉,钟华等.梅干腹综合征.临床皮肤科杂志,2010,39(8):503-504.

［25］ 王爱琴,李莉,毛立亭.Rapp-Hodgkin 综合征 1 例.临床皮肤科杂志,2003,32(7):410.

［26］ Wu M,Zhou GZ,Zhang FY,Wang CZ.A case of rombo syndrome and review of literature.J Clin Dermatol,2003,32(suppl):S122-124.

［27］ 姚志远,汪晨,蔓小红,马蕾,杨方印,陈锡唐,吴雪松,王泰龄.Rothmund-Thomson 综合征 1 例.临床皮肤科杂志,1999,28(6):380-381.

［28］ 高亮,杨瑞海,胡宗厚,等.僵硬皮肤综合征.临床皮肤科杂志,2007,7:019.

［29］ 陈柳青,曾学思,姜祎群,张学林,李阿梅,孙建方.毛发-鼻-指(趾)综合征.皮肤科杂志,2006,35(11):711-712.

［30］ 陈连军,方栩,方丽.Waardenburg 综合征 1 例.临床皮肤科杂志,2000,29(6):366-367.